Rabih Chaoui, Kai-Sven Heling
3D Ultrasound in Prenatal Diagnosis

Rabih Chaoui, Kai-Sven Heling

3D Ultrasound in Prenatal Diagnosis

A Practical Approach

2nd edition

DE GRUYTER

Prof. Dr. med. Rabih Chaoui
PD Dr. med. Kai-Sven Heling
Prenatal Diagnosis Clinic
Friedrichstr. 147
10117 Berlin, Germany

This is a translation of the original book in German:
3D-Sonographie in der pränatalen Diagnostik – Ein praktischer Leitfaden
Translated by Rabih Chaoui.

ISBN: 978-3-11-124909-4
e-ISBN (PDF): 978-3-11-124951-3
e-ISBN (EPUB): 978-3-11-124957-5

Library of Congress Control Number: 2023951974

Bibliographic information published by the Deutsche Nationalbibliothek
The Deutsche Nationalbibliothek lists this publication in the Deutsche Nationalbibliografie;
detailed bibliographic data are available on the internet at http://dnb.d-nb.de.

© 2024 Walter de Gruyter GmbH, Berlin/Boston
Cover image: Rabih Chaoui
Typesetting: L42 AG, Berlin
Printing and binding: CPI Books GmbH, Leck

www.degruyter.com

For Kathleen, Amin, and Ella Chaoui.
For Rajae, Anais, Reem, and Anna Heling.

Preface to the 2nd edition

It is with great pleasure that we present hereby the second edition of *3D Ultrasound in Prenatal Diagnosis, a practical approach*. We would like to take this opportunity to thank the readers of the German and English editions who have given us feedback on the practical approach of the book and how the book was of great value in clinical practice. We would also like to thank our colleagues in China who translated our book into Mandarin so that it was also accessible to Chinese physicians. This positive feedback, combined with our passion, inspired and motivated us to create this second edition of the book, thereby expanding the content based on our practical experience over the past eight years and building on the success of the first edition.

The first three-dimensional (3D) ultrasound demonstration of a fetal face was performed in 1989, a moment considered as the birth of 3D ultrasound. Around the year 2000, with the advent of fast processors, 3D ultrasound equipment became widely available. Today, all available high-level ultrasound systems offer the 3D/4D tool as an option with integrated software and special 3D transducers.

Although most 3D applications are similar regardless of the ultrasound system manufacturer, this book reports on our experience gained exclusively with the ultrasound systems *Voluson E10* and *Expert 22* of General Electric HealthCare, which can be adapted to all newer systems of the Voluson series.

We have divided the book into three main sections as in the previous edition: the first section describes how to acquire and navigate within a volume, the second section describes different modes of volume rendering, whereas the third section focuses on organ-specific application of 3D techniques such as e. g., brain, heart, bone, first trimester. In a total of 20 chapters, this book summarizes the essentials you need to know about the practical approach in using 3D in prenatal ultrasound.

In this new edition, we have included more than 470 new figures to illustrate different aspects of 3D ultrasound, from explaining the various render modes to illustrating the clinical applications of these tools. It was difficult to decide which images would make it into the book in the end, but we wanted to keep the spectrum broad and limit the number to 20 to 30 images per chapter. The text was adapted accordingly, considering the authors' evolving experience since the first edition.

We are indebted to several people for their significant contribution to our 3D ultrasound journey. First and foremost, our friend Dr. Bernard Benoit (Monaco), a giant in the field of ultrasound imaging, who was and is a great source of inspiration for us. Many of the 3D ultrasound tools could not have been developed without his enormous technical and artistic experience. We would also like to thank the engineering and management teams at General Electric-HealthCare in the Voluson Valley in Zipf, Austria for their close collaboration and tireless support over the years, especially during the Covid pandemic. We thank our patients who have contributed to all the images in this book and who continue to motivate us to push the boundaries of this technology. This book would not have been possible without the professional team at De Gruyter

https://doi.org/10.1515/9783111249513-201

publishing, in particular Dr. Bettina Noto, Jessika Kischke, Andreas Brandmair, and Dr. Jo Nagel (L42 AG), who have supported us tirelessly and with great dedication.

We hope that this book will motivate you to try out the great imaging opportunities that 3D ultrasound affords and to discover your artistic approach to medical diagnosis in fetal medicine.

Berlin, Friedrichstrasse   Rabih Chaoui
November 2023   Kai-Sven Heling

Technical ultrasound terms

All 3D examinations and experiences in this book are based on Voluson ultrasound equipment produced by GE HealthCare of General Electric. The images in this book were generated with Voluson e10 and Expert 22 equipment and most tools presented in this book, namely VCI®, TUI®, Magicut®, Glass-body mode®, Silhouette®, HDlive®, Omni-view®, Sono-AVC®, VOCAL®, and others are protected names. To facilitate reading we decided to omit the ® sign within the book.

Some abbreviations are listed below:

3D	Three-dimensional ultrasound
4D	Four-dimensional ultrasound
HD	High-definition
Sono-AVC®	Sonographic Automatic Volume Calculation
Sono-VCAD®	Sonographic Volume Computer Aided Diagnosis
SRI®	Speckle Reduction Imaging
TUI®	Tomographic Ultrasound Imaging
V-SRI®	Volume Speckle Reduction Imaging
VCI®	Volume Contrast Imaging
VOCAL®	Virtual Organ Computer Aided Analysis (VOCAL)

https://doi.org/10.1515/10.1515/9783111249513-202

Inhalt

Part III: Clinical Applications in Prenatal Diagnosis

Part I: **Basics of 3D Sonography**

1 Basics of 3D and 4D Volume Acquisition

1.1 Introduction

Switching from scanning with 2D ultrasound to integrating 3D ultrasound into daily work is more than just changing the transducer or activating the 3D button; rather, it is a completely different work setting. Experienced examiners scan in 3D mode in their brain and get the 2D planes from different scan perspectives by manipulating the transducer or turning the fetus, so they are more able to integrate 3D into their daily work. However, they often resist using 3D imaging because they think it is a gimmick, time consuming, or too difficult to learn. This book is designed to help change that mindset and integrate 3D ultrasound into daily scans. 3D as a technological imaging can be viewed simply as a software with many tools to learn, and learning how to use this software is the subject of this book.

Current 3D ultrasound technology is based on advanced mechanical or electronic transducers with the ability to acquire a volume (3D) or a sequence of single volumes (4D). Image information acquired in a 3D volume can then be displayed on the screen in a variety of ways: either as one or more multiplanar 2D images (see Chapters 2, 4, 5, and 6) or as a spatial volume that projects external or internal anatomic features of a volume (see Chapters 3, 7–12). The three steps for working with a 3D volume are as follows:

1. volume acquisition,
2. volume display, and
3. volume manipulation.

The quality of a volume data set which provides valuable information or a perfect 3D image depends not only on the operator's post-processing skills, but also on the adjustment of the 2D image before volume acquisition. This chapter discusses some aspects of image optimization as well as some basics of volume acquisition.

1.2 Preparing volume acquisition

Five steps should be considered during the preparation of a 3D volume acquisition. These steps are:

1. Choice of image modality (2D, color Doppler) and optimization of the image before volume acquisition
2. Choice of the best reference or starting plane with anticipation of the expected result
3. Choice of size and shape of the acquisition box (box's height and width)
4. Acquisition angle (box's depth)
5. Volume quality (resolution)

https://doi.org/10.1515/9783111249513-001

1.2.1 Optimizing a 2D image before volume acquisition

A 3D volume is a collection of adjacent 2D images, and the resolution in the entire volume improves with the resolution of each individual plane. Therefore, before acquiring a 3D, 4D, or Spatio-Temporal Image Correlation (STIC) volume, optimizing the 2D images is important in order to achieve good results. The term *reference plane* or *acquisition plane* is then used to refer to the 2D starting plane for a 3D acquisition. In addition to the choice of line density and frame rate, optimizing the image also includes the correct positioning of the *region of interest* in the volume box. In this case, both the

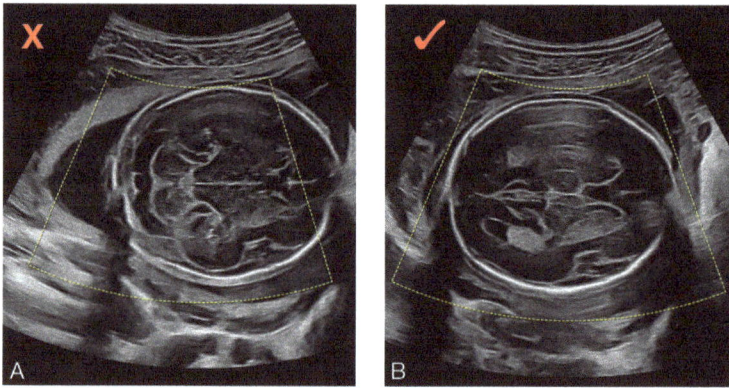

Fig. 1.1: Before capturing a 3D volume, the 2D image must be optimized and centered to include the full information. (A): the box covers only part of the head and after a volume acquisition, parts of the head and brain will be missing from the 3D volume. (B): in this image, the head is more centered and contains the full information, so it is optimized for 3D acquisition.

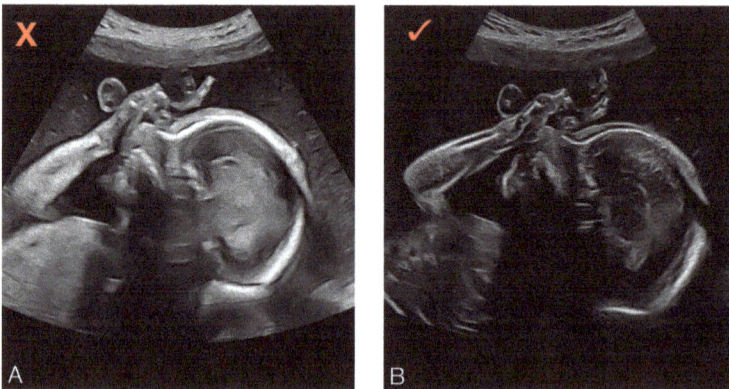

Fig. 1.2: In (A) the image is not optimized and appears too "bright" with low contrast for a 3D acquisition in surface mode. In (B), after image optimization, the amniotic fluid appears black and transparent and the surface contours are well defined.

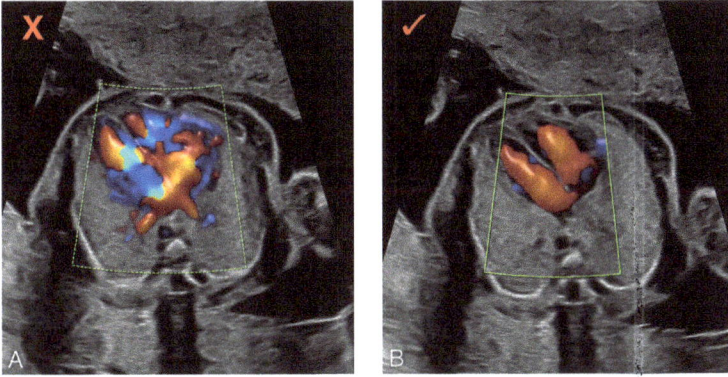

Fig. 1.3: The color Doppler settings in image (A) are not optimal for STIC acquisition because a high color gain was chosen along with a low velocity range. (B) shows the optimized image before STIC acquisition.

choice of the angle size of the box and the angle depth (acquisition angle) are important. If the volume is acquired with color Doppler, the examiner should also consider optimization of color resolution, color persistence and frame rate. Figures 1.1 to 1.3 are examples of image optimization prior to volume acquisition.

1.2.2 Choice of the best starting plane at volume acquisition

In 3D ultrasound, the best image quality within a volume is found in the reference plane and in planes parallel to this plane, while the reconstructed planes orthogonal or oblique to the reference plane have lower image quality. It is important that the operator keeps the end result in mind when preparing and performing the volume acquisition.

1.2.3 The acquisition box or volume box

The volume acquisition box, or volume box, determines two parameters of a 3D volume in the 2D image, namely the height and width (Fig. 1.4) which correspond to the x-axis and y-axis respectively (Fig. 1.5). It is recommended that the operator adjusts the size of the box to capture all anatomical components of a target volume. For a 4D acquisition, the borders of the box are chosen close to the anatomical region of interest and can be corrected directly during the live 4D rendering. However, in a static 3D image it is recommended to choose a large box size to avoid excluding structures adjacent to the anatomical regions of interest in the volume.

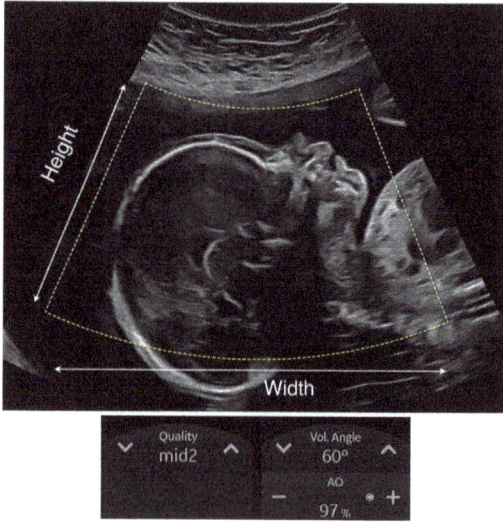

Fig. 1.4: The volume box has three dimensions: height, width, and depth. The height and width of the volume, as shown here, are determined by the choice of acquisition box size. The depth of the volume box is determined by the choice of acquisition angle on the ultrasound machine.

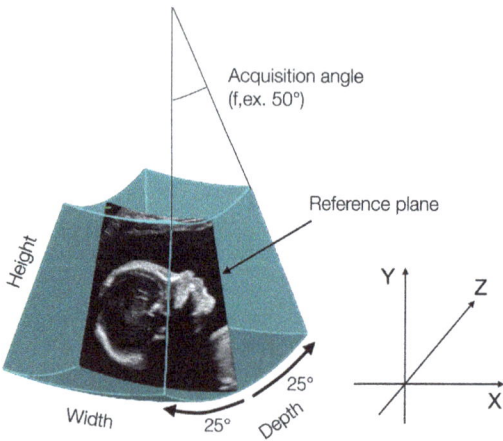

Fig. 1.5: The size of a volume box is composed of height, width, and depth. The acquisition angle is the total angle of the volume, which during acquisition is half the angle in front and half the angle behind the reference plane. The reference plane is the image that the examiner sees on the screen while activating a 3D volume acquisition.

1.2.4 Acquisition angle

The acquisition angle refers to the depth of the final volume corresponding to the z-axis and is the sweep angle of the elements within the probe during acquisition (Fig. 1.5). The acquisition angle is set by the operator prior to 3D volume acquisition. There is no gold standard for the best acquisition angle, but rather the choice depends mainly on the anatomy of the target organ and the type of acquisition. The acquisition angle is then the total angle of the volume, but during the acquisition half of the angle size is behind the reference or acquisition plane and the other half is in front of it (Fig. 1.5). The size and shape of the box varies depending on the organ being examined.

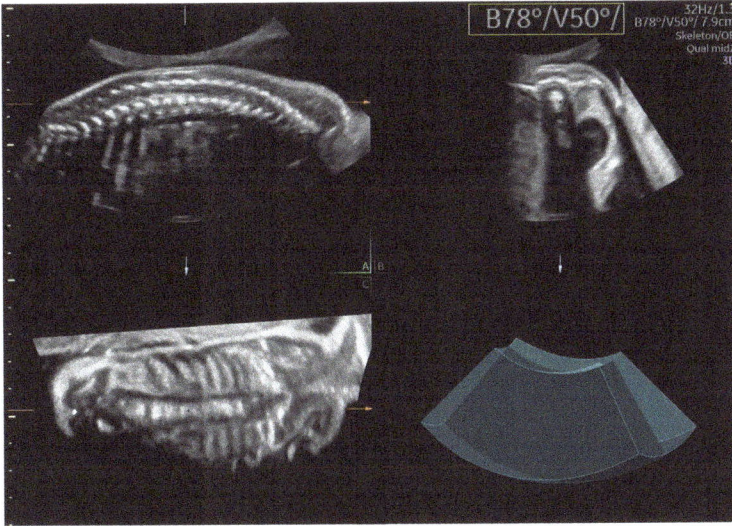

Fig. 1.6: The shape of the volume box is often determined by the shape of the examined organ. In the case of spine and ribs, the box is large and has a rather shallow depth. The size of the volume box is displayed on the screen in degrees, where B stands for width (here: 78°) and V for volume depth (here: 50°).

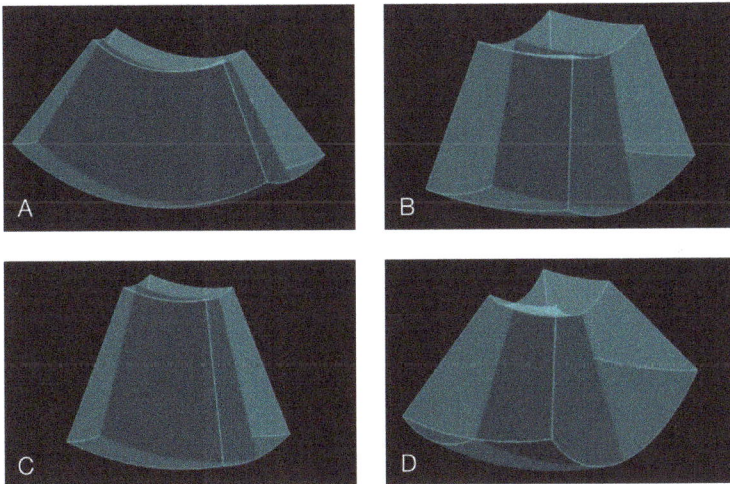

Fig. 1.7: The shape of the 3D volume box mainly depends on the region of interest being studied. (A) depicts a typical volume box of a spine in longitudinal view. (B) is an example of a box for a fetal face in 3D. The box in (C) has a flat volume depth for a STIC acquisition, and the large box in (D) is for acquisition of a large body part such as the head, abdomen with thorax, or the entire fetus in early gestation.

Figures. 1.6 and 1.7 show different types of acquisition boxes. For example, in the volume box of the fetal spine, the box is wide, but the acquisition angle is narrow (Fig. 1.6), whereas for the heart, the width and depth are almost the same (Fig. 1.7).

In a live 4D examination, the size of the volume box and the acquisition angle have a direct impact on the volume rate. The larger the box or angle, the lower the volume frame rate will be. For 4D acquisitions it is therefore advised to keep both volume width and angle as small as possible so that smooth and continuous movements can be recorded.

1.2.5 Acquisition quality

The resolution within a 3D volume is determined by the operator by choosing the *quality* of the volume acquired (low, mid, high, max). Subsequently this is translated into a duration of the volume recording. The examiner should keep in mind that within a volume box with the same acquisition angle, a slower sweep speed will result in the acquisition of more images and provide better resolution, while a faster sweep speed will acquire fewer images, resulting in a lower resolution image (Fig. 1.8). Since more images are available in a volume box for 3D calculation, the result is higher quality images of the reconstructed B and C planes in the multiplanar view. Compare the two views, as shown in the top versus bottom images in Figure 1.9. It should also be remembered that the best image is not always achieved by choosing the maximum resolution,

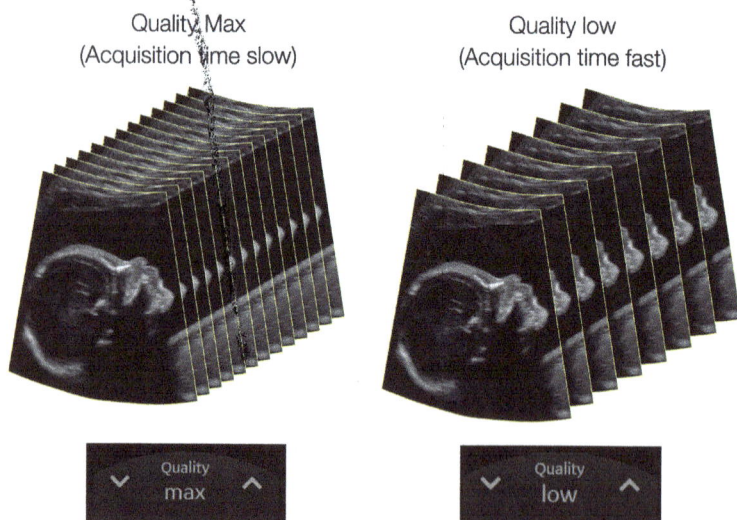

Fig. 1.8: For the same volume angle, choosing high-quality acquisition (high 1, high 2, or max) requires a little more time and results in the acquisition of many images. The result is then a high-resolution volume data set (left image). An acquisition with low to medium resolution is fast and leads to fewer images in the volume data set and thus to a lower volume quality (right image).

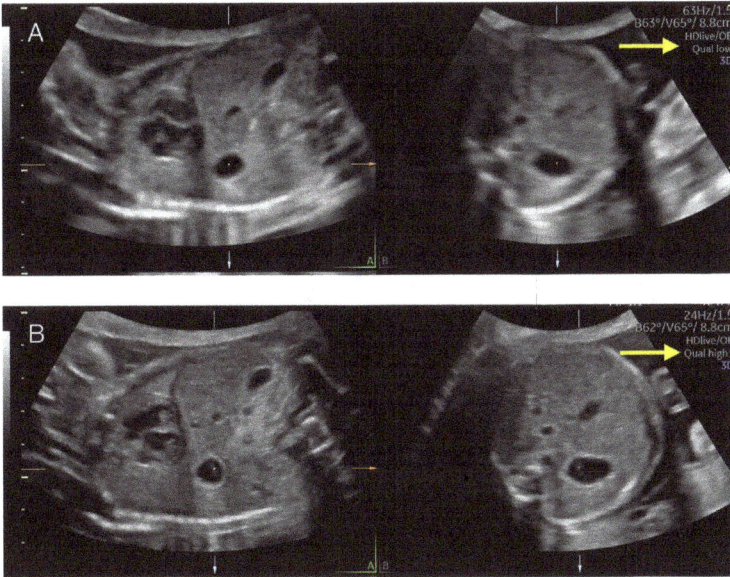

Fig. 1.9: 3D volume acquisition of the same fetus in low quality (A) and high quality (B) with recognizable different details in the two volumes, such as the liver texture and the stomach border.

and the operator should find his or her own individual preferred presets. A nice 3D face image of a mid-trimester fetus appears better if the skin surface is smooth, so a lower resolution can be chosen (Fig. 1.10). Figure 1.10 shows a fetus after a 3D acquisition in low resolution (on the left), medium resolution (in the middle), and highest resolution (on the right). In our opinion, the middle image has the best quality with a smooth face, while the right image has many details that are close to artifacts. Imaging fingers, ears, or a face in early pregnancy, however, may require higher resolution (Fig. 1.11). We use high and maximum resolution for volumes with multiplanar imaging, e. g., for tomography of anatomical details of the brain.

In 4D acquisitions, the acquisition quality has a direct impact on the volume rate. Volume rates higher than 7 to 8 volumes per second are desired in order to nicely display fetal movement in a smooth and continuous way.

For the static 3D and for the 4D examination, the acquisition quality is labeled as low, medium, high, and maximum. For the STIC acquisition, the acquisition quality is reflected in the duration of the acquisition: 7.5, 10, 12.5, or 15 seconds; for e-STIC also in low, medium, high, and maximum. Figure 1.12 shows the difference in the same fetal face after a static 3D image (left image) and after a 4D examination (right image), both acquired at medium resolution.

Quality: Low Quality: Mid 2 Quality: Maximum

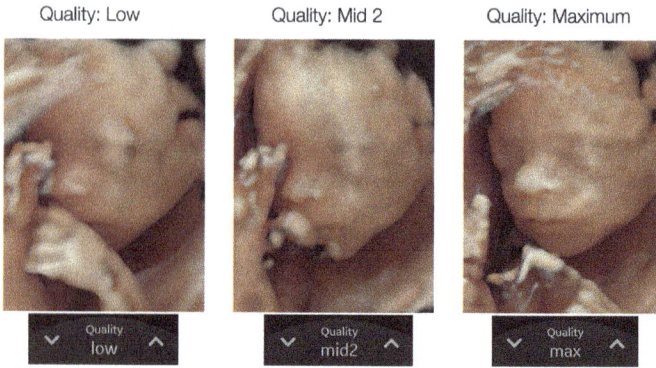

Fig. 1.10: The same fetal face after a static 3D acquisition in different resolutions, i. e., in low, mid 2, and maximum qualities. The image in the middle appears satisfactory and shows that the best result is not always obtained by choosing the highest resolution.

Quality: Low Quality: Mid 2 Quality: Maximum

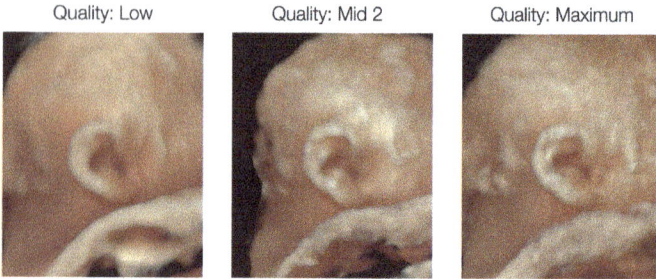

Fig. 1.11: Ear in a fetus at 31 weeks' gestation with a static 3D acquisition in different resolutions, i. e., low, mid 2, and maximum quality levels. The left image is acceptable for assessing the general shape of the ear, whereas the image in the middle appears satisfactory and shows that the highest resolution is not always required for the clinically best result. Fetal hair can also be seen on the head and around the ear.

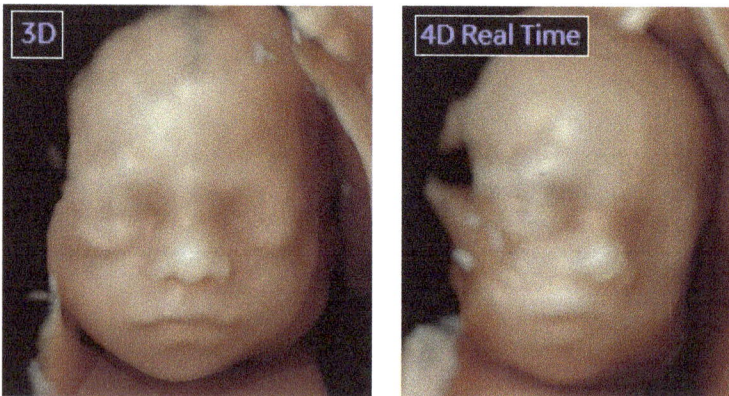

Fig. 1.12: Acquisition of a fetal face with static 3D (left image in quality mid 2, right image in live-4D). Detail detection and resolution is generally better with static 3D. Compare the resolution at the lips and nostrils in both images.

1.3 Transducers for 3D/4D acquisition

In the early days of 3D technology, conventional ultrasound probes were used with which the examiner manually acquired a series of parallel slices by simply sliding the probe over the maternal abdomen and recording a series of sequential images that were reconstructed on the ultrasound machine into a 3D image. Another approach was to attach a position sensor to the transducer, while the data receiver was in an external computer workstation. The volume was acquired by recording the spatial orientation of the planes and calculating the 3D result on the separate computer. Nowadays, volume imaging uses two types of probes, mechanical and electronic transducers, which allow fast and reliable 3D volume acquisition.

1.3.1 Mechanical transducers

Mechanical probes are the most used 3D probes (including the transvaginal probes) and consist of a single line or array of ultrasound crystals (about 200–1000) mounted on a mechanical rotation motor located in the transducer. Recording of a 3D volume data set is initiated by pressing the "3D" or "Freeze" button on the ultrasound machine. While the probe is held stationary over the region of interest, the mechanical motor rotates the array at a specific spatial interval and speed. The spatial interval is determined by the choice of acquisition angle and the velocity is determined by the volume resolution. In a 3D acquisition, a single sweep is performed resulting in one image (volume), whereas in a real-time 4D acquisition, a series of single sweeps are recorded sequentially and are then aligned as one movement cycle (cine). The major limitation of this probe is the time required for the mechanical parts to perform the sweep movement(s). Acquiring a volume at maximum resolution can take several seconds, and either fetus or mother may move during the sweep, resulting in movement artifacts. Therefore, in real-time 4D examinations, sequences are slow, reaching speeds of up to 4–5 volumes per second for a fetal face. Some transducers, called mechanical matrix transducers, have not one but an array of three or five lines of ultrasound crystals on the rotor, thus allowing better resolution.

1.3.2 Electronic or matrix array transducers

Electronic transducers are complicated, fully electronic probes without a mechanical rotor. Instead of an array of 3–5 lines of crystals, a large matrix array is aligned, resulting in more than 8000 crystals. This explains the much higher cost of these probes. Whereas for normal 2D scanning only straight beams are transmitted from the probe, 3D or 4D acquisition is achieved by electronically steering the beam into multiple directions, simulating the mechanical sweep described above. The absence of any mechanical parts enables the 4D examination in near real-time with no discernible lack of information, with a recording which is two to four times faster than with a mechanical 3D probe. The recording of a single 3D or STIC volume is also much faster than with a mechanical transducer. Chapter 14 discusses other potentials of this probe.

1.4 Types of volume acquisition

Currently three types of acquisition of a volume data set are used (Fig. 1.13), namely:
1. Static 3D
2. Spatial and temporal image correlation (STIC) with a mechanical STIC or alternatively an electronic STIC (eSTIC) with an electronic transducer
3. Real-time 4D with a mechanical 3D transducer or an electronic transducer (4D)

1.4.1 Static 3D acquisition

Principle: Static 3D refers to a single 3D volume containing many adjacent 2D ultrasound planes without regard to temporal or spatial motion. Currently, this is the most common type of volume acquisition in obstetrics and gynecology.

Potential: This type of examination is easy to learn and can be performed quickly, allowing the examiner to acquire multiple volumes and store them for later analysis. Static 3D acquisition is usually performed with a grayscale preset, but can also be combined with different color Doppler presets for vascular assessment of volume content. Post-acquisition rendering allows for different visualizations, to be discussed in detail in the following chapters.

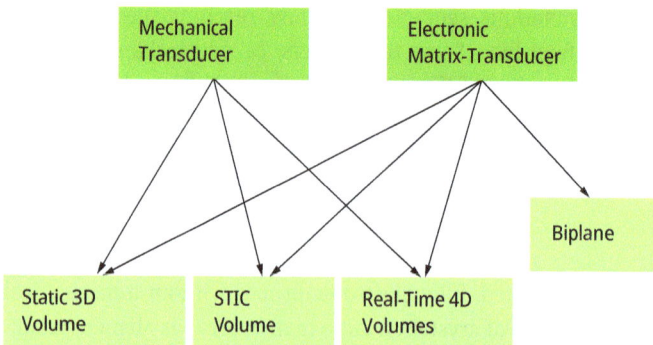

Fig. 1.13: Flowchart showing volume acquisition capabilities. With a mechanical or electronic transducer, the acquisition can be performed with either static 3D volume, STIC volume, or 4D volume. In addition, the electronic matrix transducer enables the acquisition of biplane-images.

Limitations: The main limitation of static 3D acquisition is the inability to assess mo-tion-related movement, particularly at the level of the heart in grayscale and in combi-nation with color Doppler. Valve movements, myocardial contractility, and flow events cannot be reliably assessed with static 3D images. Another limitation is the frequent occurrence of movement artifacts during acquisition, as observed in the fetal face, limbs, spine, and other areas (see Chapter 2 and Chapter 3).

1.4.2 Spatio-Temporal Image Correlation (STIC) acquisition

Principle: STIC acquisition is like slow 3D acquisition with a duration between 7.5 and 15 seconds and is mainly an acquisition of images of a beating heart or vessels with pulsation. The software allows calculation of heart rate based on tissue displacement with simultaneous cardiac motion. The acquired volume is processed by the computer, using the systolic peaks to calculate the fetal heart rate, and then rearranging the vo-lume images according to their timing within the cardiac cycle, creating a film-like loop of a single cardiac cycle. The eSTIC is the term used for a STIC volume acquired with an electronic probe that allows faster acquisition (< 5 sec.) and higher resolution. In this book, the term STIC is used to refer to both STIC and eSTIC.

Potential: Advantages of STIC volume acquisition include the ability to assess myocar-dial wall motion and valve excursion. The 4D information is available within seconds of volume acquisition. Once the reference plane is optimized, STIC acquisition can be easily performed. STIC acquisition can be performed with grayscale imaging but also in combination with other imaging modalities such as color, power, or high-resolution Doppler and B-flow. When conditions are good for grayscale and color Doppler scan-ning, STIC can be used for offline plane reconstruction and assessment. This ability to virtually examine the heart is one of the great potentials of this technique. Its clinical application is discussed in Chapter 19.

Limitations: A major disadvantage of STIC acquisition is that a single cardiac cycle is represented as a cine-loop, making this technique unable to assess arrhythmias, espe-cially ectopic beats. Another limitation, especially for STIC and less so for eSTIC, is the delayed acquisition time, which can be affected by fetal movements or maternal re-spiratory movements, introducing artifacts into the volume.

1.4.3 Real-time 4D with a mechanical or an electronic transducer

Principle: Most 4D volume imaging today is performed using a mechanical transducer with an integrated rotation motor (see Section 1.3). The principle is the same as for sta-tic 3D technology, except that the motor rotates continuously and captures a series of volumes which are presented almost as a single motion. The combination of a series of 3D volumes within a time interval is then referred to as 4D. Various terms are used to describe this method, including *real-time 3D, real-time 4D*, or *4D*. Throughout this book, the term 4D will be primarily used.

Potential: the greatest advantage of 4D acquisition is the ability to display 4D volumes in real time on the ultrasound screen as they are acquired. This is particularly impressive when displaying the face, hands, and feet of a moving fetus. Opening eyes, yawning or other movements make the fetus appear much more real and human to the parents. This technique is ideal for many examiners, including beginners, because the 3D image appears directly on the screen and can be adjusted accordingly. The speed of 4D examination is much faster with an electronic transducer, and future devices with faster processors may increase this speed.

Limitations: The main limitation of this type of acquisition is the challenge of finding a balance between good quality 4D image on the one hand, and the speed of rotation of the motor on the other hand in order to give a near-live impression. A routine, good-resolution image of a fetal face in 4D displays four volumes per second, which is not close to the 15 frames per second or more required for a "live" impression of images to the human eye. As a result, the image flow often does not appear smooth unless the fetal movements are slow. Slow movements of the fetus's arms and legs or grimaces, yawns, and eye openings can be tracked well with this technique. The major limitation is the time required for mechanical rotation of the probe. Therefore, the advent of faster processors in the future is expected to improve 4D imaging produced by electronic rather than mechanical transducers.

1.5 Display of a volume data set

Once recorded, the volume data set can be displayed on the screen in different ways, depending on the question of interest, as shown in Figure 1.14, and explained in the following chapters. In general, two main groups can be distinguished, either as planes, known as *multiplanar reconstruction,* or as a spatially rendered 3D volume image. In multiplanar reconstruction, one has the choice between demonstrating three perpendicular planes, known as *orthogonal mode* (see Chapter 5), parallel slices, known as *tomography mode* (see Chapter 6), or selecting a single plane. The single plane can either be extracted from the volume data set after navigating within the volume, as explained in Chapter 2, or it can be created after "cutting" the plane out of the volume by tracing a straight or curved line with the Omniview tool (see Chapter 5). On the other hand, if the expected result is to be a spatially rendered 3D image, different views can be chosen: visualizing the surface of a region of interest (see Chapter 7), or making the volume more transparent and looking through it, highlighting bones (see Chapter 8) or

Static 3D Volume	STIC Volume	Real-Time 4D Volumes

Multiplanar display	Volume rendering

Planes:
- Single plane
- Orthogonal mode
- Tomography mode
- Omniview planes

Volume-Images:
- Surface mode
- Transparency mode
- Glass-body mode
- Volume calculation

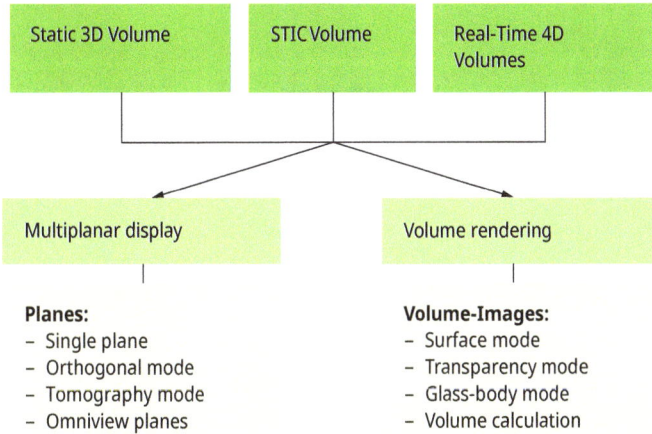

Fig. 1.14: After a volume data set is acquired as either a 3D static volume, a STIC volume, or a 4D volume, as shown in Figure 1.13, the result can be displayed on the screen in a variety of ways. This flow chart shows the different options for volume rendering and display. A volume data set can be displayed either as planes, known as multiplanar reconstruction, or as a spatial volume, called volume rendering.

the anechoic regions (see Chapters 9–11). If the examination was combined with color Doppler, the *glass-body mode* can be selected (see Chapter 12). Finally, the volume data set can also be used for volume calculation (see Chapter 13).

1.6 Conclusions

Nowadays, acquisition of 3D volumes can be performed either with a mechanical 3D or with an electronic matrix transducer (Fig. 1.13). Before starting the recording, the examiner should decide which region to examine and what result to expect, and adjust the image presets and type of volume acquisition accordingly. Often, the display of the image on the screen is chosen by selecting the presets prior to acquisition, but this can also be changed after a volume has been recorded and saved. This chapter briefly introduced the different transducers, acquisition types, and display types. The following chapters will discuss in detail the different ways of displaying and editing 3D volume data.

2 Orientation and Navigation within a Volume Data set

2.1 Introduction

Acquiring a 3D volume data set and displaying it on the screen are the first steps in offline processing of raw volume data. The display of the image can be done in two different modalities, either in multiplanar or 3D rendering mode, as described in Chapter 1. In this chapter, we will show how to display the result of a 3D volume on the screen in orthogonal mode and how to navigate within the volume and extract different 2D images. Most examiners save the volume during the examination to edit it at the end of the examination or later. To get the expected result from the volume data, the examiner needs to know how to navigate through the volume and use the different tools of the 3D software. In other words, 3D volume manipulation is purely an application of digital software that must be learned. This expertise can only be acquired by hands-on use of this software, as well as by reading literature and attending courses on 3D ultrasound. The goal of this chapter is to provide the user with helpful tips on how to navigate through the volume to achieve the best result. Spatial 3D rendering of a volume will be discussed in Chapter 3.

2.2 Storing and exporting volume data sets

Often, the acquired volume is directly manipulated by the operator during the examination. This poses the risk of losing the volume if one of the knobs is accidentally pressed. For this reason, we recommend saving a good volume directly to the hard drive of the ultrasound machine before processing the volume further. When saving the data set to the hard disk, care should be taken to ensure that the correct file format is selected. This is usually achieved by adjusting the configuration of the "save buttons" when the ultrasound unit is installed in an ultrasound lab. A volume can be saved (incorrectly) as an image (TIFF, JPEG, PNG) or correctly as a volume data set (3D). Acquired STIC or 4D volumes should be saved as "volume cineloop" and not as 3D. If a volume is saved in the wrong format, later editing will be impossible. To determine if a volume or image is stored correctly on the device, it is best to capture different images and volumes and open and edit them at the end of the examination. STIC and 4D volumes have a timeline icon that is used to illustrate a series of volumes.

When working with a volume, the "Export" function allows you to export the result as an image (e. g., the figures in this book), as a video clip (e. g., for patients or for use in scientific lectures), or as a digital data set. To export a volume or collection of volumes from a patient examination to an external drive, it is recommended to export the data set as "uncompressed volume data" and in the ".4dv" format. Saving in this format makes it easier to select the data for re-import into an ultrasound system of the

https://doi.org/10.1515/9783111249513-002

same series or for use on a remote computer with the PC 4D-view® software. Exporting in digital 3D format size (.obj, .xyz, .stl, .ply and others) for the use on a 3D printer or 3D software is also possible.

2.3 Orientation in the three orthogonal planes

After a volume acquisition, the 3D display on the screen is in most cases in a multiplanar mode, usually in the three orthogonal planes (Fig. 2.1). These planes are labeled A, B and C, respectively. Plane A is displayed at the top left of the image and refers to the reference plane during volume acquisition (see Chapter 1). Planes B and C are digitally reconstructed planes and perpendicular to plane A. Plane B is the 90° rotation, and C corresponds to the horizontal plane. The acquisition angle corresponds to the aperture angle of plane B, while the width of the box corresponds to the width of image A. The image in plane A has the best quality because it was generated directly during the volume acquisition, while the images in planes B and C are of lower resolution because they were calculated from the digital information. However, the display of the 3D vo-

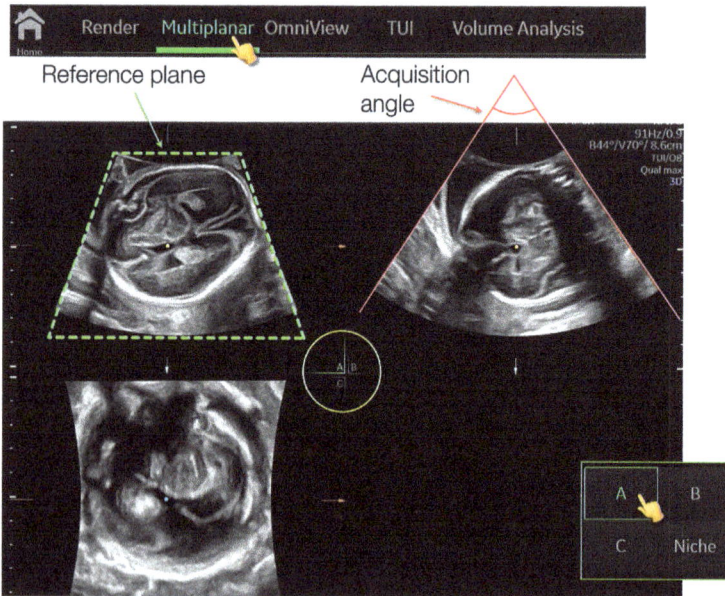

Fig. 2.1: In orthogonal mode (called multiplanar), the volume data set is displayed as three planes that are perpendicular to each other. The reference plane A is shown in the upper left (circle), the 90° vertical rotation plane B in the upper right, and the 90° horizontal rotation plane C in the lower left. In plane B, the acquisition angle (volume depth) is recognized by the size of the image. Note that in the center of the image, planes A, B and C are displayed (circle); the active plane is shown in green and the non-active planes are faded. The activation of the plane is done via the touch panel of the ultrasound machine as shown in the lower field on the right.

lume can be saved differently by the user as a preset, so that a 3D rendering, a tomographic image, or any other result appears on the screen immediately after a volume has been acquired.

2.4 Navigation within the orthogonal planes

Navigation within a volume allows the creation of new planes and can thus simulate an ultrasound examination. Navigation usually requires four buttons and the trackball, as shown in Figure 2.2. These functions are activated as soon as the volume is opened in any 3D mode. In orthogonal mode, the planes visible on the screen are interrelated and any change in one plane affects the other two (Fig. 2.3–2.7). The so-called active plane is selected as the start plane, which can be recognized by the green color of the letter A, B or C for the corresponding active plane (Fig. 2.3). When navigation is performed in the active plane, the images in the other two orthogonal planes change. The operator can switch to another plane to continue navigation, which then becomes the active plane. In general, navigation in a 3D volume can be done in three ways:
1. By moving the intersection point in one plane (called navigation),
2. by rotating the axes (called rotation), or
3. by scrolling through the volume and obtaining parallel images (called translation).

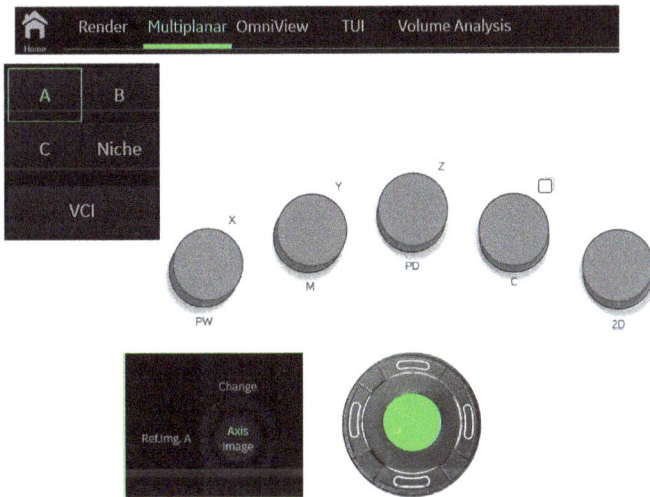

Fig. 2.2: By choosing the multiplanar mode on the touch panel, a submenu opens that shows the A, B and C planes. If desired, Volume Contrast Imaging (VCI) can be activated. The buttons on the keypad can be used to rotate the x, y, or z-axis; a button (C) additionally allows scrolling through the selected plane. The trackball can be used to change the position of the intersection point on the screen.

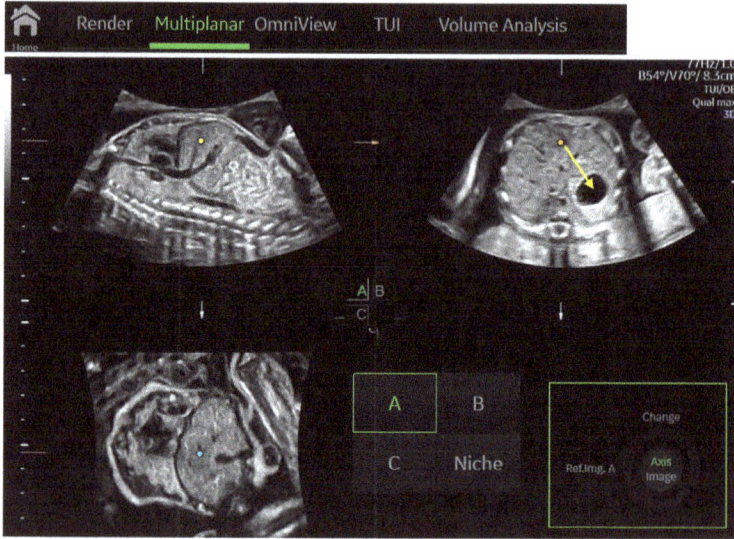

Fig. 2.3: This figure and Figure 2.4 show how the intersection point can be used for navigation within the volume. The multiplanar mode (orthogonal display mode) is selected. In panels A, B, and C the point is shown at the same position in the three planes. In A (upper left), it is displayed in yellow, in B (upper right) in orange, and in C (bottom left) in cyan. In this example, all three planes intersect in the liver. In plane B, the stomach is detected. Select panel B and move the point in plane B (arrow) to place it on the stomach. The images in layers A and B change accordingly with the result shown in Figure 2.4.

The planes are labeled A, B or C (Fig. 2.1), whereas the axes are labeled x, y and z and are displayed in different colors (Fig. 2.8, 2.9).

Navigation with the intersection point: In the orthogonal mode, the three planes A, B, and C are perpendicular to each other and the intersection of all three planes is the intersection point displayed on the screen (Fig. 2.3). This point can be actively clicked and moved from its position by the examiner, resulting in a change in the other two planes (Figs. 2.3, 2.4, 2.5). Since the point always indicates the same structure in all three planes, it can be placed and changed in any plane depending on the region of interest. Such navigation can always be done in any of the A, B, or C planes. Figures 2.3 to 2.5 illustrate a step by step navigation using the intersection point.

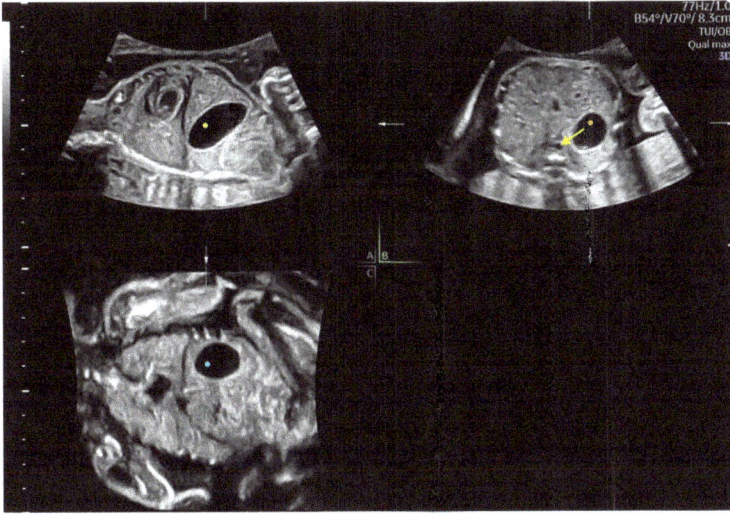

Fig. 2.4: See Figure 2.3. After moving the intersection point in plane B (upper right) to the stomach, the images in plane A (upper left) and plane C (bottom left) have changed to reveal new images showing the stomach (colored dot). The dot always shows in the same place in all three planes. Now imagine the examiner wants, e. g., to visualize the descending aorta. In plane B, the dot is moved to the descending aorta (arrow) and two new planes, A and C, appear, as shown in Figure 2.5.

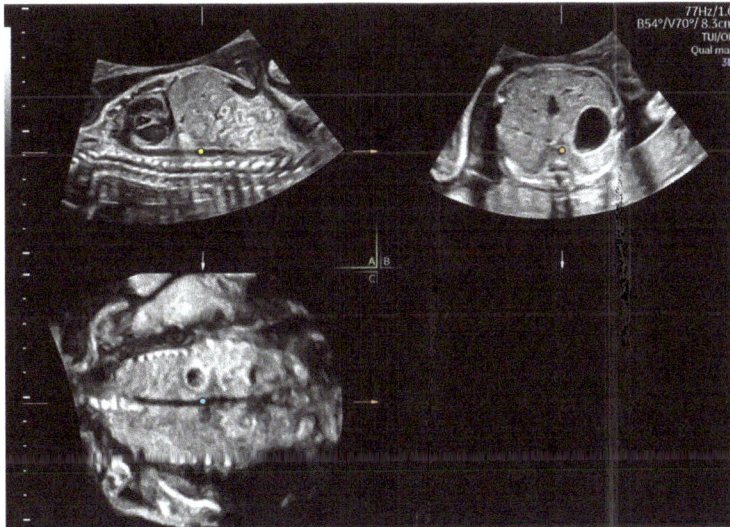

Fig. 2.5: See Figures 2.3 and 2.4. In this figure, the intersection point is now in plane B (upper right) in the aorta, which can also be seen in planes A (upper left) and C (bottom left). Plane A has additionally been rotated to show the aorta horizontally.

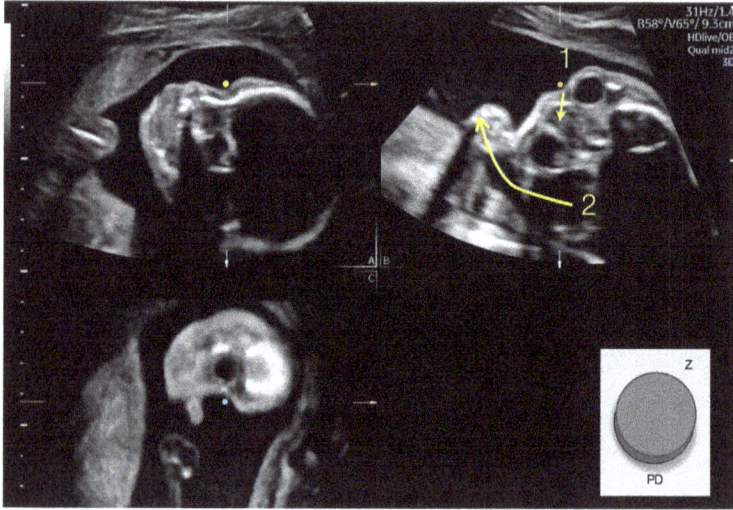

Fig. 2.6: 3D volume of a fetal face in orthogonal display mode. Plane A (upper left) gives the impression that the fetal profile is visible, but planes B (upper right) and C (bottom left) show that the plane is oblique. To adjust the volume, the intersection point in plane B is moved so that it is on the nose (1, short arrow) (as explained in Fig. 2.1). The image is then rotated (2, curved arrow) about this point by turning the rotation knob (Z) (bottom right) until both eyes are horizontal and the profile in plane A can be seen exactly in the midline, as shown in Figure 2.7. This step of the manipulation is called rotation.

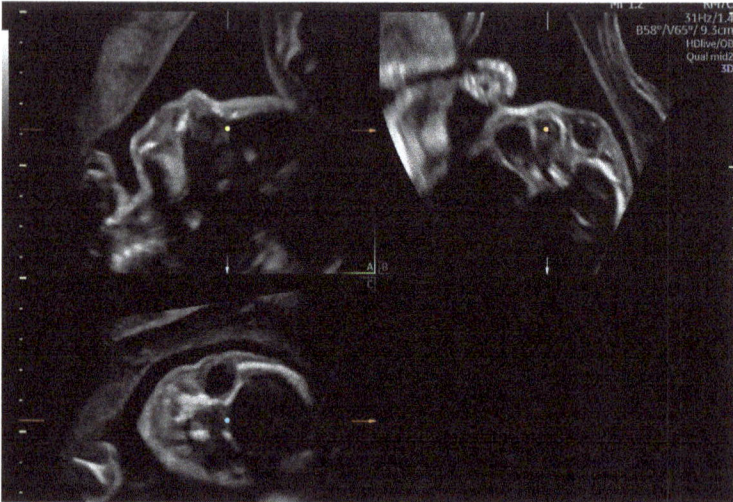

Fig. 2.7: The 3D volume in Figure 2.6 was adjusted so that both eyes in plane B (upper right) are horizontal. In the next step, plane C (bottom left) was adjusted to align the facial axis and obtain the profile in plane A exactly in the midline.

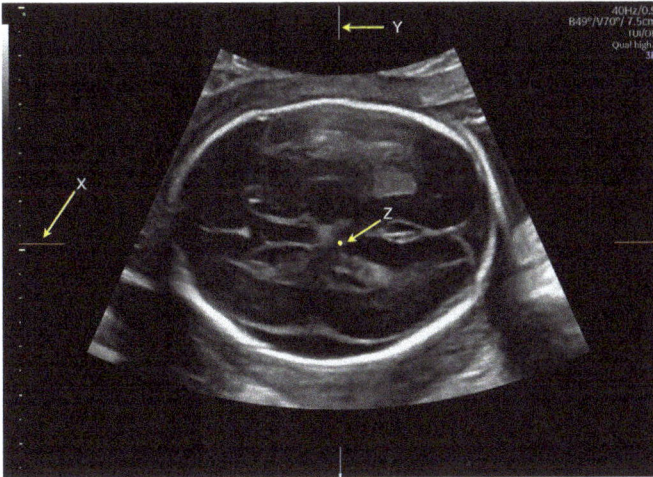

Fig. 2.8: This image is part of a 3D volume in orthogonal display mode where plane A shows the three axes x, y, and z as a horizontal line, vertical line, and a dot, respectively.

Rotation: Selecting one of the x, y, or z-axes allows the image to be rotated along that axis (Figs. 2.6, 2.7, 2.8). The axes can be rotated either by using one of the three knobs on the machine (Fig. 2.2) or by selecting one of the lines on the screen with the track-ball. Rather than trying to figure out which knob results in which rotation, most beginners will take a trial-and-error approach by turning a knob and seeing what happens on the screen.

Translation: After selecting an active plane on the screen, turning the translation knob results in scrolling through parallel planes to the active plane (Figs. 2.9, 2.10). This scrolling is like a sliding movement with the transducer during a live examination.

INIT, the initial position and starting point: Occasionally, the examiner may lose orientation after turning various knobs and moving the intersection point (Fig. 2.11). The easiest way to restore orientation is to press the "INIT" button, which will return the volume display to the initial position (Figs. 2.11, 2.12) when it was acquired and saved.

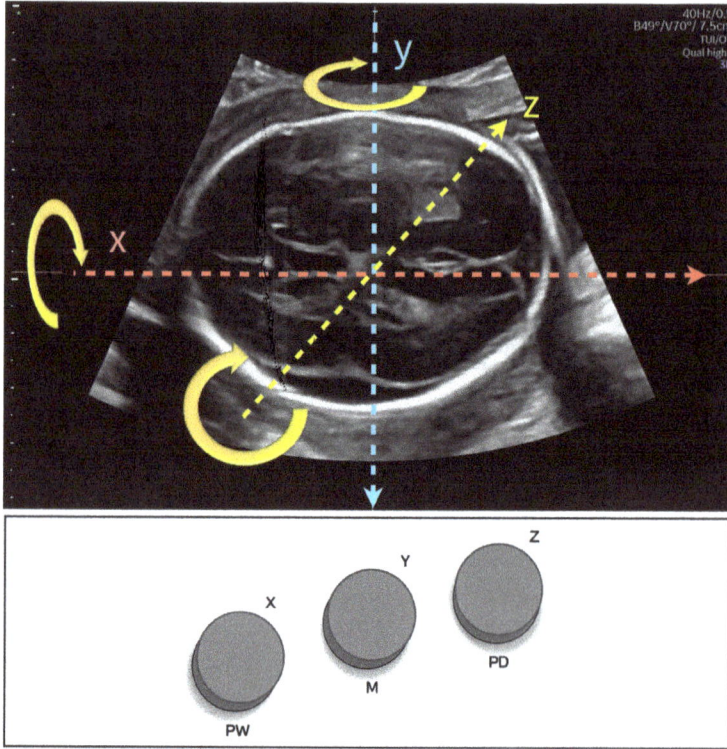

Fig. 2.9: Orthogonal display mode with the lines of the x, y, and z-axes drawn for better understanding. The arrows show the directions of rotation that result when the x, y, or z buttons are rotated in either direction. The bottom panel shows that the Pulse Wave Doppler (PW), M-Mode (M) and Power Doppler (PD) buttons change their function when a 3D volume is acquired and they become the x, y, and z-axis rotation buttons.

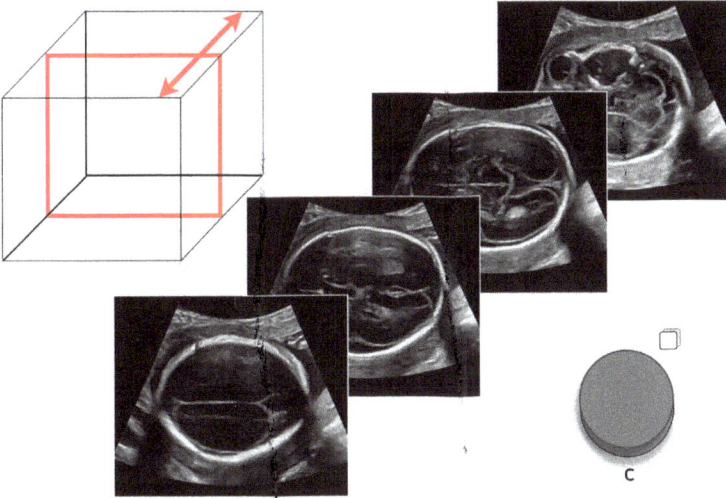

Fig. 2.10: Scrolling through a volume means that the displayed images are parallel to the initial plane and the scrolling corresponds to a translational motion. It is a sliding along a horizontal axis (upper left shape). The bottom right panel shows that the color Doppler button (C) changes its function when a 3D volume is acquired and becomes the button used for scrolling. Turning it to the left and right scrolls the volume up and down. In addition to the navigation tools already explained, such as the intersection and the x, y, and z rotations, translation is the third tool used to navigate within a 3D volume data set.

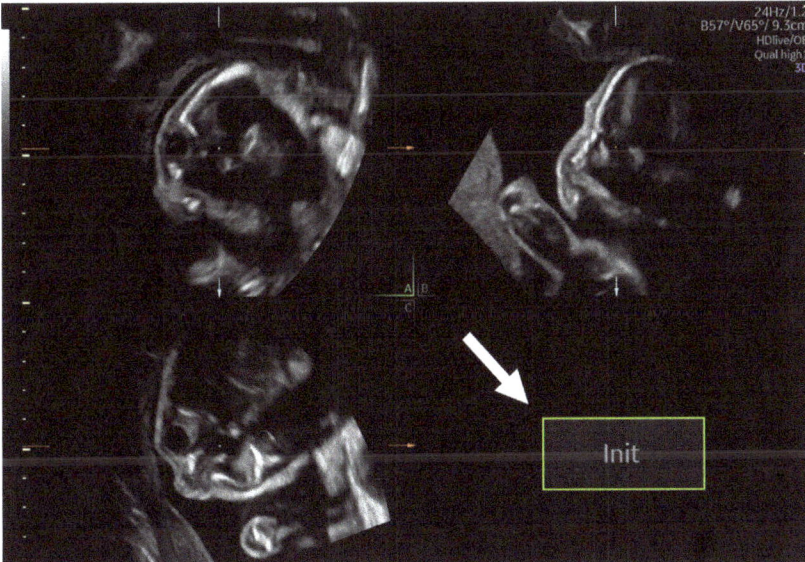

Fig. 2.11: During navigation through a volume with axis rotation and translation, orientation was lost, as shown in this case. By activating the INIT function on the touch panel, the user can return to the original version of the images as acquired in the volume, similar to an "Undo" function.

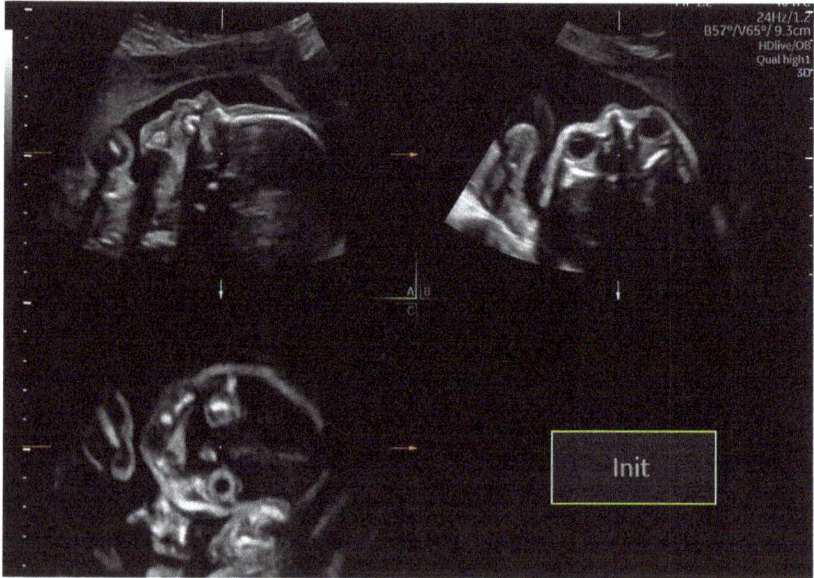

Fig. 2.12: The figure shows Figure 2.11 after activating the INIT function. Now the frontal view of the face can be seen as captured in the original volume.

2.5 Artifacts in the multiplanar mode

Artifacts occur more frequently in 3D sonography than in 2D sonography. They occur during 3D volume acquisition and are either due to maternal movements, such as breathing, laughing etc., or more commonly due to fetal movements. Artifacts that occur during volume acquisition are best detected in the B or C plane in orthogonal mode (Figs. 2.13, 2.14). While significant movements are easily detected, small movement artifacts result in only a slight distortion of the image that can escape detection. Subtle artifacts in volume acquisition of regions such as the brain, heart, abdominal organs, or skeleton often remain hidden. The examiner should therefore always bear in mind that a 3D examination is a reconstructed examination of acquired planes; this may become relevant when performing measurements.

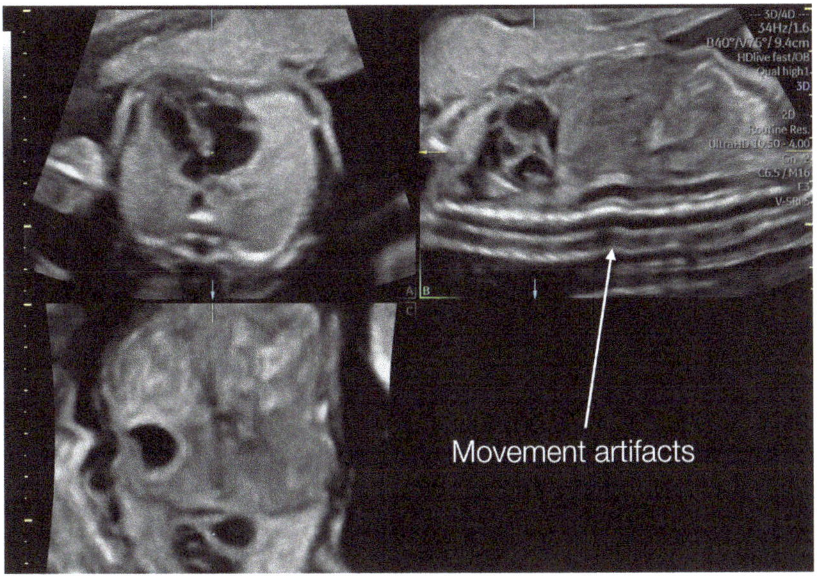

Fig. 2.13: Images in plane A (upper left) are captured directly during volume acquisition and are rarely subject to motion artifacts. Images in planes B (upper right) or C (bottom left) are digitally reconstructed images from adjacent images in plane A and may therefore reflect movement artifacts during acquisition. The artefacts may originate from fetal or maternal movements. Artifacts during volume acquisition are therefore best detected in layers B and C.

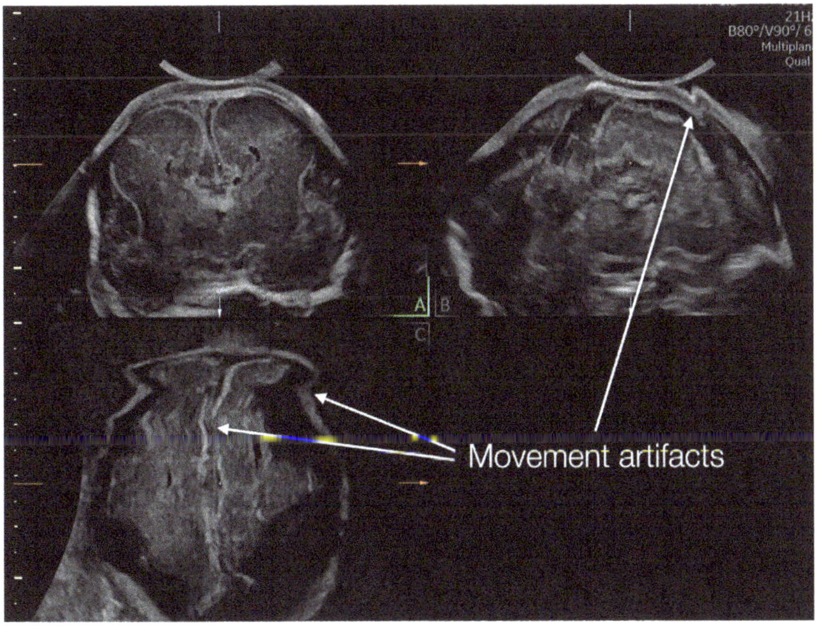

Fig. 2.14: Movement artifacts can be recognized in planes B (upper right) or C (bottom left) as seen in this 3D volume acquisition of a fetal brain.

2.6 Conclusions

Post-processing a volume is a prerequisite for understanding 3D volume ultrasound. The two most important steps are orientation and navigation within a volume. Navigation within a volume is better in the multiplanar mode than in the volume rendering mode. The best orientation is achieved in the three orthogonal planes, called A, B and C planes, with the intersection point directed to the same point in the three planes. The intersection point can be used to navigate within the planes, while the x, y, and z axes are used to rotate the images within the volume. The scrolling button can be used to move from one plane to the next in translation. These basic steps allow to generate planes out of a volume, especially if they were not ideally visualized in the live scan, thus opening a new field of imaging. Navigation also makes it possible to simulate an examination from a stored volume data set, which can be used to share volumes between examiners or to save them on storage drives for later assessment.

Part II: **3D Display Methods**

3 3D Rendering and the Rendering Modes

3.1 Introduction

Spatial reconstruction of a volume data set with the projection of a 3D image onto the screen is synonymous with 3D ultrasound for many users. Ideally, this involves documenting the face of the fetus or other body parts, such as hands and feet. In the language of 3D software and terminology, this spatial reconstruction and projection is referred to as *rendering*. The 3D rendering of an ultrasound volume data set is done according to some principles and with different tools which will be explained in this chapter. Understanding some of the basics of volume rendering and volume manipulation can be very helpful in obtaining good quality results in the various render modes. These modes are described separately in Chapters 7 to 13.

3.2 The render box and the orientation within a 3D volume

In any multiplanar mode, 3D volume rendering can be selected by activating the "Rendering" function on the touch panel. A rectangle then appears in the three planes (A, B and C), and an additional fourth, computed 3D image is displayed in the lower right corner (Fig. 3.1). This volume rendering box, referred to as the *render box* throughout this book, can be changed in height, width, and depth. In the render box, the operator can select the information to be included in the 3D calculation (Figs. 3.2–3.6). The result is immediately visible on the rendered 3D image. All sides of the box are white, except for one side shown in green in two planes (Figs. 3.2 to 3.6). This is the *projection line* or *green line* (like a camera) from which the perspective of the 3D image is seen. To facilitate orientation, the box has two landmarks, namely a rectangle and a diamond, which are also displayed in the 3D box (Fig. 3.7). As experience increases, orientation in the 3D image becomes easier and the green box with the landmarks can be removed from the 3D image; the perspective from which the image is viewed in 3D can also be changed (Figs. 3.3–3.5). To visualize the face, the line is often placed directly in the amniotic fluid in front of the face (Fig. 3.2). Figures 3.3 to 3.5 show examples of how changing the projection line affects the result. Under certain anatomical conditions, e. g., when imaging the heart (Fig. 3.6), it may be necessary to change the line into a curve (Fig. 3.3). This can be achieved by changing the position of a point to obtain a curved line. Figure 3.3 shows how the straight line can be transformed into a curved line.

https://doi.org/10.1515/9783111249513-003

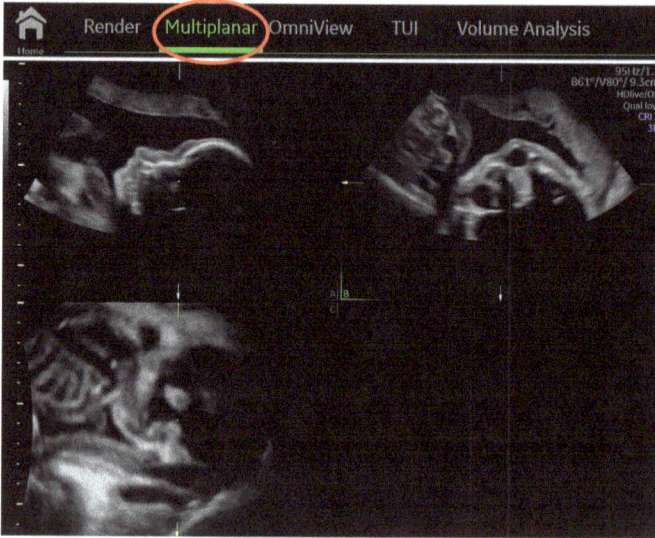

Fig. 3.1: 3D volume acquisition was performed on this fetal face; it is displayed in the orthogonal mode, as shown in the top panel labeled "Multiplanar". To display the 3D rendering of the face, the "Render" function should be activated on the touch panel (top panel).

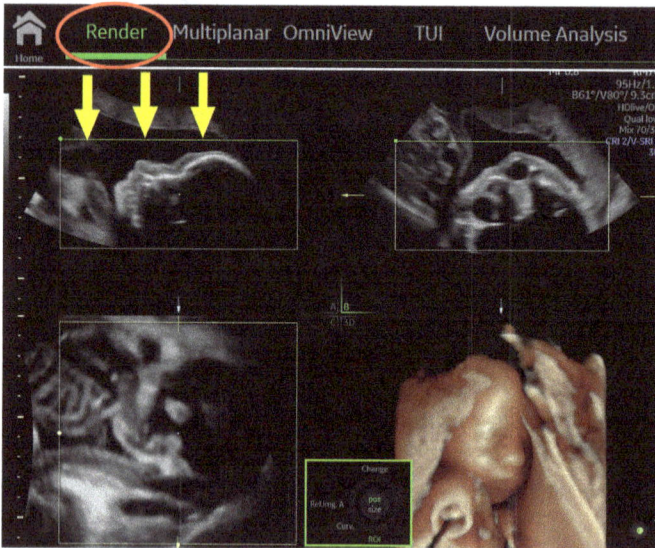

Fig. 3.2: By activating the "Render" function on the touch panel (circled in the top panel), the examiner can switch from orthogonal rendering mode to volume rendering mode. A render box appears in planes A, B, and C and the 3D image is generated and displayed in the bottom right panel. The size of the render box can be changed with the trackball by changing the position of one of the six edges of the box, thus defining the ultrasound information to be displayed in the volume (see Fig. 3.3). The green projection line (arrows) shows the perspective of the view into the volume. The green rendering line can be changed in its shape and position, as shown in Figures 3.3 through 3.8.

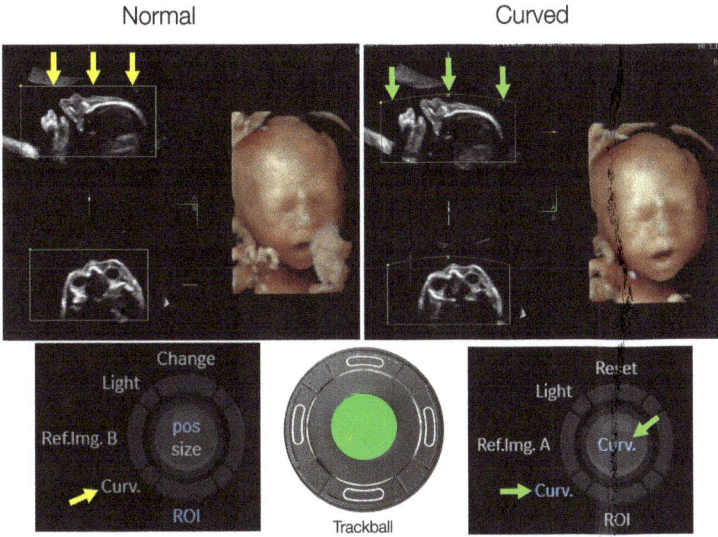

Normal   **Curved**

Fig. 3.3: The render box line is a straight line by default but can be changed with the trackball to a curved line to better fit certain situations, as shown in the upper right image. The lower left button near the trackball activates the curved line and the upper button labeled "Reset" can deactivate the curved line so that it becomes a straight line again.

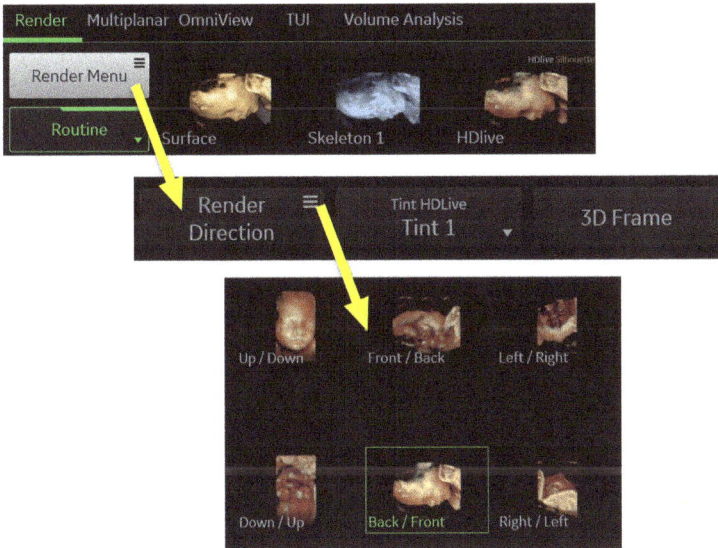

Fig. 3.4: The touch panel shows how to change the render direction. The position of the render line in the 3D render box can be changed according to the desired viewing direction into the volume. By default, the top/bottom view is selected. To select a different render direction, the "Render Menu" panel is selected (top panel) and the "Render Direction" menu is chosen in the submenu (middle panel), retrieving six options. See Figures 3.5 and 3.6 for different views.

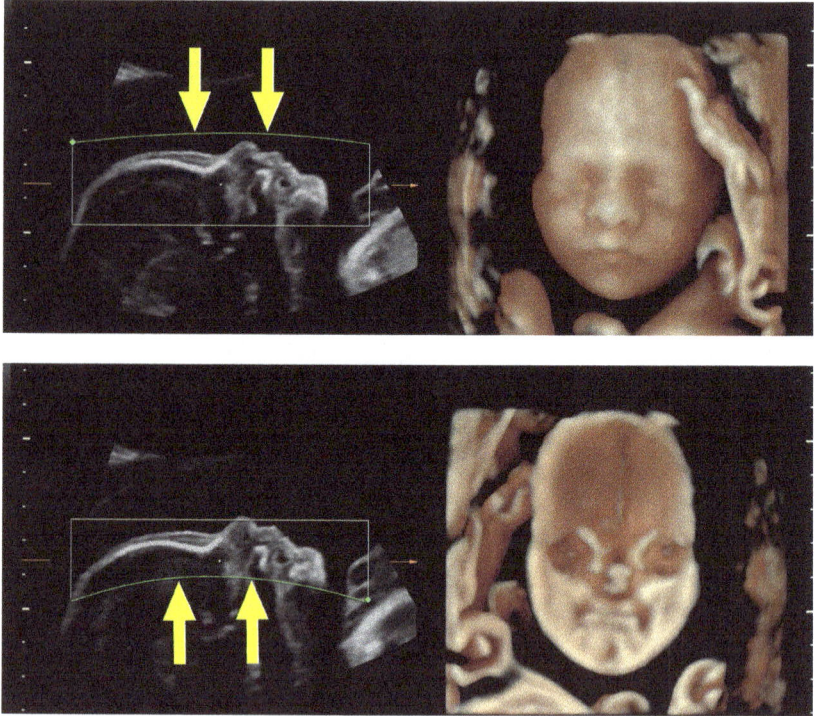

Fig. 3.5: In the upper image the projection line is placed in the amniotic fluid in front of the face (up/down line). In the lower image, the projection line is placed behind the face (down/up), and the so-called reverse-face view is displayed. See Figure 3.4 for explanation.

Once the render box is placed in its final position in the volume and contains the required information, it can be "fixed" for further manipulations. With this selection, the orientation lines disappear (Fig. 3.8). In other words, out of the entire acquired volume, only the information placed inside the render box is then available for further 3D volume manipulations; the adjacent information is no longer displayed in the 3D image. After this step, the *Magicut tool* (electronic scalpel) can be used to remove parts of the image, the 3D result can be rotated, and different display modes can be selected. These actions are called *volume manipulation*.

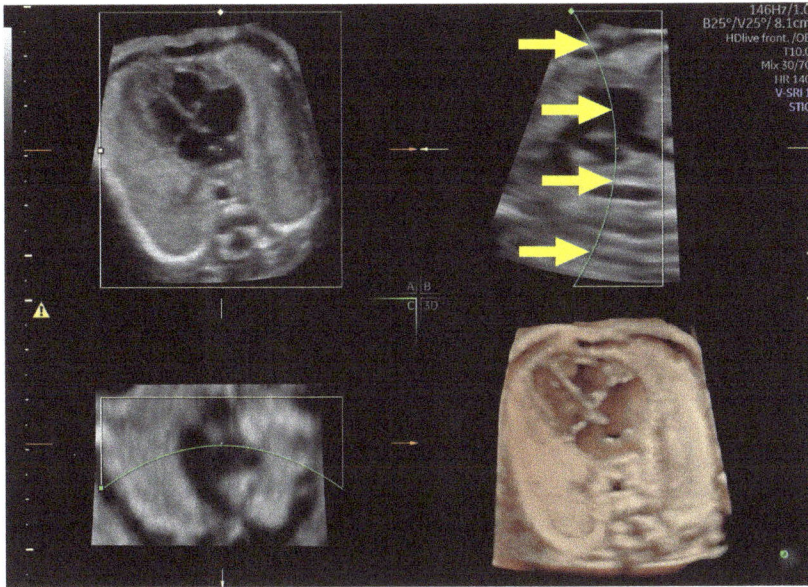

Fig. 3.6: In this STIC volume, the projection line (arrows) is placed in the thorax just inside the heart and below the aortic root (plane B) with a curved line (see Fig. 3.3); the direction line has been chosen as front/back (see Fig. 3.4). This allows demonstration of the four-chamber view in STIC and can also be used for color Doppler STIC.

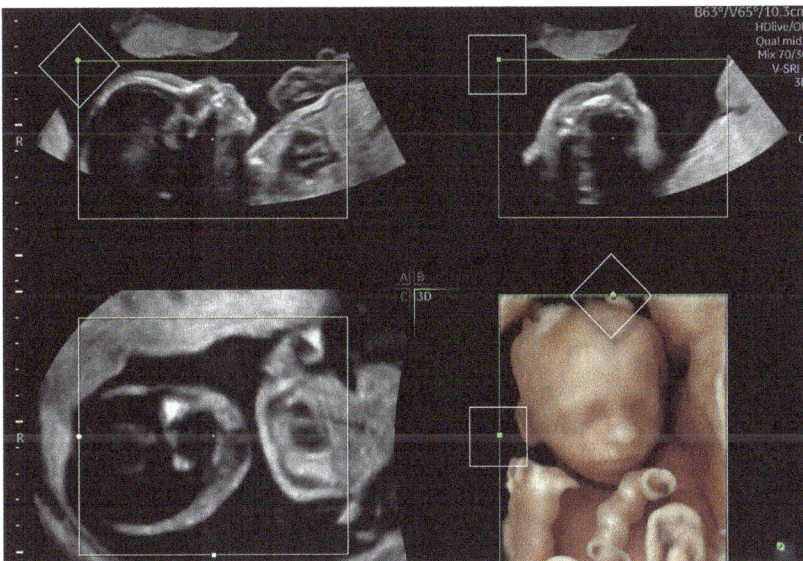

Fig. 3.7: The 3D image (bottom right) shows only the information contained in the render box. Here, the upper part of the head is outside the box and therefore not visible in 3D. For better orientation, two markers are displayed in the render box, namely a square and a rhombus.

3.3 Artifacts in 3D rendering

Artifacts in 3D are often the result of fetal movements during volume acquisition; occasionally they are caused by maternal movements. These artifacts can be identified during 3D rendering directly on one of the displayed 2D images or on the rendered 3D image (Fig. 3.9). While large movements cause obvious artifacts that render the image useless for further interpretation, some smaller fetal movements cause slight image distortions that may not be detected. Small artifacts in the face are often recognized immediately, whereas smaller artifacts in other regions may remain undetected. In a real-time 4D examination, the examiner can immediately switch to the image without artifacts, whereas in a 3D examination, the examiner must repeat the volume acquisition. Figure 3.9 shows some 3D movement artifacts.

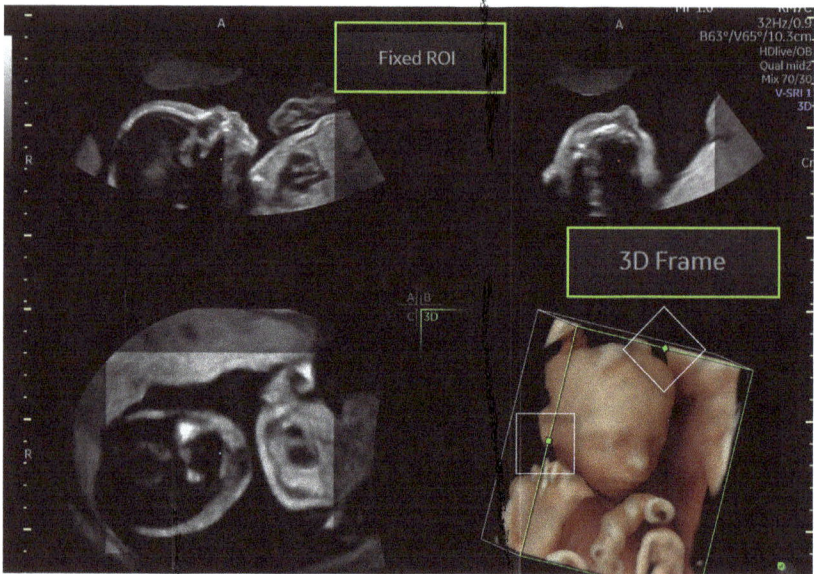

Fig. 3.8: In this case, the render box has been "fixed" or "confirmed", meaning that the contents of the 3D image, as shown in the bottom right image, are the result that can be manipulated. The lines of the render box in planes A, B, and C are no longer shown. The 3D frame is shown only in the 3D image, but as you gain experience, the 3D frame can be disabled, as displayed in all the figures in this book.

3.4 Different rendering modes and mixture of modes

The render box provides the ability to display information from the acquired volume data set using various rendering modes. The rendered 3D image then appears as a 2D projection on the monitor with the impression of a 3D effect (like all 3D images in this book). The render box often contains information from different fetal structures that have different ultrasound properties: fluid is anechoic, bony structures are hyperechoic, and tissue is hypoechoic. Once the render box and projection line are selected, the ultrasound system evaluates all signals in the depth of the box seen from the projection line, and the selected mode displays the desired information. In general, there are two algorithms for 3D rendering with different types of visualization: surface rendering or transparent rendering.

Movement artifacts

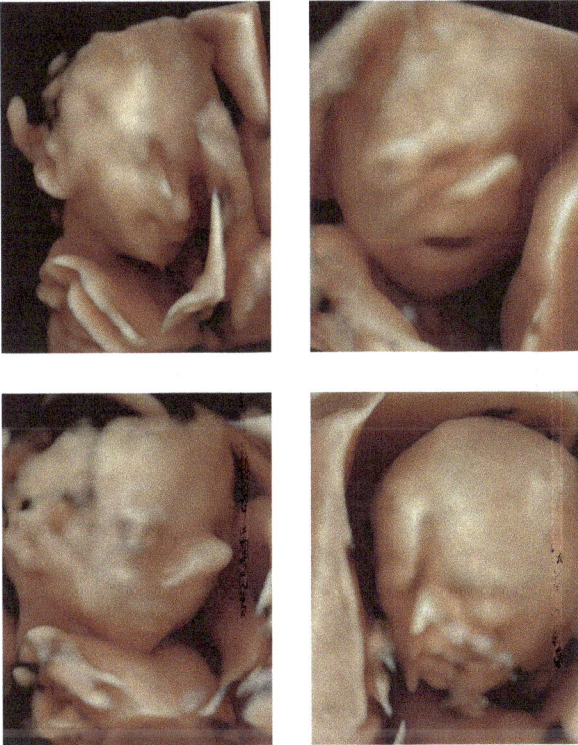

Fig. 3.9: During 3D volume acquisition these fetuses moved, resulting in obvious motion artifacts in the imagery.

3.4.1 Surface mode rendering

Surface mode rendering (Fig. 3.10) mainly analyzes the ultrasound signals located directly behind the projection line. Generally, the projection line is placed in the amniotic fluid so that the fetal skin is visible. Chapter 7 discusses in detail the surface mode. Several rendering algorithms available for surface mode visualization are discussed in this section. Their selection depends on the object to be visualized but also on aesthetic or taste aspects. The following rendering and display modes are available:

Surface smooth, surface texture: In these modes only the area next to the projection line is displayed (Figs. 3.10, 3.11). In surface texture, the exact grayscale information of the images is displayed; in surface smooth, the grayscale information is slightly blurred with a filter and displayed softly. This render mode is often used, but it is almost replaced by the HDlive mode.

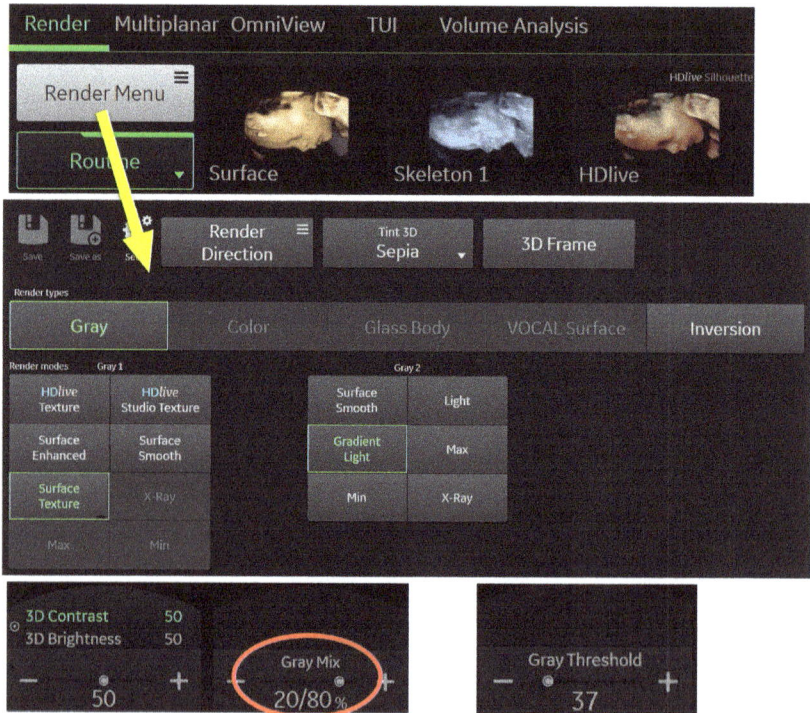

Fig. 3.10: Once the 3D rendering mode is selected, the examiner can choose a mixture of two gray modes for the displayed image (red circle at the bottom). The selectable modes can be found in the submenu of the "Render Menu" (arrow). Figures 3.11–3.13 show the available renderings.

Surface smooth   Surface texture

Maximum   Light

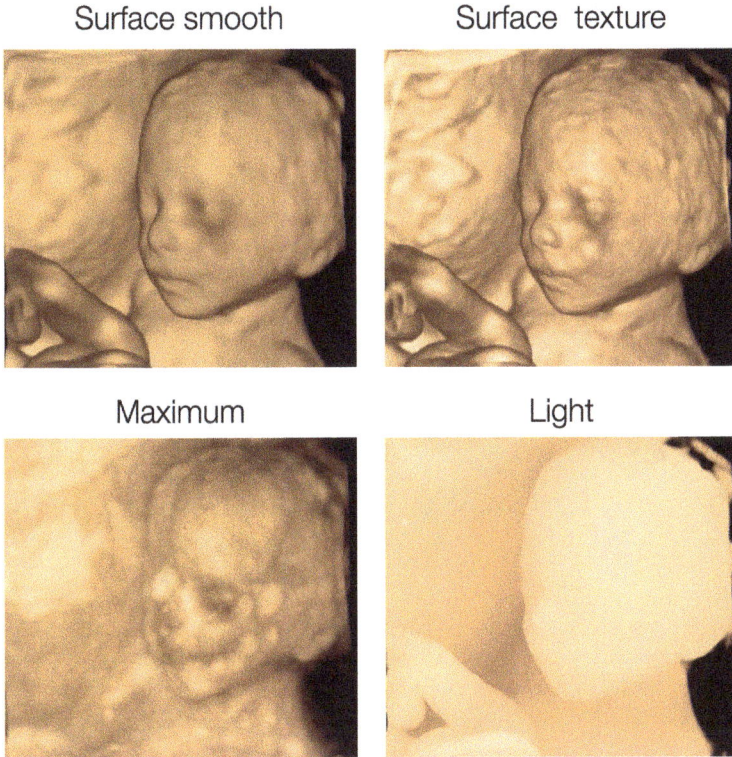

Fig. 3.11: The 3D rendered image of the same fetus is displayed in different render modes, such as "Surface smooth", "Surface texture", "Maximum" or "Light" (see Fig. 3.10). For these fetuses, 100%/0% was selected.

Light: In this display, light and dark modes are predominantly rendered in such a way that structures near the projection line are rendered light and deeper structures are rendered dark (Fig. 3.11, bottom right). The light mode is hardy used anymore though it might be used occasionally with the inversion mode.

Gradient light: In this display, the surface is shown as if it is illuminated by a light source with depth effect (Fig. 3.12, upper left). Structures that are perpendicular to the insonation are displayed brighter than others. Gradient light gives the best results when there is sufficient fluid around the structure. This render mode has been often used until recently but is now almost replaced by the HDlive display.

HDlive: The High-Definition (HD) live mode was introduced years later to improve the surface image and produce a more realistic, skin-like image (Figs. 3.5, 3.7, 3.12). HDlive can be used by selecting HDlive texture or HDlive smooth, but usually a mixture of both, depending on the desired organ and softness. This mode has become the most

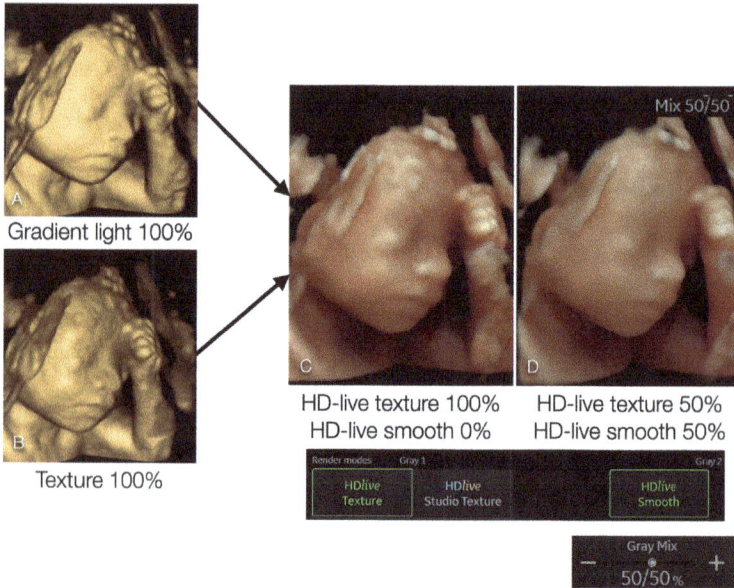

Gradient light 100%

Texture 100%

HD-live texture 100% HD-live texture 50%
HD-live smooth 0%   HD-live smooth 50%

Fig. 3.12: A mixture of two gray modes is often selected for 3D image display. The figure shows in (A) a fetal face in Gradient light mode (100%) and in (B) in Surface texture mode (100%). The introduction of HDlive has improved the skin-like appearance of the face, resulting in the images (C) and (D) with a mixture of HDlive surface and smooth at different proportions.

popular for surface mode. In addition, HDlive rendering mode has since evolved and an additional transparency mode, called *silhouette mode*, has been introduced. The silhouette mode can only be used in combination with the HDlive mode. Chapter 11 describes in detail how to use the various tools in the silhouette mode.

3.4.2 Transparency mode rendering

While only the first layer is displayed in surface mode, the various transparency modes provide the ability to highlight specific details within the entire box according to their echogenic properties. Depending on the object of interest, all signals contained in the render box are analyzed and displayed accordingly.

Maximum mode: In this transparency mode, all hyperechogenic information in the render box is calculated and projected (Fig. 3.13, upper left) (see also Chapter 8). This render mode is used to visualize bones and is ideal for examining the fetal skeletal system (see Chapter 17). This tool is often used to visualize bones in live 4D examination in combination with VCI-A.

Maximum

Minimum

Inversion

X-Ray Contrast

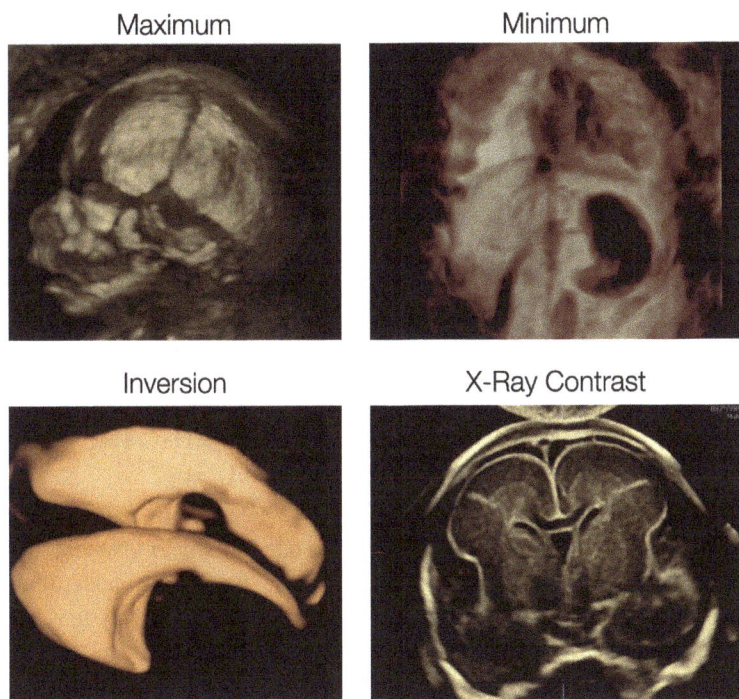

Fig. 3.13: Demonstration of different organs and regions using different transparent modes, such as maximum mode (100%), minimum mode (100%), inversion mode, and X-Ray contrast mode. See text and corresponding chapters for the different modes.

Minimum mode: In this transparency mode, anechoic information is calculated and displayed throughout the volume (Fig. 3.13, upper right) (see also Chapter 9). This approach is ideal for visualizing fluid-filled organs as well as the lumen of heart and great vessels. This method is rarely used by now.

Inversion mode: In this transparency mode, components with anechoic information (black) are displayed in inverted color (bright) and become echogenic visible. Signals from neighboring structures are suppressed (Fig. 3.13, bottom left) (see Chapter 10). This rendering mode is still used occasionally.

X-Ray mode: This mode is a contrast mode used for visualization of tissue and is calculated as a mixture of the minimum and maximum transparency modes. The ideal regions to use this mode are the lungs, abdominal organs, brain (Fig. 3.13 bottom right), placenta, and other regions. The X-Ray mode is most often used in combination with a thin slice, as it is the case in Volume Contrast Imaging (VCI) (see Chapter 4). It is rarely used as a stand-alone rendering mode.

HD-live   + Silhouette

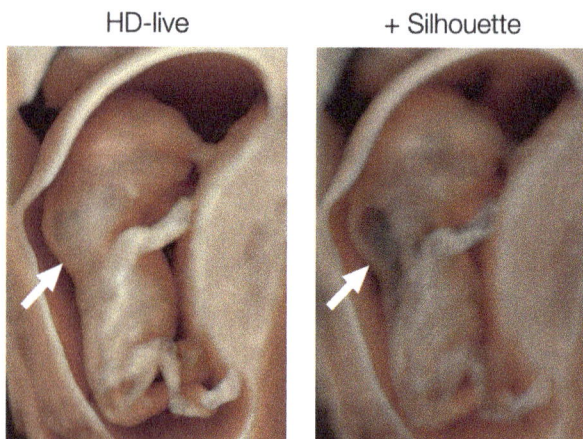

Fig. 3.14: The left image shows this first trimester fetus with increased nuchal translucency in surface mode and HDlive. By activating the silhouette mode and increasing it to a certain value, the skin becomes transparent and the fluid in the neck region becomes more obvious.

Silhouette mode: This recently introduced rendering mode is used to visualize the contours of internal structures. This mode is an add-on to the HDlive mode, with which the gradual transparency is selected by the operator (Fig. 3.14). This tool, together with the surface mode in HDlive, is the most frequently used render mode today and will be discussed separately in Chapter 11.

3.5 Special effects in 3D: dynamic depth rendering and light source

The 3D display on the screen is a projection of a 3D image onto a 2D surface and does not require stereoscopic glasses (as is common in consumer electronics today). To increase the spatial perception of the 3D image, additional image enhancements have been developed. Three functions are of particular importance:

3D Dynamic Depth Rendering: This software can be used in combination with sepia colored display modes such as surface smooth, texture, and gradient light. It renders structures that are deep in the volume with the colors blue, gray, or black; a depth rendering can be perceived with the color change between sepia and blue. However, the degree of depth can be adjusted. These colors can then be shaded, depending on the depth of the regions being examined: nearby areas are rendered lighter and deeper areas are rendered darker. Figure 3.15 shows an example without depth rendering (A) and with depth rendering in gray (B) and blue (C). In early pregnancy, the entire fetus with the amniotic cavity can be easily displayed and highlighted with this depth rendering.

Normal   Dynamic Depth Rendering

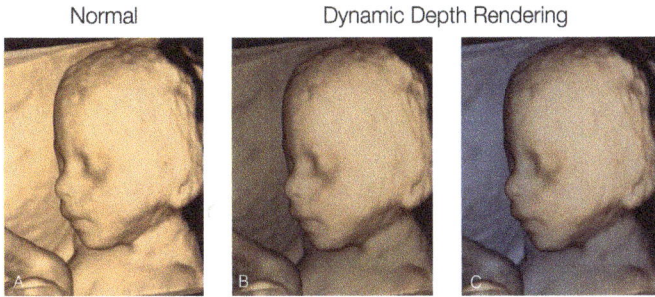

Fig. 3.15: The depth effect can be enhanced by using the "Dynamic Depth Rendering" tool which adds a blue or black color to the structures in the depth of the volume. The image in (A) is the raw image and images (B) and (C) are the result after adding black and blue, respectively. The degree of coloring can be adjusted according to the depth information in the image.

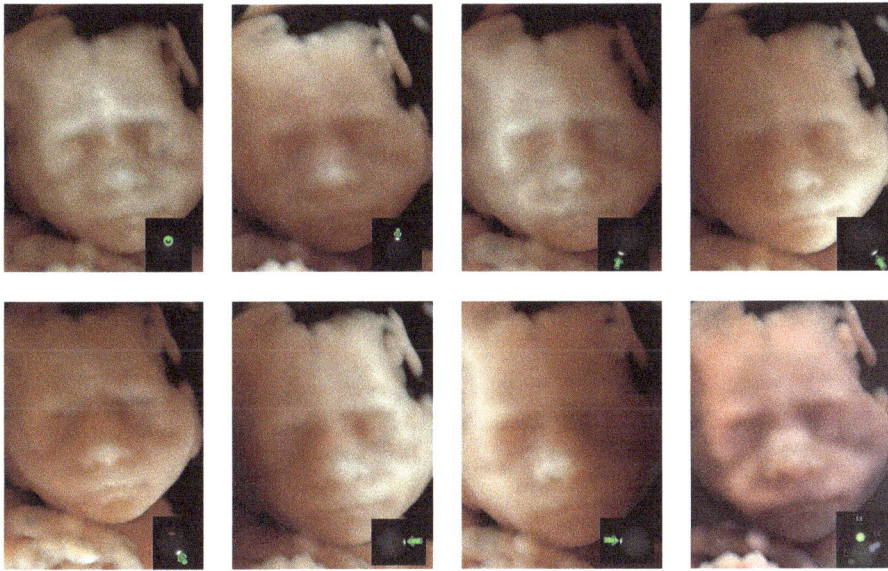

Fig. 3.16: With the current software, the 3D effect can be enhanced by using a light source. Like a flashlight, the light source can be placed in different positions to give the image a different aspect or "mood". For a fetal face, placing the light source in the upper part of the image is ideal. The image in the bottom right was taken with studio light, which consists of a combination of up to three light sources.

HD-live Studio

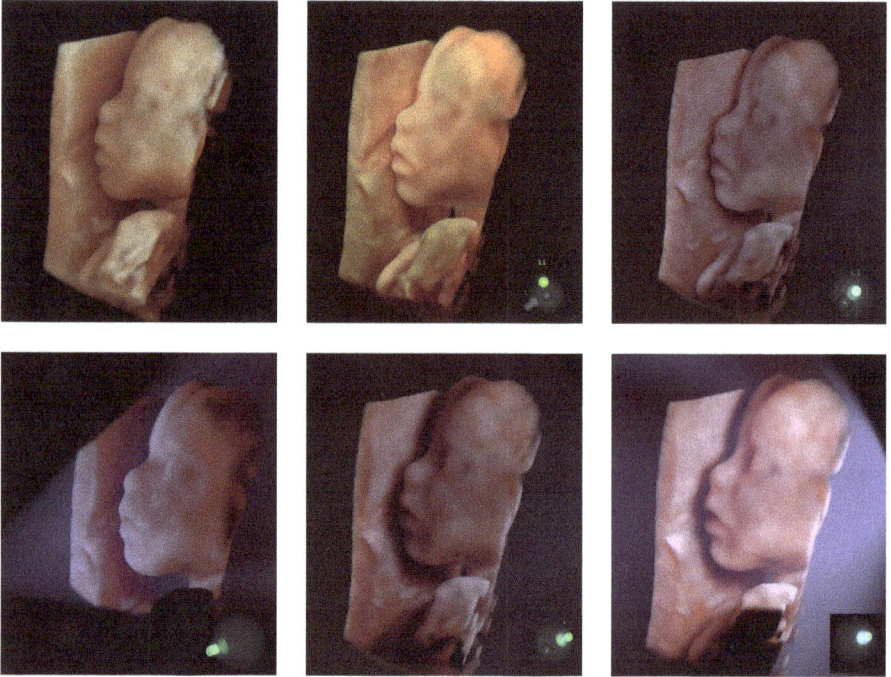

Fig. 3.17: The same fetal face shown in HDlive, but with one light source (upper left). When the HDlive studio tool is activated, three light sources are available that can be placed separately, as shown in the other images. The light sources in use are shown in the bottom right corner of each image, respectively.

Light source function: This software can be used in combination with HDlive and silhouette mode. It allows the 3D image to be illuminated by a light source. Normally, the 3D image appears as if light is projected directly onto the image from the front. The light source software allows the user to move a light source around a virtual sphere in order to illuminate the image from different perspectives, even from behind (Figs. 3.16, 3.17). This can produce impressive results, especially in early gestation (Figs. 3.18, 3.19).

Multiple light sources with "HDlive studio": The introduction of a new light source a few years ago (Fig. 3.16) offered a new option to improve the 3D effect in many render-

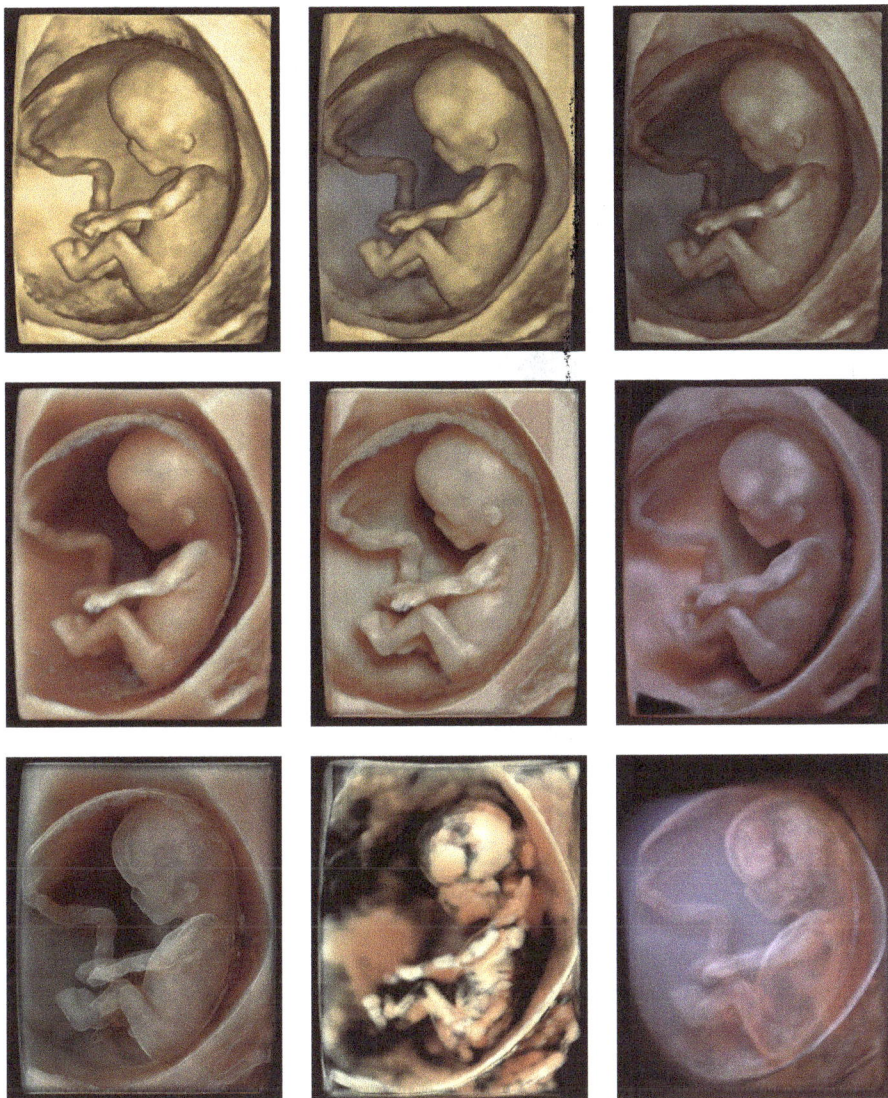

Fig. 3.18: The same 3D volume of this fetus at 12 weeks' gestation is shown in different combinations of displays, such as surface mode, gradient light, HDlive, silhouette and light sources, etc. See also Figure 3.19.

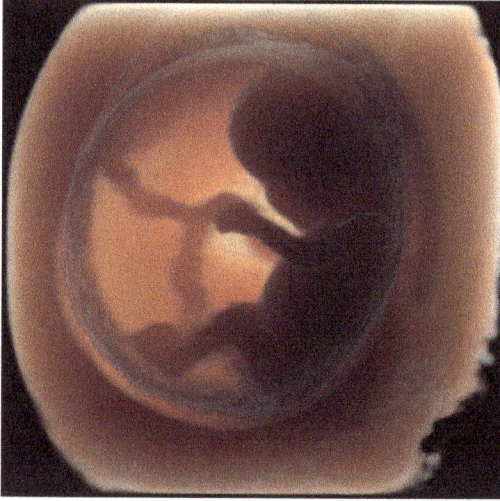

Fig. 3.19: 3D volume of the same fetus as in Figure 3.18, here shown in a combination of surface mode with HDlive surface and combined with the silhouette tool. The light source has been placed behind the image to create this backlight effect.

ing images, especially in combination with HDlive. A more recent software version has improved this light effect by using up to three light sources simultaneously, similar to photography studios. It is therefore called *HDlive studio* (Figs. 3.17, 3.18). The examiner must have some understanding of how to use these light sources since the position of each light source, its distance from the object, and its type can be manipulated separately.

3.6 Threshold, transparency, brightness, and color scales

The quality of a rendered 3D image depends mainly on the 2D image that preceded the volume acquisition (Chapter 1). During 3D volume rendering and manipulation, some tools can be used to improve the quality of the 3D image.

Threshold: The "threshold" or "gray threshold" function defines the degree of gray scale used when displaying the 3D image calculation (Fig. 7.1). This knob can be used mainly to eliminate faint artifacts and speckles in order to highlight structures with real signals. A very low threshold (< 20) may be required to visualize fine structures such as the amniotic membrane or umbilical cord. A medium threshold (25–40) is used to show a wide range of grayscale information as in fetal skin, while a high threshold (> 50) may be applied to highlight bones in maximum mode or other structures in inversion mode. The operator is encouraged to play with this button and see the result on the screen.

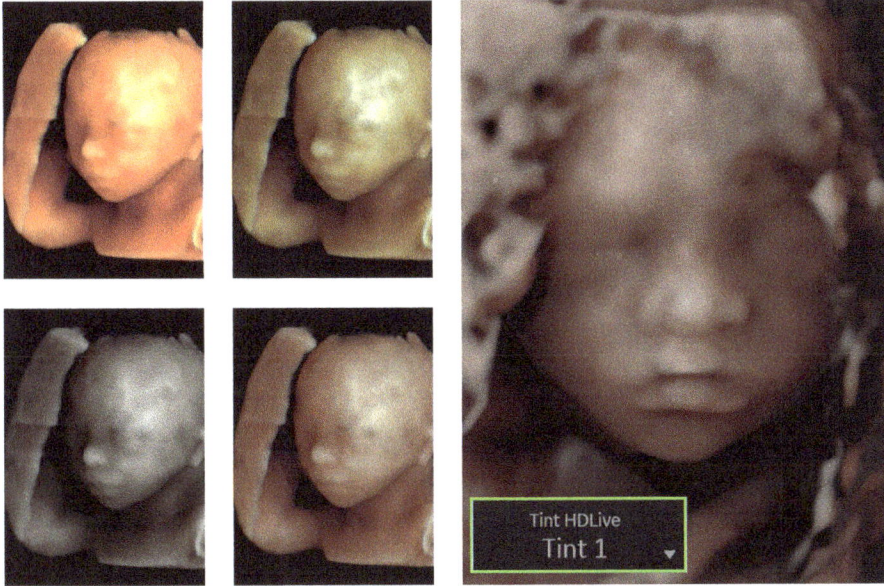

Fig. 3.20: In the 3D rendering modes, different colors can be selected and changed by the examiner. The skin color shown in the images in this book is the popular tint, but occasionally it can be interesting to try other skin tones by opening the "Tint" folder in the HDlive submenu.

Transparency and gain: Gray transparency level can be increased so that the image appears transparent in its depth. More grayscale information can also be obtained by increasing gain, but this often results in more artifacts and less detail.

Brightness and contrast: These can be changed only slightly in most 3D systems and are used to improve the image.

Color tints: Various color tones can be selected to colorize the 3D image, such as the familiar sepia, but also gray, ice or various skin tones. This coloring is often used to enhance the 3D effect (Fig. 3.20). Most examiners will have only a small number of colors in regular use. Various customizable color tones also exist for HDlive.

3.7 Magicut, the electronic scalpel

Magicut basics: Only rarely does the examiner succeed in obtaining such a good 3D image that it does not require any further corrections or post-processing manipulation. In most cases of static 3D volumes, the image can be improved after some retouching and the use of some of the manipulation tools described above. This is often necessary in order to make certain areas better visible, or simply for aesthetic reasons. The elec-

Magicut: simple case

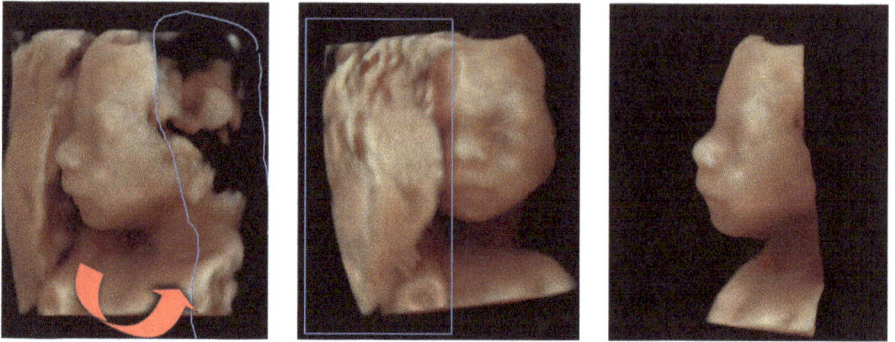

Fig. 3.21: The electronic scalpel is also known as "Magicut". After a volume data set is frozen, the volume can be rotated in all directions and information that is not needed can be deleted. In this simple case, details behind the head have been removed. After rotating the volume, the area behind the face is also deleted, creating this profile view. See also Figure 3.22. The lines are drawn either with the trackball or by hand on the touch panel.

Magicut: challenging case

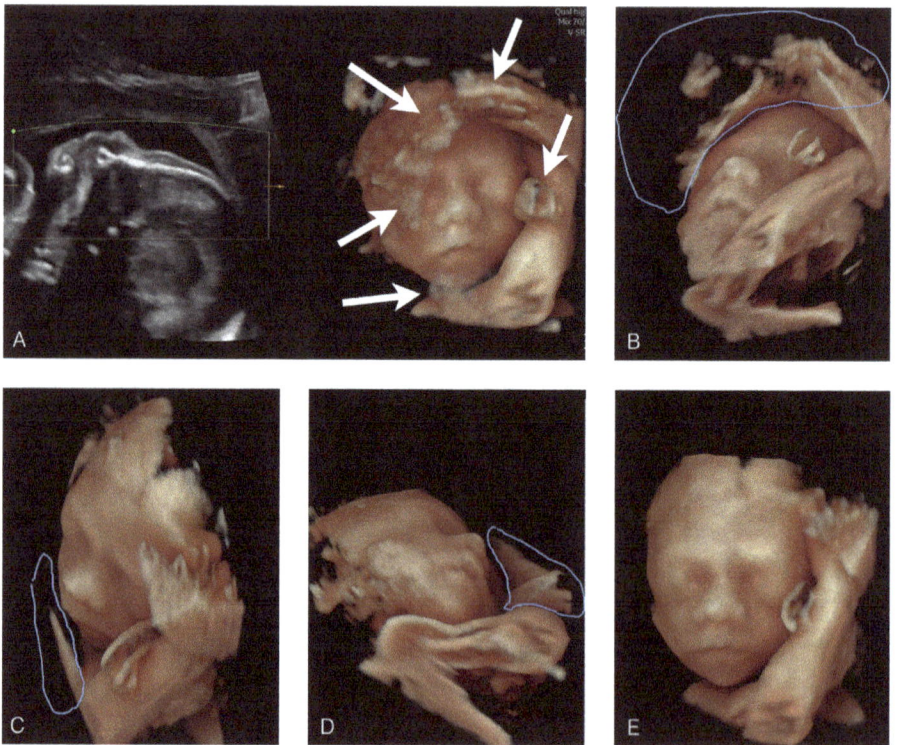

Fig. 3.22: Using Magicut to delete unneeded structures that obscure the face (A). In this complex case, the volume is firstly fixed (see Fig. 3.8); by rotating the volume step by step, different areas are selectively cut out, as shown in panels (B) through (E).

Before   After Magicut

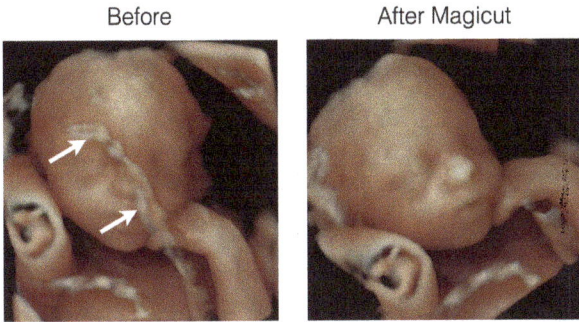

Fig. 3.23: Another example of a face before and after using Magicut to delete the umbilical cord covering the face.

Before   After Magicut

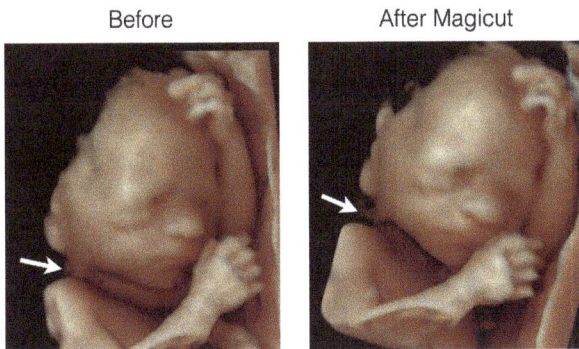

Fig. 3.24: Another example of a head with an umbilical cord before and after using Magicut to delete the umbilical cord around the neck.

tronic scalpel, called *Magicut*, can be activated after the image has been fixed ("Fixed Region of Interest" button). Magicut offers various forms for erasing information within the 3D volume, such as the "eraser small or big", cutting in the "box inside/outside", or free drawing with "trace inside/outside". The depth of the erased information can also be selected between "full" and "defined", and additional functions are available in the color Doppler glass-body mode. Figures 3.21 to 3.24 show examples where the Magicut tool was used to obtain the optimal image.

Full depth Magicut: In most cases, the operator chooses as default the "full depth" Magicut. After fixing the region of interest, the operator rotates the volume so that the structure to be removed is floating without a structure behind. The area to be removed is traced and immediately deleted after confirming. Figures 3.21 to 3.24 show examples of both simple and challenging cases using the Magicut tool to obtain the optimal image.

Defined depth Magicut: The other type of Magicut is the "defined depth" (or selective) erasing which allows the user to select a specific region and erase layer by layer without completely removing the structures behind it (Fig. 3.25). In such a situation, after selecting "defined depth", the area is outlined (Fig. 3.25, Step 1) and the knob is rotated

Step 1   Step 2

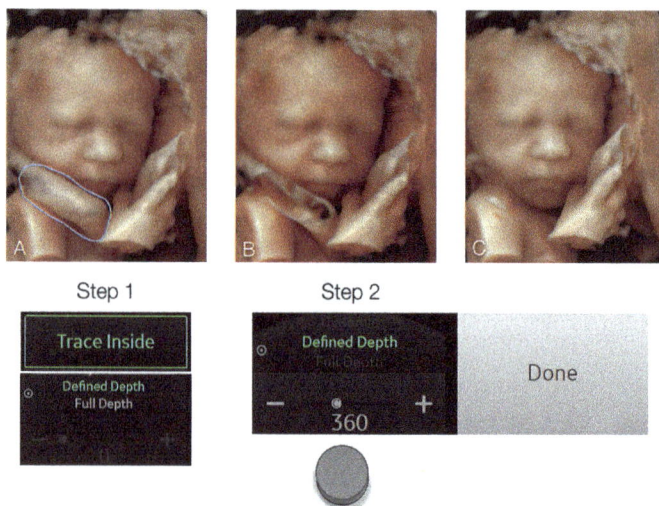

Fig. 3.25: When using Magicut, the default is set to "full depth" with all structures behind the selected region erased. In situations like the one shown in (A), the cord to be removed is close to adjacent structures. In such cases, "defined depth" can be selected instead of "full depth", as shown in the box labeled Step 1, and the region to be removed is traced. As shown in the box labeled Step 2, the button or slider can be used to gradually increase the erasing depth; the result can be tracked directly until the desired result is achieved. The "Done" touch field (bottom right) is pressed to confirm. In such an example, the volume had to be rotated to cut the umbilical cord from a different perspective with "defined depth".

to erase the depth layer by layer (Fig. 3.25, Step 2) until the desired result is achieved and confirmed (Button "Done"). Fig. 3.25 shows an example of defined depth erasure.

Magicut in color Doppler glass-body mode: Of particular interest is the use of Magicut with 3D volumes acquired with color Doppler and displayed in glass-body mode. In such cases, it is possible to delete only the structures on the grayscale image, or only those on the color Doppler, or both. This tool is discussed in detail in Chapter 12.

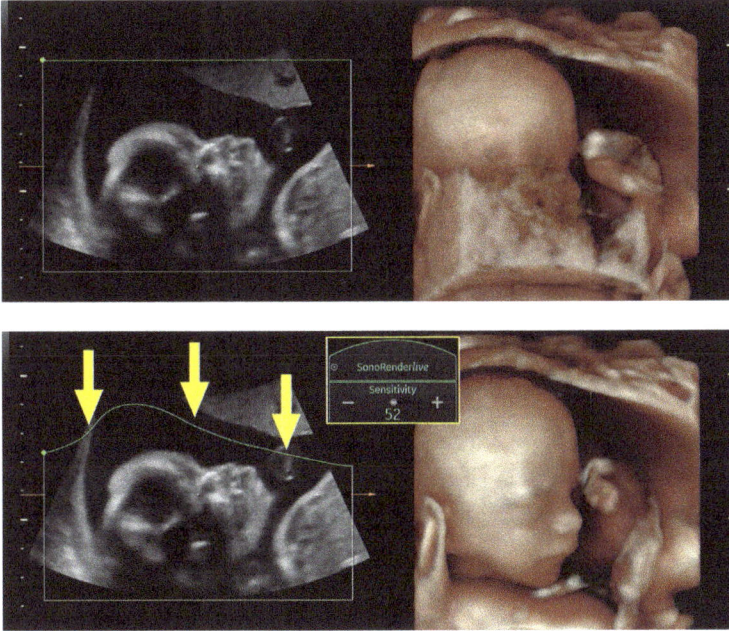

Fig. 3.26: Instead of manually using Magicut to remove structures in front of the face, the SonoRender live tool automatically detects the amniotic fluid and deletes the information in front of the amniotic fluid, revealing the face. As can be seen in the panel (bottom left), the green line changes from a straight to a curved shape (arrows) to fit the area of interest. The sensitivity of this tool can also be adjusted. This tool is very interesting for use in a 4D real-time examination when using Magicut is cumbersome owing to fetal movements. See also Figure 3.27.

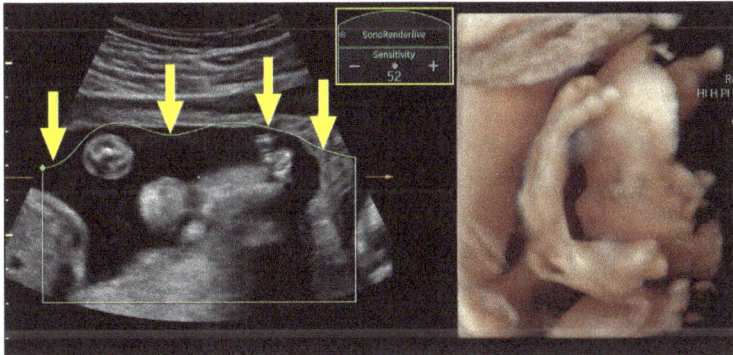

Fig. 3.27: The use of SonoRender live is interesting in such situations because it adjusts the curve to the limb in front of the face, as seen in the curved green line (arrows).

3.8 SonoRender live

A newly introduced feature, called *SonoRender live* (Fig. 3.26), allows the shape of the green line to be changed automatically during volume rendering. Instead of a complicated removal of some structures with Magicut, as shown in Figure 3.26, the software identifies the free fluid between the face and the anterior wall or placenta and places the projection line (also curved) in this area so that the face appears immediately. This tool is especially important in a live 4D examination when using Magicut can be difficult. This tool can be of big help in irregular structures, as shown in Figure 3.27.

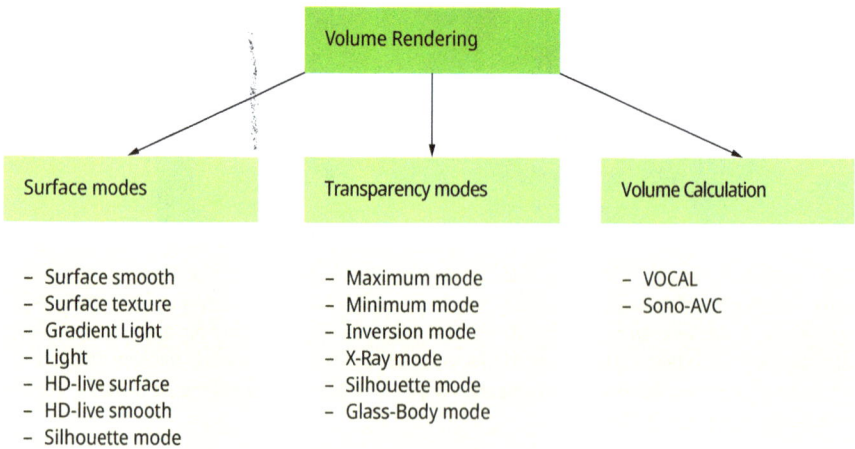

```
                        ┌─────────────────────┐
                        │  Volume Rendering   │
                        └─────────────────────┘
             ┌──────────────────┼──────────────────┐
             ▼                  ▼                  ▼
    ┌─────────────────┐ ┌─────────────────┐ ┌─────────────────┐
    │  Surface modes  │ │ Transparency modes│ │ Volume Calculation│
    └─────────────────┘ └─────────────────┘ └─────────────────┘
```

– Surface smooth	– Maximum mode	– VOCAL
– Surface texture	– Minimum mode	– Sono-AVC
– Gradient Light	– Inversion mode	
– Light	– X-Ray mode	
– HD-live surface	– Silhouette mode	
– HD-live smooth	– Glass-Body mode	
– Silhouette mode		

Fig. 3.28: Flowchart of the different volume rendering modes either in surface mode or in the various transparency modes with different displays.

3.9 Conclusions

3D rendering of a volume is far more complex than navigating the various planes; it requires intensive training in the 3D software and its various manipulation tools. The use of the render box, the green line, and orientation are the basics that must be learned before applying other steps of volume manipulation. The ultrasound information contained in the render box can be displayed in 3D either in a surface or in a transparent display (Fig. 3.28). The Magicut tool is used to clean up the image and highlight the structures of interest, while the light source can be used to enhance the spatial impression. The different render modes and other tools will be discussed in the next chapters.

4 Volume Contrast Imaging (VCI)

4.1 Introduction

In a 3D/4D examination with a multiplanar display, it can be of great additional benefit to obtain a 3D slice instead of a simple plane. This is the principle of *Volume Contrast Imaging* (VCI), the advantage of which is increasing resolution and contrast by reducing artifacts. VCI is routinely used for a static 3D volume and in STIC acquisition. It can also be used in real-time 4D by creating a slice of the A-plane (VCI-A), or the C-Plane (VCI-C), or an Omniview plane (VCI-Omniview). The rendering information within this slice can be selected by the operator, as the volume rendering displays explained in the previous chapter, choosing between X-Ray, maximum, minimum, or surface modes (Fig.4.1). Recently, VCI has been developed to add color Doppler volumes and can now be combined with multiplanar color Doppler reconstruction. In this chapter, we will discuss the technical background of the VCI tool and encourage the reader to use this tool when planes of a 3D volume are displayed. Cases with VCI are also presented across the chapters of this book.

4.2 Principle of VCI

A single reconstructed 2D image from a 3D volume contains both real information and artifacts, called *noise* or *speckles*. By activating the VCI tool and choosing a thin slice, image resolution is increased, contrast is enhanced, and artifacts are reduced (Fig. 4.1). Figure 4.2 illustrates the principle of VCI. In this figure, high amplitude peaks represent the actual ultrasound information, whereas low amplitude peaks represent speckles and artifacts. Comparing two adjacent image planes, the true information is found at the same locations with the same intensity on the images, while the artifacts differ in intensity and position. Superimposing successive images improves the required information about the anatomical structures while reducing, sometimes eliminating, randomly generated noise and speckles in different slices (Fig. 4.2). VCI is activated via the touch panel of the ultrasound system (Fig. 4.3) and, once activated, a new submenu is available to select the render menu.

   Examples are shown in Figures 4.1, 4.4, and 4.5. In these cases, two planes of the fetal lung with liver and brain are visualized in tomography mode. The images on the left are the original raw volume images, whereas the images on the right are the result after activating VCI with increase in contrast.

https://doi.org/10.1515/9783111249513-004

Raw image

with VCI

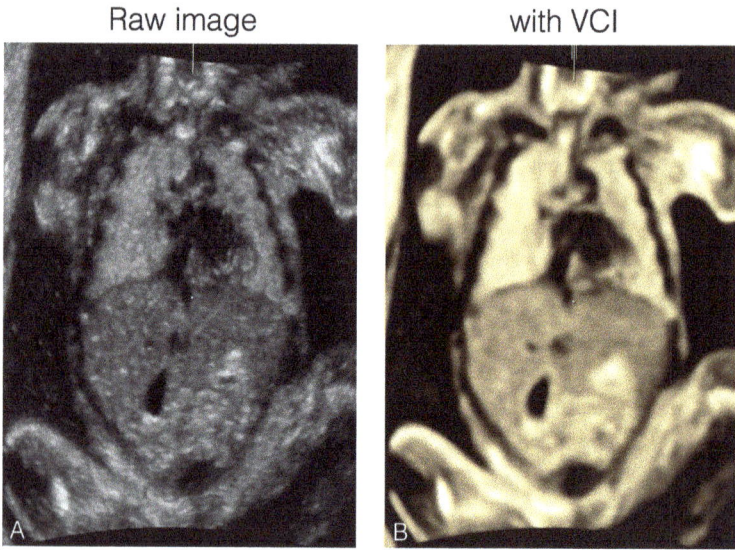

Fig. 4.1: 3D volume showing a coronal visualization of the lungs, heart, diaphragm, and liver. The left image shows a raw image in tomography mode. The right image shows the image result after activating Volume Contrast Imaging (VCI), which increases contrast and detail detection.

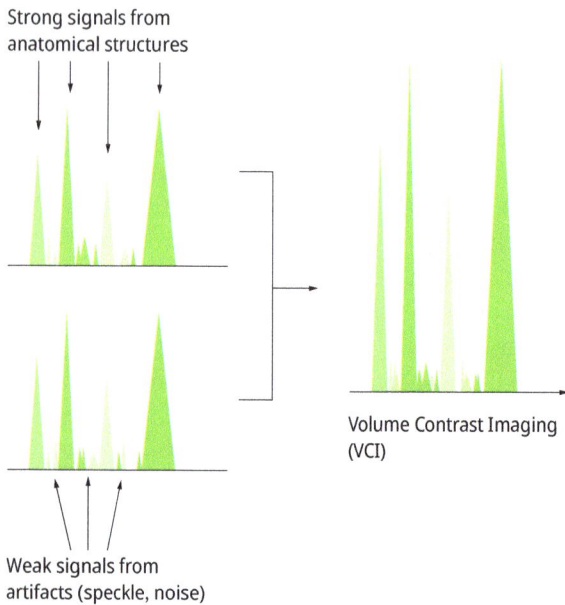

Strong signals from anatomical structures

Weak signals from artifacts (speckle, noise)

Volume Contrast Imaging (VCI)

Fig. 4.2: Principle of VCI. The image in VCI is reconstructed from several adjacent images, of which two are shown here. The signals of true tissue information are high and present in the same location in the neighboring images, whereas the signals of noise and speckles are weak and appear in different locations. The sum of two adjacent images (VCI) increases the intensity of the true signals and the information of noise and speckles almost disappears.

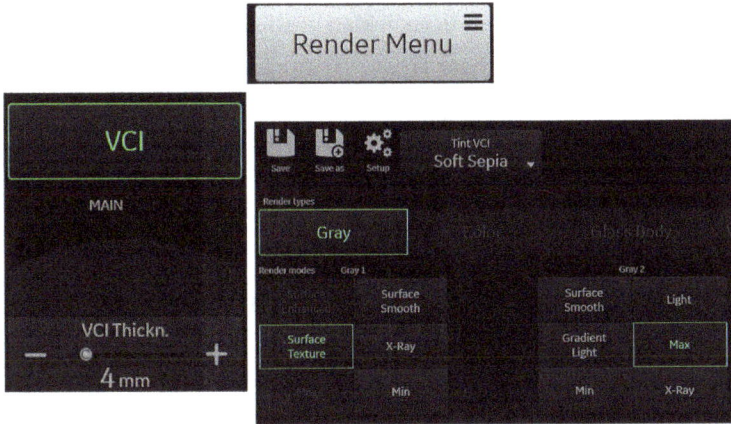

Fig. 4.3: Once the VCI function is activated on the touch panel (left panel), the VCI layer thickness appears and can be increased from 1 to 20 mm. The display of the VCI information can be selected in the submenu of the render menu (right panel). Four surface modes are available: Light, Minimum, Maximum and X-Ray. Maximum mode is used for bone, while X-Ray mode is used for tissue enhancement.

4.3 Static VCI

VCI can be applied to any orthogonal, tomographic, or selected plane display (as in Omniview) to improve image quality and contrast (see examples in Chapter 5 and Chapter 6). The image appears to be a plane but is a thin slice. The layer thickness can be selected between 1 and 20 mm, depending on the information to be displayed. In this book, most of the images showing examples with tomography or Omniview modes were created by adding VCI, often with a slice thickness of 1–3 mm.

The rendering type of the slice can be selected as X-Ray, maximum, minimum, surface, or a mix of two of these modes (Fig. 4.3), just like 3D rendering discussed in Chapter 3. The results are shown in Figures 4.4 to 4.10.

X-Ray mode: This mode is ideal for enhancing tissue information and is used in brain, lung, kidney, nuchal translucency, and other imaging. In most cases, a thin slice of 1–5 mm is selected (Figs. 4.1, 4.4–4.8).

Maximum mode: This mode is ideally used to image the spine, extremities, long bones, or cranial bones (Figs. 4.6, 4.9, 4.10). A good slice thickness is selected between 5–20 mm.

Minimum mode: This mode is ideal for echolucent structures and can be used in combination with the X-Ray mode.

Surface mode: This mode is rarely used in combination with static VCI because thin slice is rarely required to image a surface (Fig.4.9). Instead, a standard 3D or 4D image is usually more useful because the 3D effect of surface mode is enhanced when the volume is larger. Occasionally, surface mode is combined with X-Ray mode and maximum mode (Figs. 4.9, 4.10).

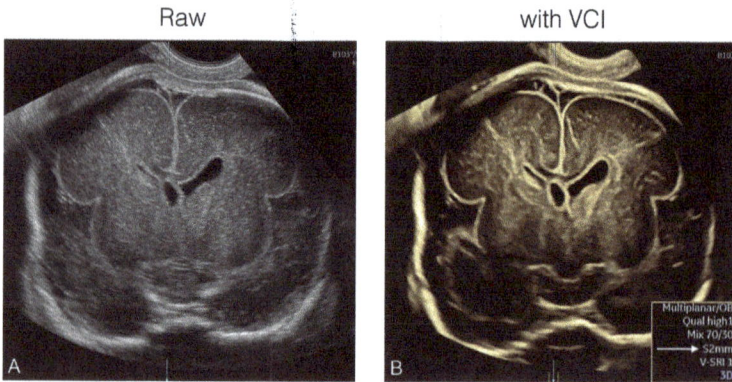

Fig. 4.4: Two images of a static 3D volume of a brain in tomography mode. The left panel (A) is the raw image. The right panel (B) shows the image after activating VCI (here 2 mm thickness) (arrow) with the result of a more detailed image with better contrast.

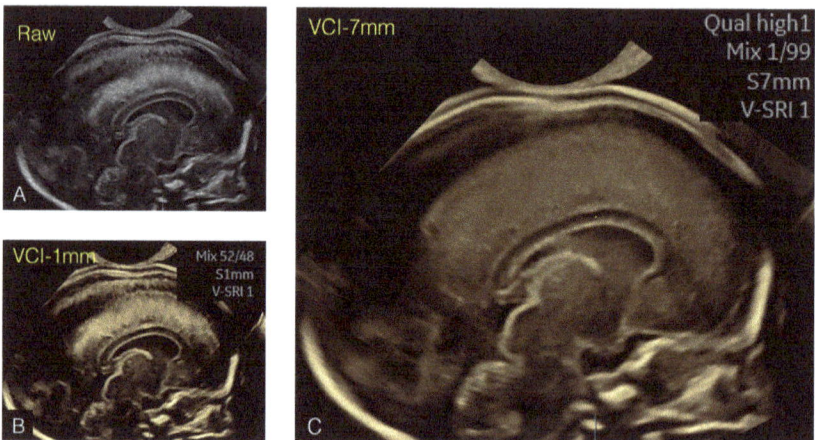

Fig. 4.5: Three images of a static 3D volume of a brain in tomography mode, where the raw image is shown in the upper left panel (A). Panel (B), bottom left, shows the result after activating VCI (here 1 mm) with a mixture of X-Ray and surface smoothing, making the image clearer and with better contrast. In panel (C), the thickness of the VCI layer has been increased to 7 mm and the X-Ray component to almost 100%, resulting in a smoother image.

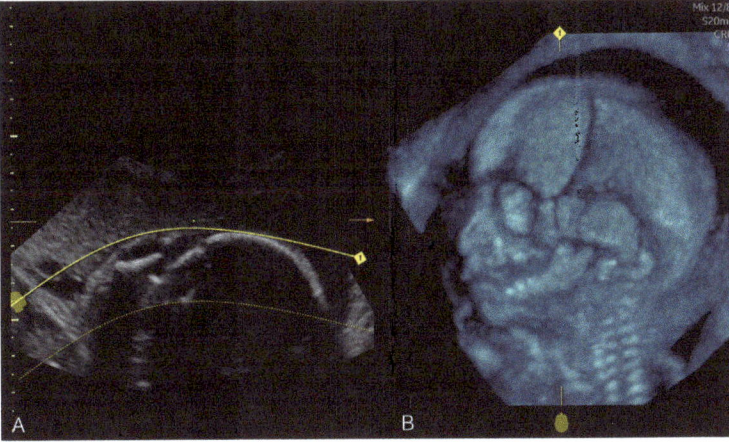

Fig. 4.6: VCI with maximum mode. Lateral static 3D image of the fetal head with a VCI of 20 mm and maximum mode (panel B) shows the cranial bones with the corresponding sutures.

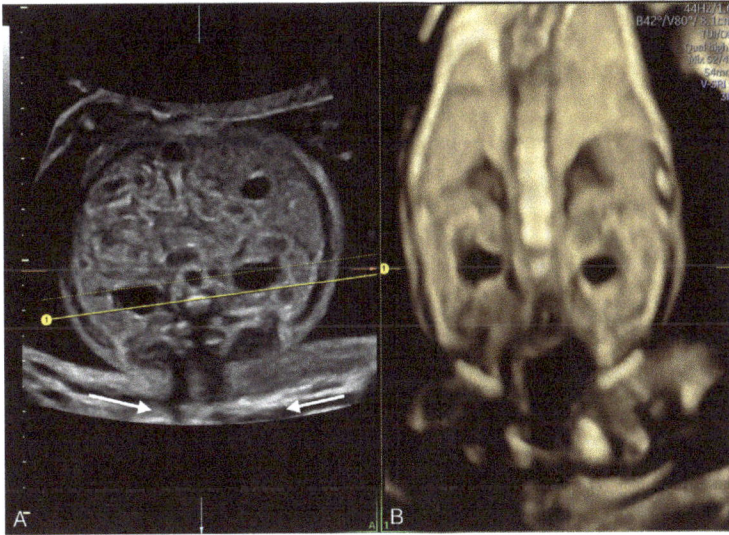

Fig. 4.7: VCI with minimum mode. Acquisition at the level of the abdomen shows the kidneys in tomography mode. The combination of a 2 mm VCI slice with minimum mode (panel B) highlights the hypoechoic renal pelvis and shows the presence of mild pyelectasia.

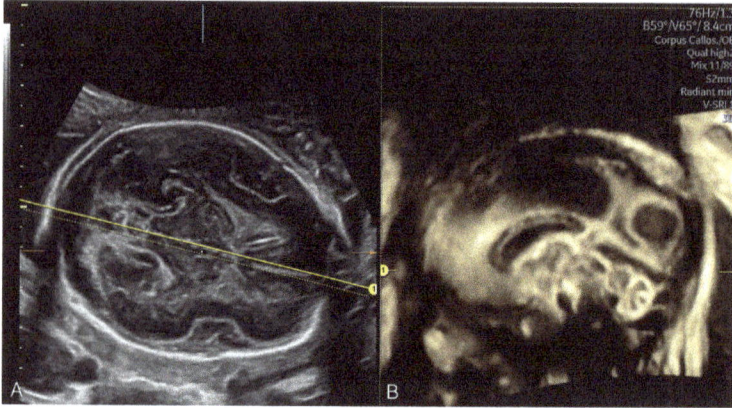

Fig. 4.8: VCI with X-Ray mode. Corpus callosum and vermis are reconstructed with the Omniview tool and the result is improved by choosing a VCI thickness of 2 mm in X-Ray mode.

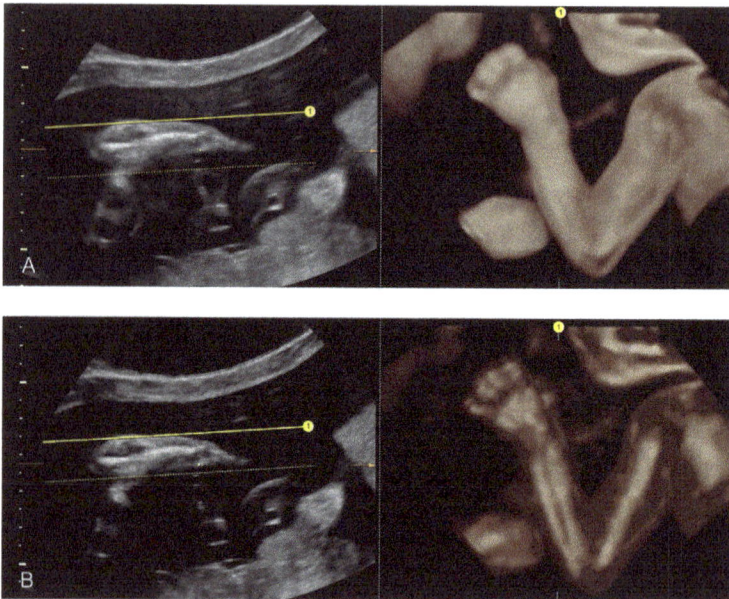

Fig. 4.9: VCI with surface and maximum modes. Top Panel (A): 3D volume of the fetal arm showing the arm with Omniview and a VCI slice thickness of 14 mm with surface texture and gradient rendering. Bottom Panel (B): the same view with slice thickness reduced to 11 mm and maximum mode rendering.

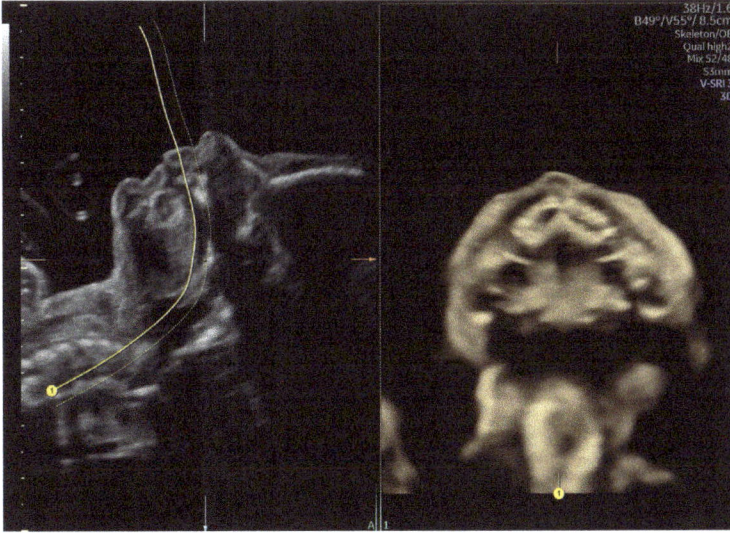

Fig. 4.10: Demonstration of the hard palate with a curved Omniview line and a VCI of 3 mm. The display was chosen as a mixture of maximum and surface mode.

4.4 VCI with color Doppler

Since a few years it has been possible to apply VCI to color Doppler 3D and STIC volumes as well. Creating a layer of grayscale and color Doppler information gives a more spatial aspect to the image, as known from glass-body mode (Figs.4.11–4.13). If a thin slice (1–5 mm) is chosen (Fig. 4.11), the color simply appears as spatial 3D from the background, but the selection of a large slice (10–20 mm) allows visualization of more depth (Figs.4.12, 4.13); in a cardiac volume, for example, the crossing of the great vessels can be well demonstrated (Fig. 4.12). Figure 4.13 shows two fetuses with aneurysmal malformation of the vein of Galen with the vascular lesion well demonstrated by a thick layer of VCI.

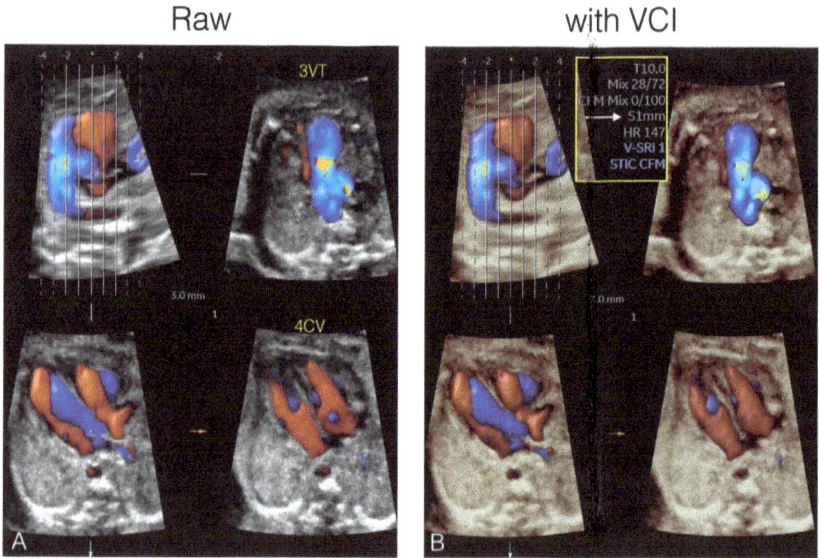

Fig. 4.11: STIC volume in tomography mode in color Doppler displaying a four-chamber view (4CV) and a three-vessel trachea view (3VT). As of recently, VCI can be added to color; the right panel (B) shows 1 mm thickness, revealing not only increased resolution and contrast of 2D image information, but also a volumetric appearance of the color Doppler. Compare with Figure 4.12.

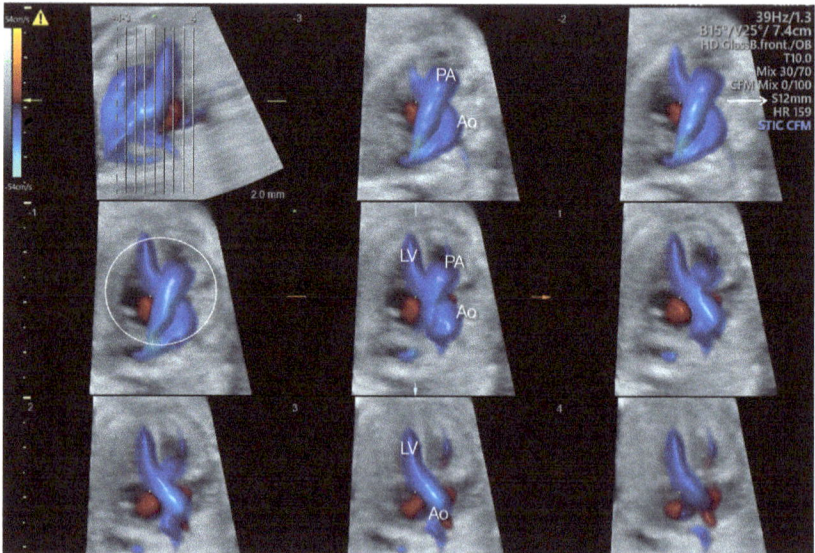

Fig. 4.12: STIC volume in tomography mode with color Doppler in systole, showing the aorta (Ao) in the five-chamber view and the pulmonary artery (PA) in the three-vessel trachea view. In this case, VCI with a thickness of 12 mm (arrow) was chosen, resulting in simultaneous visualization of the crossing of vessels in multiple planes (circle). Left ventricle (LV).

4.5 4D with VCI-Omniview

In a 4D examination, the examiner can also directly draw a straight or curved line along the region of interest to obtain an appropriate slice or view. The result can be enhanced by combining it with VCI of a corresponding thickness (Fig.4.15). The 4D result can be displayed directly next to the 2D image. The authors have had good experience with this technique and use it in screening examinations. In a fetus with vertex presentation, online reconstruction of the corpus callosum and vermis can be achieved directly by selecting a straight line with a thin slice of 1–3 mm and the X-Ray mode. Another option is to combine VCI with the maximum mode for imaging skull bones with sutures (Fig. 4.14) or the spine with ribs (Fig. 4.15). Chapter 14 discusses further the potential of the electronic transducer.

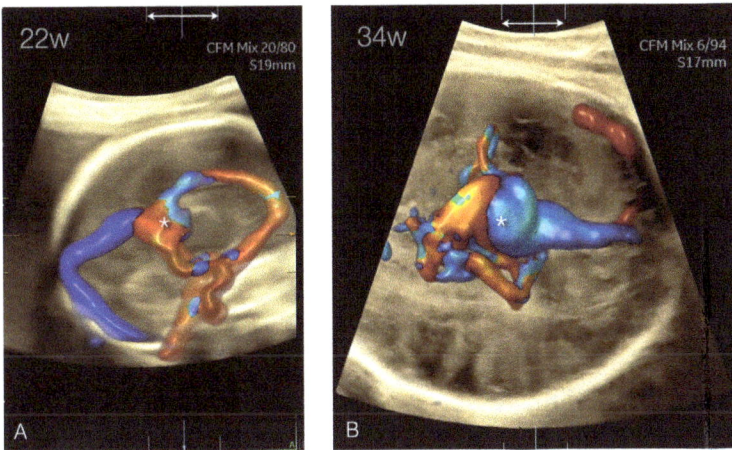

Fig. 4.13: Abnormal fetal cerebral vessels in two fetuses with aneurysm of the vein of Galen (*) at 22 weeks (A) and 34 weeks of gestation (B) with multiplanar mode and VCI of 19 mm and 17 mm, respectively (double arrow), improving the spatial appearance of the abnormal cerebral vessels. VCI in color is easier to apply than 3D glass-body mode.

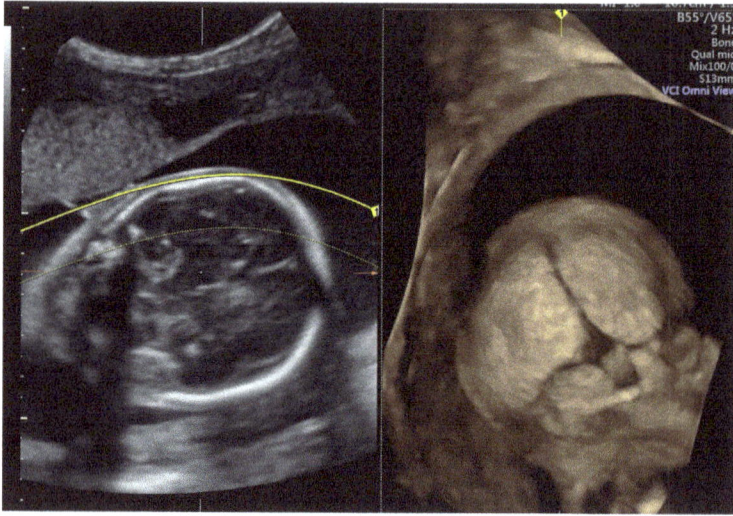

Fig. 4.14: VCI in real-time 4D: lateral view of the fetal skull in 4D. A curved Omniview line was drawn laterally to the skull and a slice of 13 mm thickness was selected. The maximum mode view then allows direct visualization of the skull bones with the coronal suture.

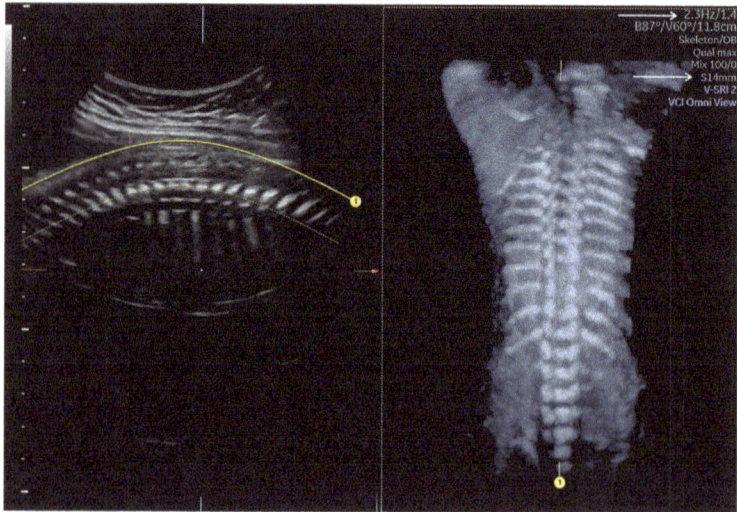

Fig. 4.15: VCI in live 4D. Direct visualization of spine and ribs with 4D ultrasound, curved Omniview line, and VCI of 14 mm.

4.6 4D with VCI-A

VCI of the A-plane is a technique of scanning with a slice instead of a 2D plane. This technique can be used with a mechanical probe but has a low frame rate and poor resolution. Resolution has improved with the introduction of the electronic matrix transducer (see Chapter 1), which allows the quick calculation of images (Figs. 4.16–4.20). Slice thickness and rendering display can be adjusted as needed. The VCI-A can be used to examine the fetal lungs, heart, kidneys, face, brain, placenta, and other organs. In our experience, combining this technique with X-Ray mode can be used to improve contrast discrimination between adjacent regions, such as the heart-thymus, myocardium-lumen (Fig. 4.16), corpus callosum-cortex, or kidney-bowel. The skeletal system can be well highlighted during live examination when combined with maximum mode (Figs. 4.17–4.20). See also Chapter 14 for more examples.

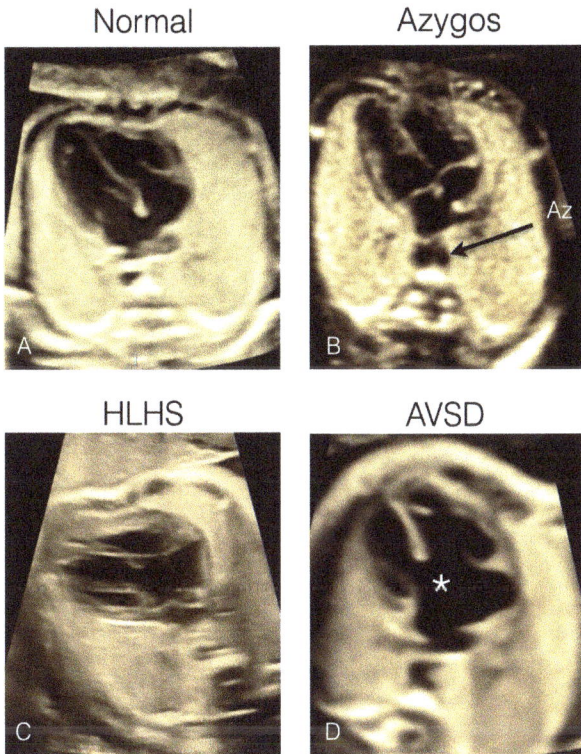

Normal | Azygos

HLHS | AVSD

Fig. 4.16: VCI-A in live 4D with tissue mode rendering. Examination of the four chambers in VCI-A with X-Ray tissue rendering. In (A) a normal heart; in (B) a heart with azygos (Az) continuity behind the heart; in (C) a fetus with hypoplastic left heart (HLHS); and in (D) with atrioventricular septal defect (AVSD) (*).

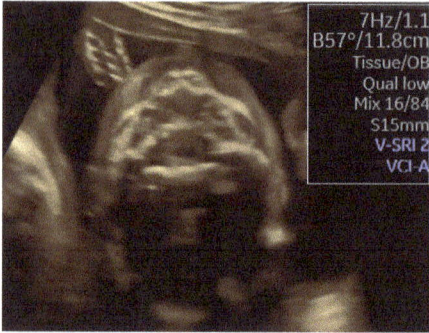

Fig. 4.17: VCI-A of the axial view of the jaw in real-time 4D at a slice thickness of 15 mm in maximum mode with maxillary and mandibular region and the hard palate.

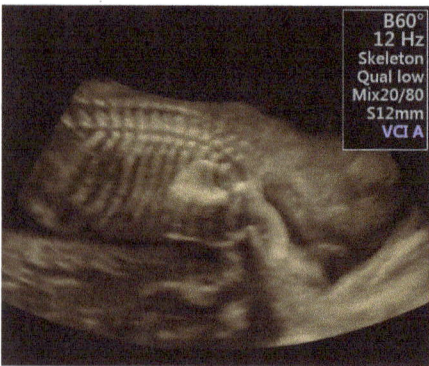

Fig. 4.18: VCI-A of the spine and scapula in real-time 4D at a VCI slice thickness of 12 mm in maximum mode.

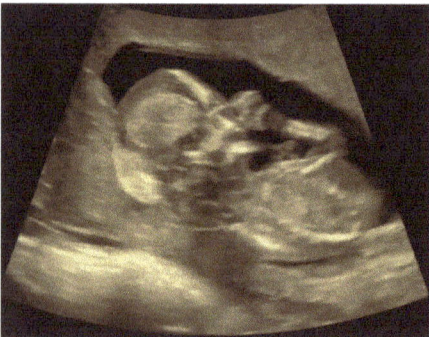

Fig. 4.19: VCI-A in real-time 4D with a slice thickness of 12 mm in maximum mode in a first trimester fetus showing the skull, face, and limb bones in one image.

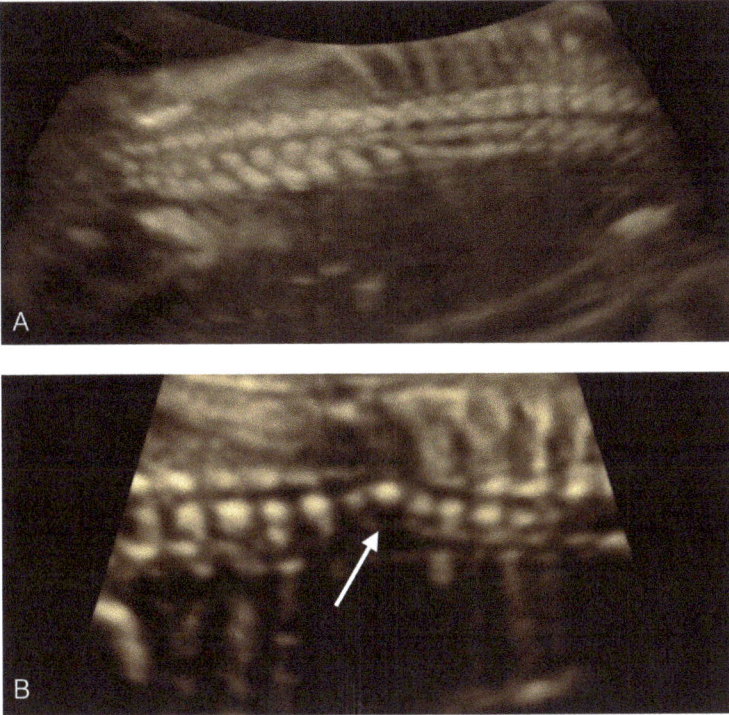

Fig. 4.20: VCI-A of the spine in a coronal view in a normal fetus (A) and in a fetus with a hemivertebra (arrow) in (B).

4.7 Conclusions

VCI is an important additional tool for 3D and 4D examinations with any of the multiplanar displays, allowing rapid use of a 3D slice rather than going through the many steps of volume acquisition and rendering. In combination with Omniview, the potential for use increases, especially when curved lines are applied. The authors recommend that the user applies VCI to all multiplanar reconstructed planes, to increase contrast and reduce artifacts of reconstructed planes.

5 Multiplanar Display I: Orthogonal Mode and Omniview Planes

5.1 Principle

An ultrasound examination is still based on the demonstration of standard 2D cross-sectional images of the examined organ or area. Therefore, most examiners try to visualize such "standard" planes during their ultrasound examination, and some examiners do not yet feel familiar with the series of images displayed in orthogonal or tomographic mode. For the specialist, the fetal profile, four-chamber view, sagittal view of the corpus callosum, and other regions are all standard planes to be visualized during a routine examination. However, due to fetal position or other reasons, some views may not be directly visualized during a routine fetal ultrasound examination. As the examiner gains experience with 3D ultrasound, he or she realizes that one of the main advantages of a digital volume data set is the offline post-processing of the data. Rather than trying to find the optimal 2D plane during the live scan, it can be helpful to acquire a volume data set and extract the desired plane from the volume block plane. Navigation within a volume, explained in Chapter 2, is of great help for this purpose and VCI, explained in Chapter 4, improves image quality. This chapter discusses two modes – orthogonal mode and Omniview – which allow typical slice planes to be obtained from a volume data set. Tomography mode will be discussed in the next chapter.

5.2 Multiplanar reconstruction and different displays of cross-sectional images

The demonstration of single images from a digital volume data set can be displayed in a variety of ways. In imaging, the general term for such a technique is *Multiplanar Reconstruction* (MPR). In 3D ultrasound, the used nomenclature differs slightly from one manufacturer to another. In the system used by the authors, the term *multiplanar* is often used as a synonym for *orthogonal mode*. In this book, we will use the term *multiplanar reconstruction* or *multiplanar imaging* in a broader sense and treat the different modalities separately.

Currently, the following three modalities of MPR are available in volume ultrasound:

- Single or multiple images in orthogonal mode (3 perpendicular images) (Figs. 5.1–5.4)
- Multiple images in tomographic mode (multiple parallel images)
- Single image slices obtained by selective slicing within the volume using tools such as Omniview.

https://doi.org/10.1515/9783111249513-005

With the latter, it is possible not only to cut within the volume with a straight line, but also to fit a curved line or draw any multipoint line and obtain an "any plane".

To improve the quality of the reconstructed images and reduce speckles, the authors recommend using the VCI function in all modalities (Figs. 5.3–5.5), as described in Chapter 4, or using the 3D- volume speckle reduction imaging (3D-VSRI) filter, if available.

5.3 Practical approach in orthogonal mode

Before acquiring a volume, the preset can be selected on the touch panel to display the result in either orthogonal or tomographic mode (or in a 3D render mode). Once the volume is acquired, the three perpendicular images are displayed (Figs. 5.1, 5.2). The examiner first looks for the best-known structure to begin manipulation. In some situations, it is helpful to scroll through the volume or navigate the different planes using the intersection point as explained in Chapter 2. Once the image closest to the ideal plane is obtained, the examiner uses rotation (spinning) in the other planes to align the structure of interest along one of the typical fetal axes (falx, spine, aorta, etc.), thus facilitating orientation.

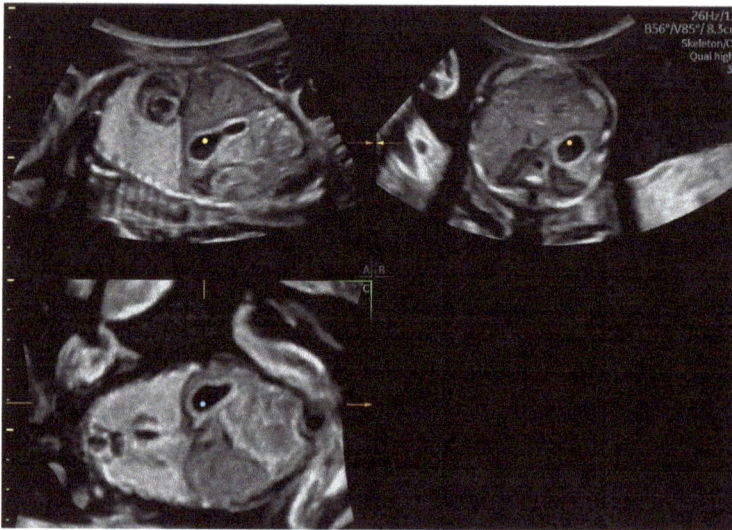

Fig. 5.1: Fetal thorax and abdomen in orthogonal 3D view. To have a good orientation, a well recognizable structure – such as the stomach here – was chosen. In plane A (upper left), the intersection point was moved to the stomach; images B (upper right) and C (bottom left) were modified so that the stomach is now visible. The intersection point always points to the same place in all three planes and can be used for navigation.

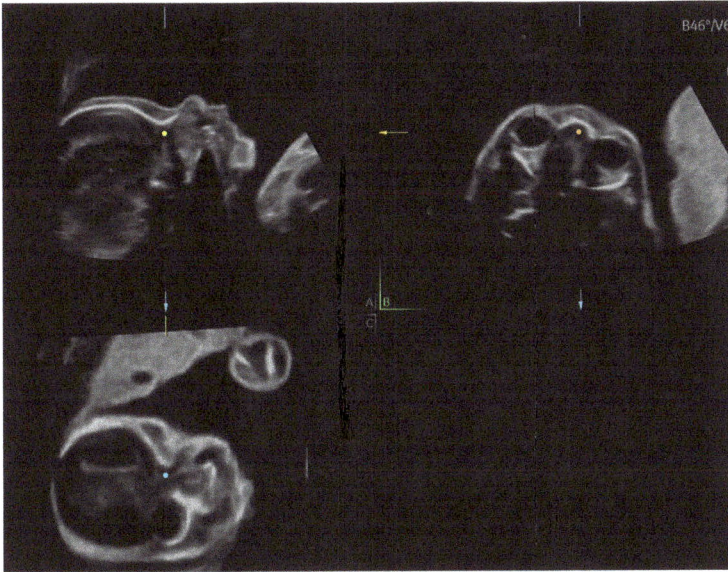

Fig. 5.2: Fetal face in orthogonal 3D view. The intersection point was placed in plane A (upper left) near the nose and is also shown in the other two images after correction of the figures.

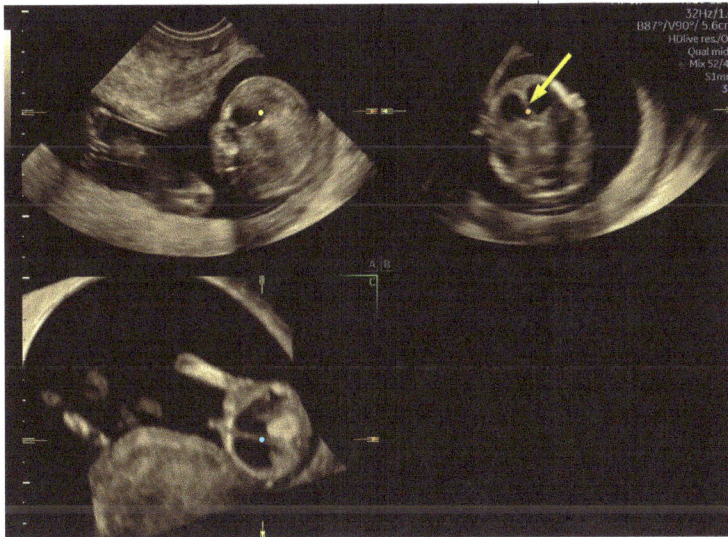

Fig. 5.3: Step by step reconstruction of a plane from a 3D volume data set, using the nose and nuchal translucency as an example. In a transvaginal examination, it is often difficult to obtain the ideal midsagittal view with profile. The acquisition of the fetal face was taken from the side. VCI is activated (see Chapter 4) and the intersection point is placed on the falx cerebri (arrow in plane B), a readily identifiable structure. In plane C (bottom left), the falx is oblique. The lower image is then rotated until the cerebral falx is horizontal, as shown in Figure 5.4.

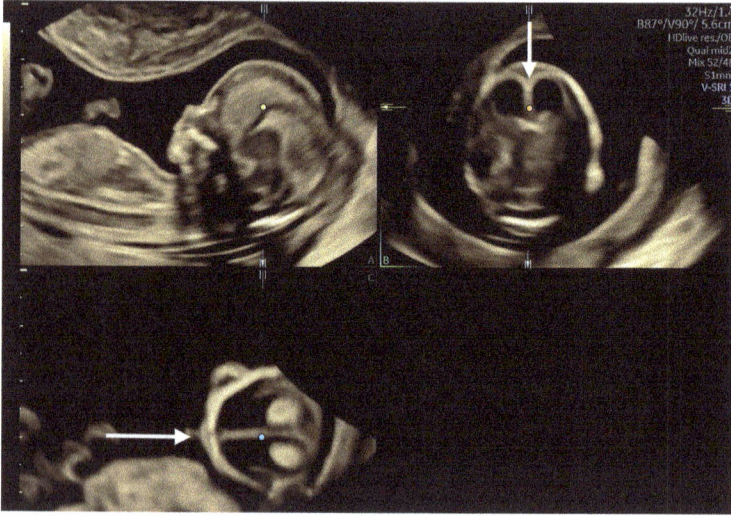

Fig. 5.4: Continuation of Figure 5.3. Now the falx is well aligned in all three planes and the intersection point can be seen on the falx cerebri in all three planes. In plane A (upper left), the profile can now be seen clearly, and Figure 5.5 shows the final result.

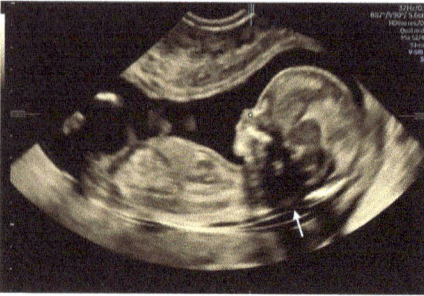

Fig. 5.5: Result of a fetal profile reconstructed from the 3D volume data set of an oblique view of the fetal face. Now the nasal bone and nuchal translucency are clearly visible, and the nuchal translucency can be measured.

Figures 5.3 to 5.5 show how an ideal midsagittal view with the nuchal translucency and the nasal bone is generated step by step from a transvaginal volume of the fetal face. Due to the limitations of transducer manipulation, the profile could not be visualized initially, so a 3D volume was acquired. After activation of the VCI, the falx cerebri was searched for in a first step (plane B in Fig. 5.3) and aligned along the Y-axis. In plane C, the falx is still oblique and is aligned along the X-axis in the next step (Fig. 5.4, 5.5). In this plane, the profile is clearly visible and visualization of the plane (Fig. 5.5) now allows measurement of the nasal bone and nuchal translucency.

Figure 5.6 shows how intracranial translucency is visualized by manipulating a volume of a fetal head at 12 weeks' gestation taken in cross-section. Figure 5.7 shows visualization of the maxilla by manipulating a volume of a fetus in the second trimester and combining with VCI (1 mm) to highlight the findings. Figures 5.8 to 5.10 show the use of orthogonal mode to visualize a double bubble sign in duodenal atresia, cerebellar vermis, and aortic arch, respectively. In all these cases, we navigated with the intersection point, rotated to the ideal plane of interest, and added VCI for contrast enhancement.

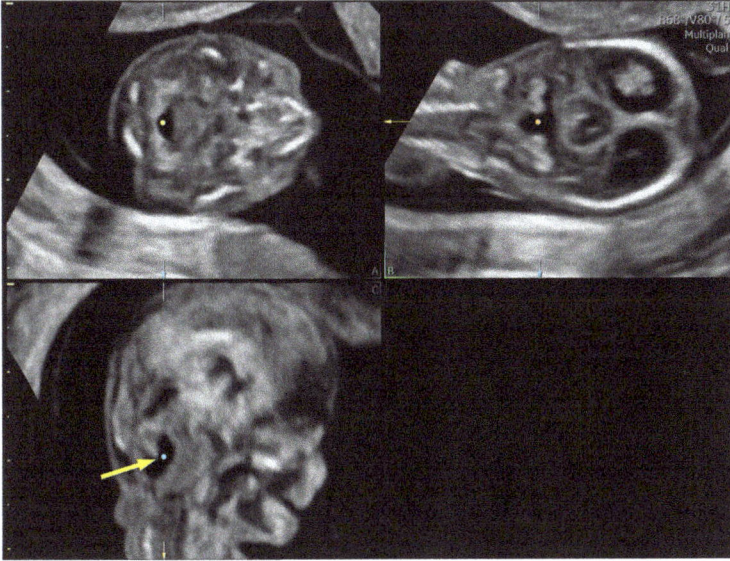

Fig. 5.6: Reconstruction of the intracranial translucency (arrow) from an axial view of the brain at 12 weeks' gestation with volume rotation and navigation.

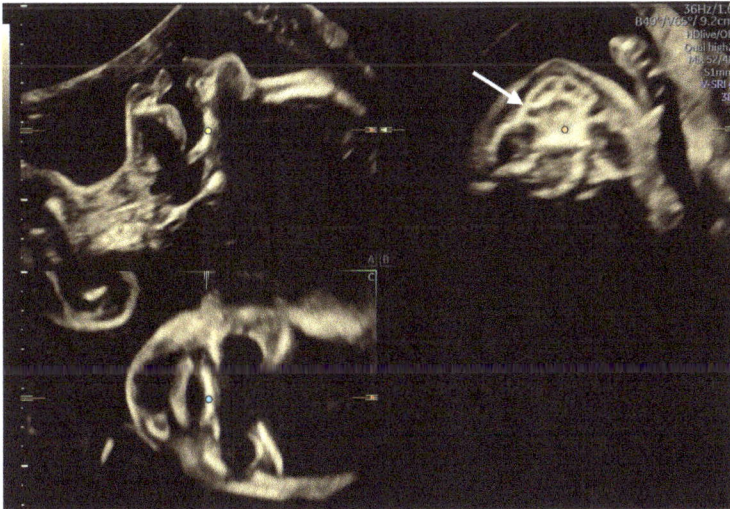

Fig. 5.7: 3D reconstruction of the maxilla with hard palate in orthogonal mode. After moving the intersection point on the hard palate in the image in (A), the face is adjusted in (C) so that it is horizontal. With these shifts, the maxilla and hard palate then appear clearly visible in plane B (arrow).

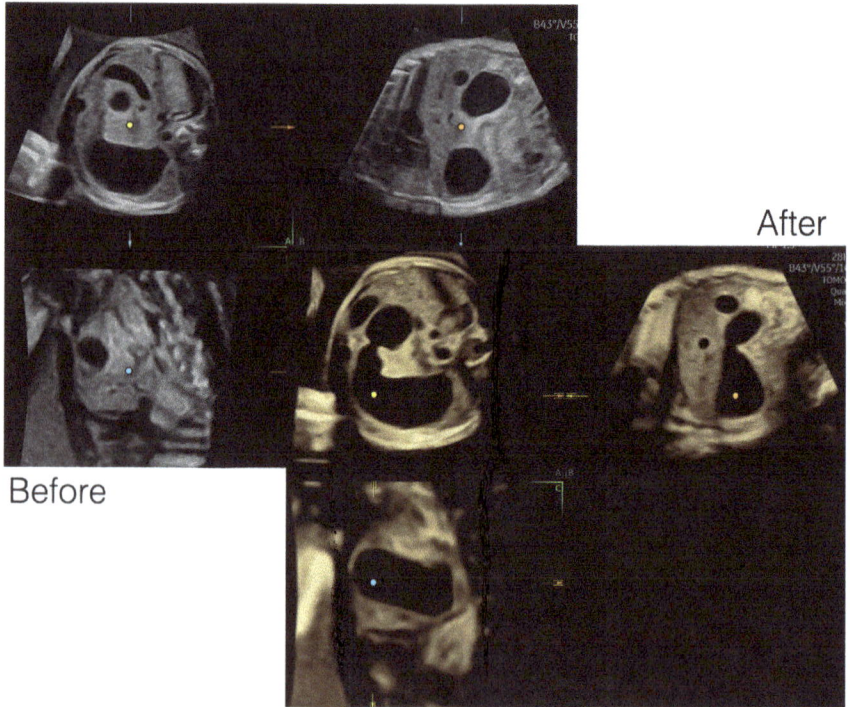

Fig. 5.8: 3D volume of the abdomen in a fetus with duodenal atresia and double bubble. In the raw image on the left ("Before"), the double bubble is not quite visible, but when the intersection point is moved in planes A and then B, the typical image appears with the stomach connected to the duodenum ("After").

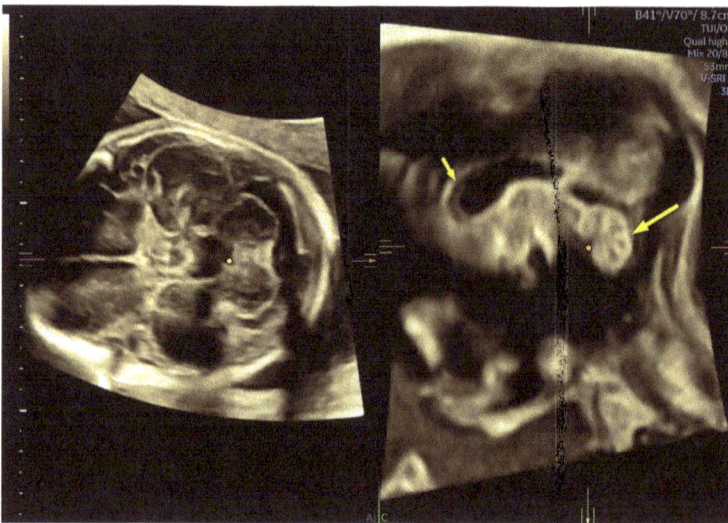

Fig. 5.9: Reconstruction of the cerebellar vermis (long arrow) and corpus callosum (short arrow) in the midline of the brain from an axial 3D volume acquisition and navigation with the intersection point.

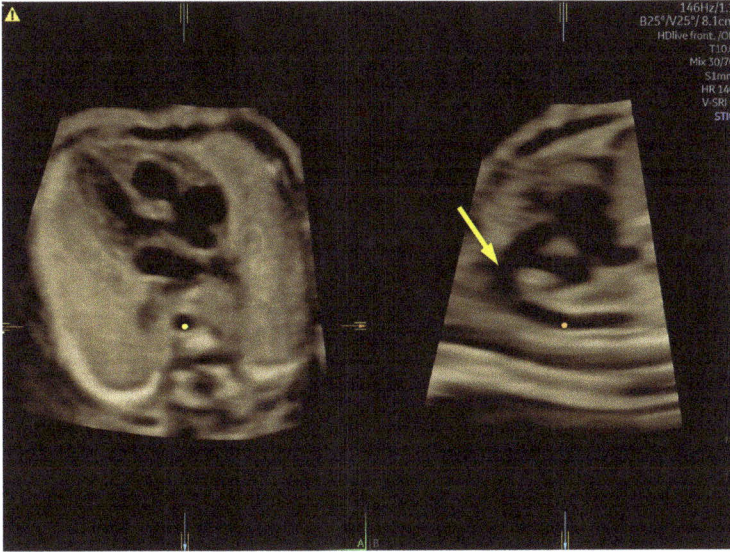

Fig. 5.10: Reconstruction of the aortic arch (arrow) from a STIC volume of the heart acquired in a four-chamber axial view plane. The intersection point was placed on the descending aorta to facilitate volume rotation.

5.4 Practical approach in obtaining an "anyplane" using Omniview mode

A good alternative for the display of a single plane (called *anyplane*) is to use the Omniview mode. The Omniview mode is activated on the touch panel (Fig. 5.11). After making some adjustments to the image to identify parts of the structure of interest, the examiner can draw a line directly in the volume and obtain the reconstructed image at the same time. Since the reconstructed Omniview image appears simultaneously, an adjustment to the drawn line can be made directly. Up to three lines can be drawn on the same image and can be identified by different colors and the numbers 1, 2 and 3 (Figs. 5.12, 5.13). After a line has been drawn and fixed, it can be shifted in a parallel, tilted or rotated manner. An Omniview line can be drawn as a straight line, curved, traced, or polyline (Fig. 5.11, right panel). The resulting image can be used either as a projected line or, in some cases, with a curved line that can also be displayed as a stretched line. To improve the image quality, it is recommended to reduce the speckles by either using the 3D-VSRI filter or combining it with the VCI tool. It is important to emphasize that the use of the Omniview mode is not limited to a static 3D volume but can also be used in a 4D or STIC volume.

Submenu of the Omiview tool

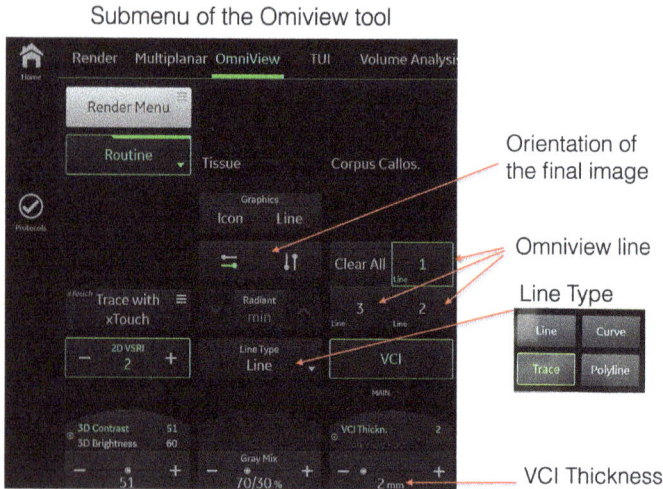

Orientation of the final image

Omniview line

Line Type

VCI Thickness

Fig. 5.11: Touch panel and submenu of Omniview. When the Omniview function is selected, the panel shown in this figure appears. It consists of selecting one of the three Omniview lines (1, 2, 3), activating VCI with its thickness (see Chapter 4) and selecting the line shape, whether a straight line, a curved, or a polyline. In the submenu of the Render menu, the various gray mixtures can be selected, as explained in Chapter 4.

5.5 Typical applications of the Omniview mode

The use of the Omniview mode can be applied to all types of volumes and all organs to be examined, as shown in the examples in Figures 5.12 to 5.23.

Thorax and abdomen: Figure 5.12 shows that Omniview is ideal for visualizing thoracic and abdominal organs, documenting typical cross-sectional planes. Figure 5.13 shows a simple way to visualize the kidneys in a volume by using Omniview planes.

Fetal skeleton: the fetal spine and cranial bones can also be visualized quite well by combining Omniview with VCI and maximum mode, as shown in Figures 5.14 and 5.15. Depending on the organ examined and the fetal position, it can be decided whether a straight or a curved line should be selected. The maxilla with the hard and soft palate can often be visualized with the orthogonal mode (Fig. 5.7), but in some cases it is more reliable to use Omniview for targeted visualization with either a curved or a traced line (Fig. 5.16).

Fetal brain: Figures 5.17 to 5.19 show examples of fetal neurosonography where Omniview mode allows rapid reconstruction of the corpus callosum, vermis, and a coronal view of the cavum septi pellucidi, cerebellum, and other structures.

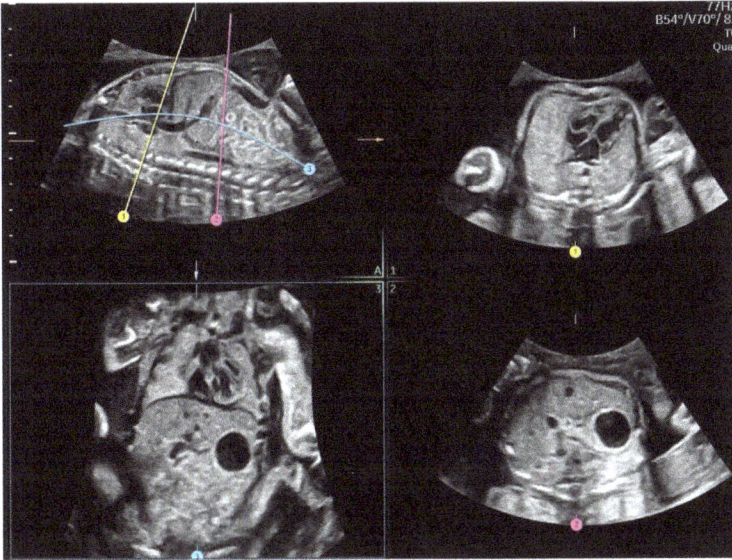

Fig. 5.12: Application of Omniview to a 3D volume of thorax and abdomen. The user can draw up to three lines. In this case, two lines created axial planes above the heart (yellow line, 1, upper right panel) and at the level of the stomach (magenta line, 2, bottom right panel). The third horizontal line (cyan) is a frontal view of the thorax, lungs, diaphragm, stomach, liver, and intestines (3, bottom left panel). While planes 1 and 2 result from straight lines, line 3 was chosen as a curved line.

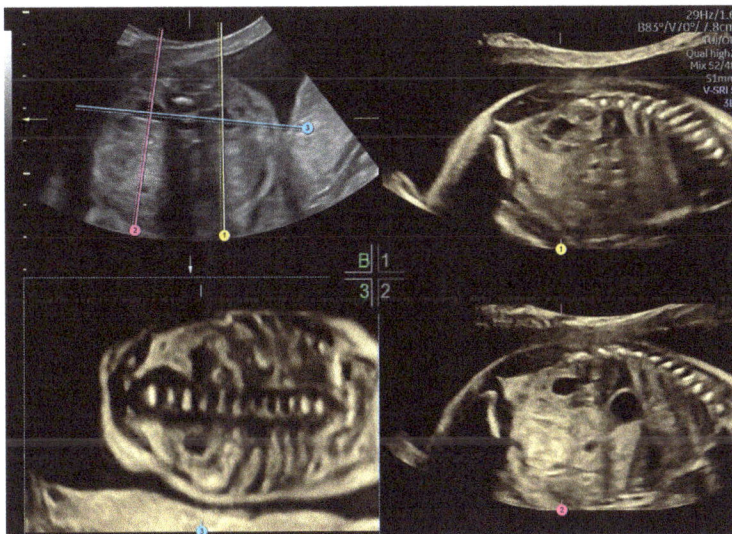

Fig. 5.13: Use of Omniview in the visualization of kidneys. The 3D volume was acquired in the fetal dorsoanterior position, and the kidneys are located to the left and right of the spine. Two Omniview lines were drawn parasagittally (1, yellow line, 2, magenta line) and one coronally (3, cyan line), thus highlighting the kidneys from different perspectives.

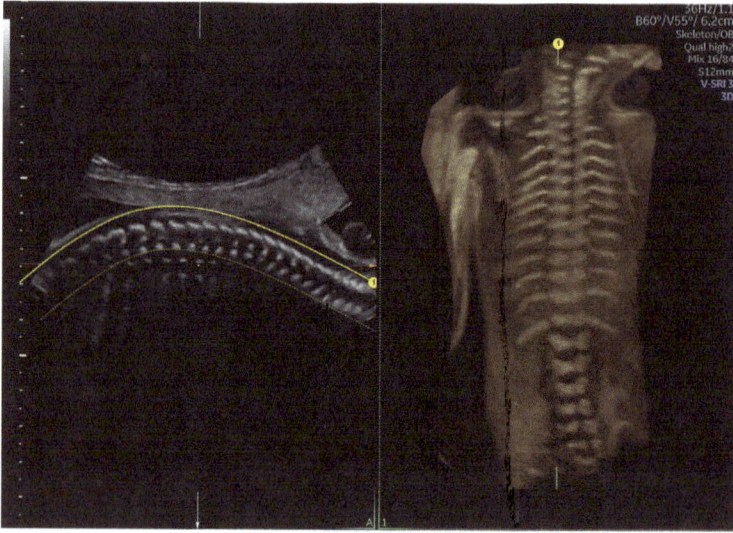

Fig. 5.14: A curved Omniview line (trace) was drawn on a 3D volume and the VCI tool was activated with a 12 mm slice. For the bones, the maximum display mode was selected in the rendering menu, which in this case visualizes the spine and ribs.

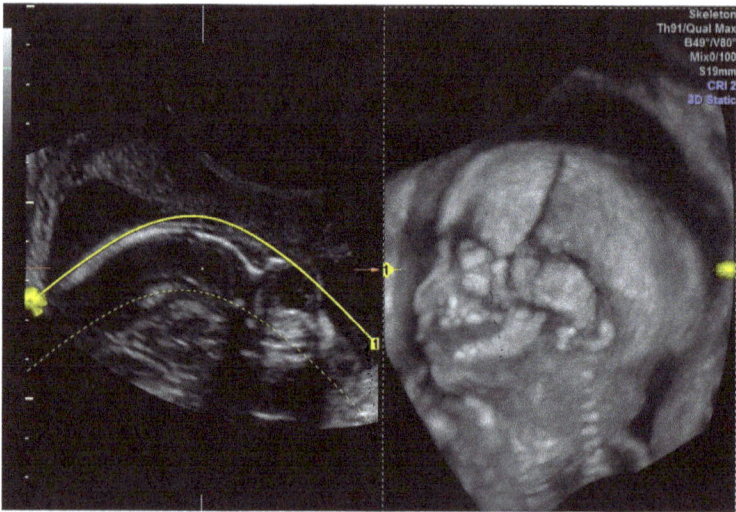

Fig. 5.15: Skull bones can be well visualized after a lateral acquisition of a fetal head and the use of Omniview, here as a curved line with 19 mm width and maximum rendering.

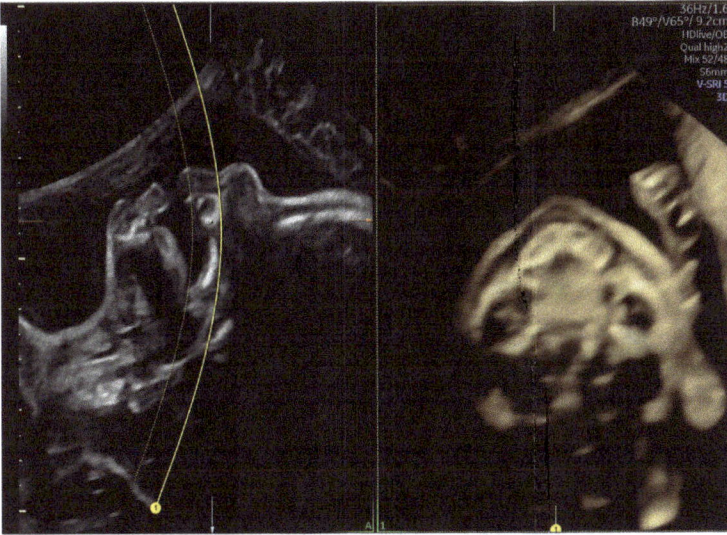

Fig. 5.16: After a 3D volume acquisition of a face from below, the maxilla with hard palate can be visualized by using a curved Omniview line, a VCI of 6 mm and maximum mode display in this case (compare with Fig. 5.15).

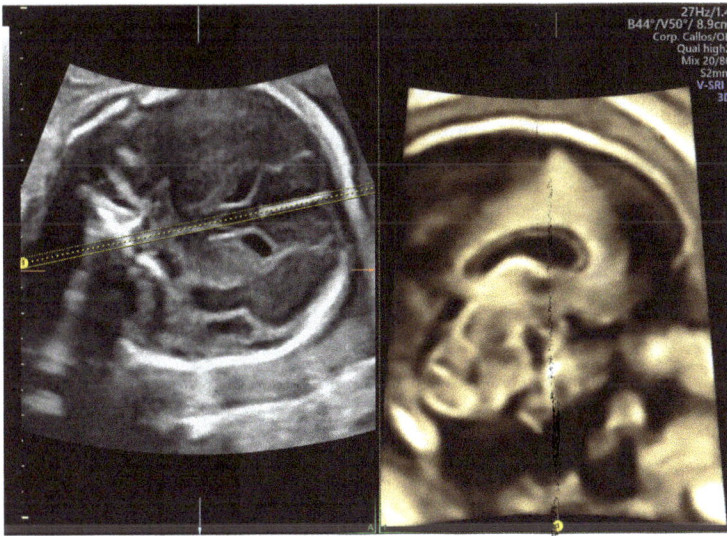

Fig. 5.17: Omniview with VCI demonstrating the corpus callosum. The falx cerebri and cavum septi pellucidi are used as landmarks.

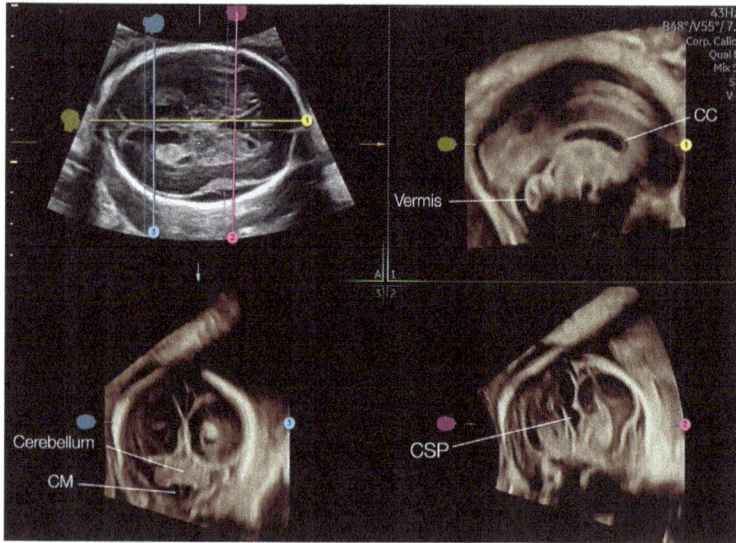

Fig. 5.18: After a lateral static 3D acquisition of a fetal head, three Omniview lines were drawn to visualize the corpus callosum (CC) in a sagittal plane (upper right), a coronal plane to visualize the cavum septi pellucidi (CSP) (bottom right), and another posterior coronal plane to visualize the cerebellum and cisterna magna (bottom left).

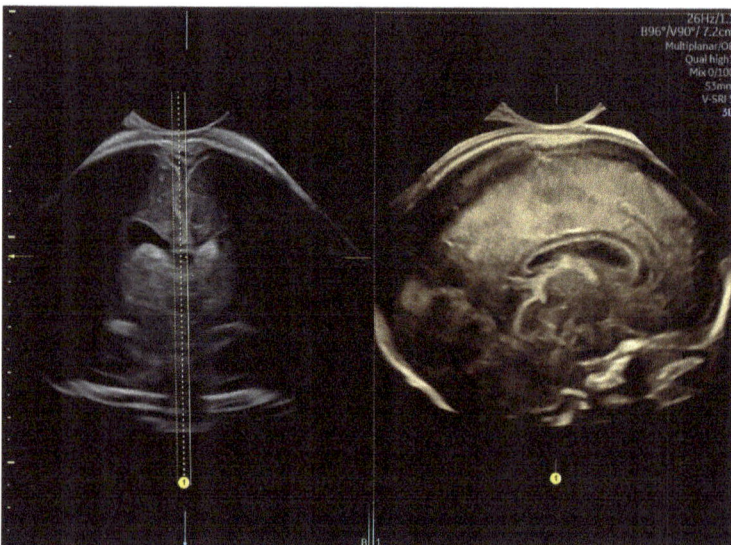

Fig. 5.19: Omniview with VCI (3 mm) for the visualization of the corpus callosum after a transvaginal volume acquisition.

Fetal heart: Omniview mode can be applied on the fetal heart with either STIC in grayscale (Fig. 5.20) or color Doppler (Fig. 5.21). Standard views, such as the four-chamber view and the three-vessel-trachea view can be displayed well and quickly with this tool (Figs. 5.20, 5.21). A direct view of the atrioventricular valves can demonstrate the "en-face" view and valve apparatus.

Early pregnancy: In early fetuses and embryos examined before 14 weeks' gestation, there is limited ability to manipulate the transducer during transvaginal scan. In such situations, Omniview mode helps to obtain reconstructed planes of some typical regions of interest. Figure 5.22 shows an example of intracranial translucency reconstructed. Of interest, but not yet of clinical value, is the freehand drawing of an Omniview line, as shown in the example of a stretched embryo in Figure 5.23.

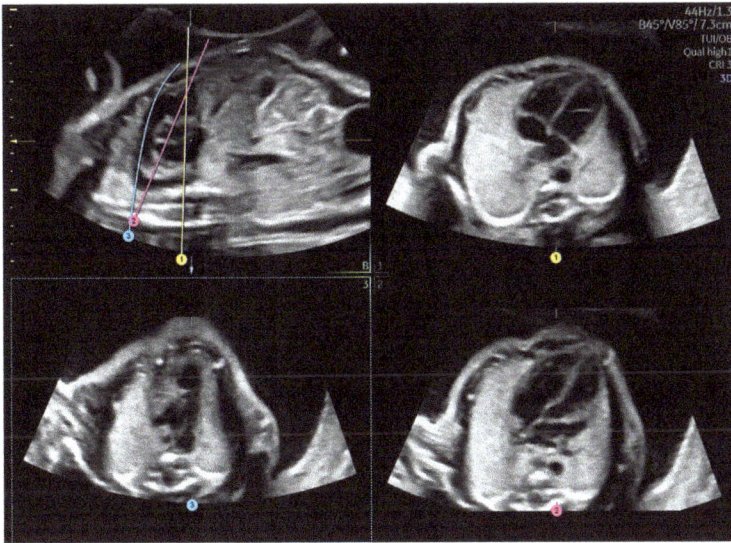

Fig. 5.20: Omniview can also be used for the fetal heart. In this case, the orientation plane is displayed in the upper left panel, three lines are drawn, and the result is displayed in the other three panels. The yellow line is the axial view of the four-chamber view (1), the magenta line intersects at the level of the five-chamber view (2), and the curved cyan line intersects at the level of the three-vessel trachea view (3).

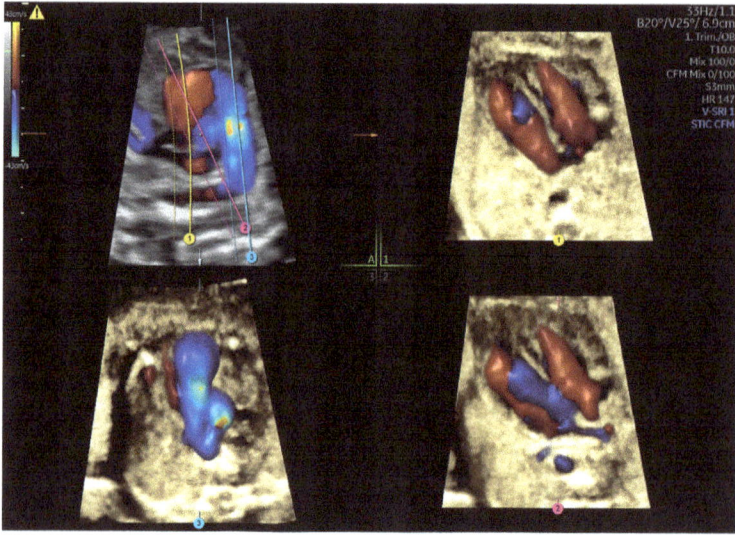

Fig. 5.21: Omniview can also be used here with STIC in combination with color Doppler. Three lines are drawn in the orientation plane in the upper left panel and the result is shown in the other three panels as the four-chamber view (yellow, upper right), five-chamber view (magenta, bottom right), and the three-vessel trachea view (cyan, bottom left).

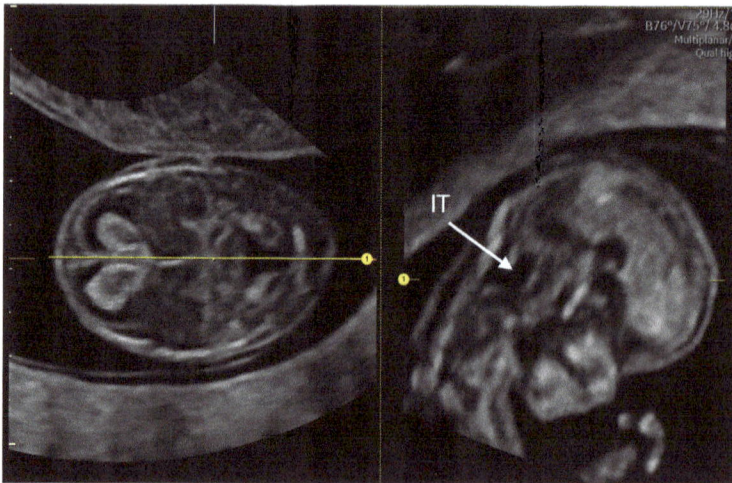

Fig. 5.22: On a volume of a fetal brain in early gestation, the Omniview line can show intracranial translucency (arrow).

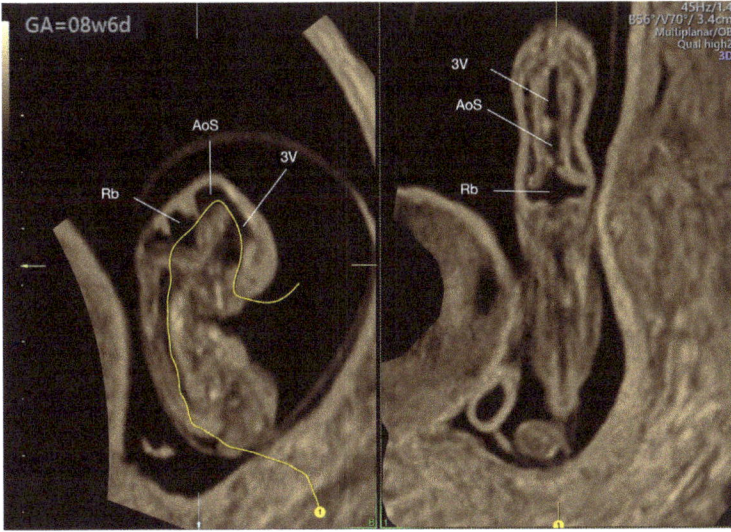

Fig. 5.23: An interesting application of Omniview is the freehand line. Using an embryo at 9 weeks' gestation as an example, the drawn line can show a stretched and projected fetus with brain and body. Third ventricle (3V), Sylvian aqueduct (AoS), rhombencephalon (Rb).

5.6 Conclusions

Navigating within a volume in the different planes requires a learning curve. By scrolling and rotating within the volume, one can understand how to easily reach the plane of choice and highlight the needed details. In our teaching experience, we found that once the examiner becomes accustomed to navigating within a volume, he or she can easily use it for routine scans. In particular, the use of Omniview can be rapidly integrated into a live examination, either on an acquired 3D volume or during a 4D examination. Some examples of the use of the various multiplanar or Omniview modes are presented in this book.

6 Multiplanar Display II: The Tomography Mode

6.1 Principle

The previous chapter discussed multiplanar reconstruction of orthogonal (perpendicular) views and single planes, and this chapter focuses on the other display mode, the *tomography mode*. Tomography mode, also called Tomographic Ultrasound Imaging (TUI) (or multiplane or multislice), is one of the most often used multiplanar reconstruction modes in the fetus because it displays serial adjacent parallel planes side by side. Its frequent use in neurosonography has promoted its use in fetal medicine. In recent years, increasing experience in 3D ultrasound has shown that one of the main advantages of a digital volume data set is post-processing, which allows any 2D plane (see Chapter 5) or series of planes to be obtained from the volume block, especially if that region is not easily accessible during a live scan. Furthermore, storing such a volume block enables the display of parallel slices of an area, similarly to CT- and MR imaging. Although an ultrasound examination is still a dynamic online examination in which live planes are immediately visualized and analyzed, we believe that tomographic ultrasound will become increasingly important in the future. This applies not only to the documentation of a finding, but also to the growing field of ultrasound image standardization and automation. The latter is the basis on which tools such as Sono-CNS or Sono-VCAD are built, generating typical CNS or cardiac images from a volume data set. In this chapter, various aspects of imaging in tomography mode are discussed. The Sono-CNS software will not be discussed in this chapter. Sono-VCAD is discussed shortly in Chapter 19.

6.2 Practical approach

Chapter 5 introduced the orthogonal mode with the display of three planes and the intersection point for navigation within the volume (Fig. 6.1). One of the other important navigation tools is "translation" within the volume, also known as *scrolling* (see Chapter 2). The user interested in parallel planes scrolling can alternatively apply the tomography mode. TUI is a multiplanar display of the volume in parallel planes, similar to the tomographic images of the workstations CT and MR. After activating tomography mode on the touch panel (Figs. 6.1, 6.2) and selecting the region of interest, the examiner controls the number of planes (slices) to be displayed on the screen as well as the interslice distance (Fig. 6.3). Once the region of interest is defined, tomography mode is activated and parallel slices are displayed on the screen next to the reference image, which is in the upper left corner (Figs. 6.2, 6.4). The adjustable interslice distance is displayed in the orientation image in the upper corner (Figs. 6.4, 6.5). In tomography mode, all the manipulation tools of the orthogonal mode can be used, such as intersection point, planes rotation, scrolling within the volume, and VCI.

https://doi.org/10.1515/9783111249513-006

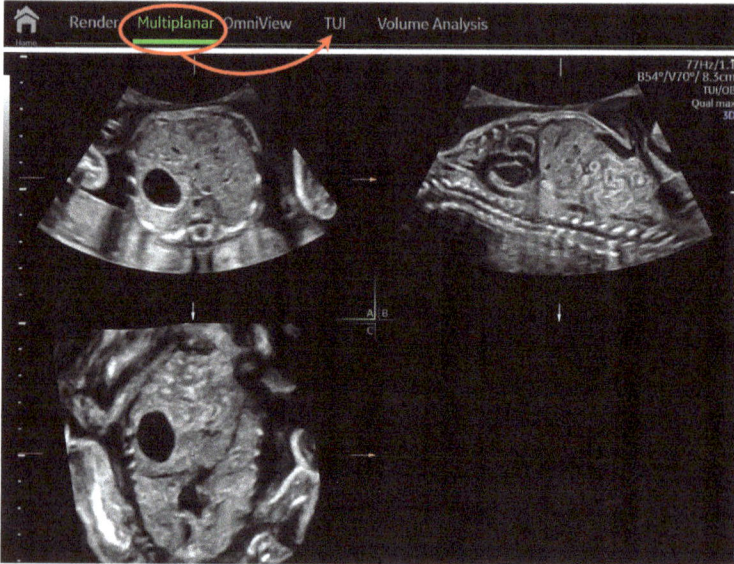

Fig. 6.1: A 3D volume of the thorax and abdomen displayed in orthogonal mode (called multiplanar here). The tomography mode described in this chapter, called Tomographic Ultrasound Imaging (TUI), can be activated on the touch panel (arrow), resulting in Figures 6.2 through 6.9.

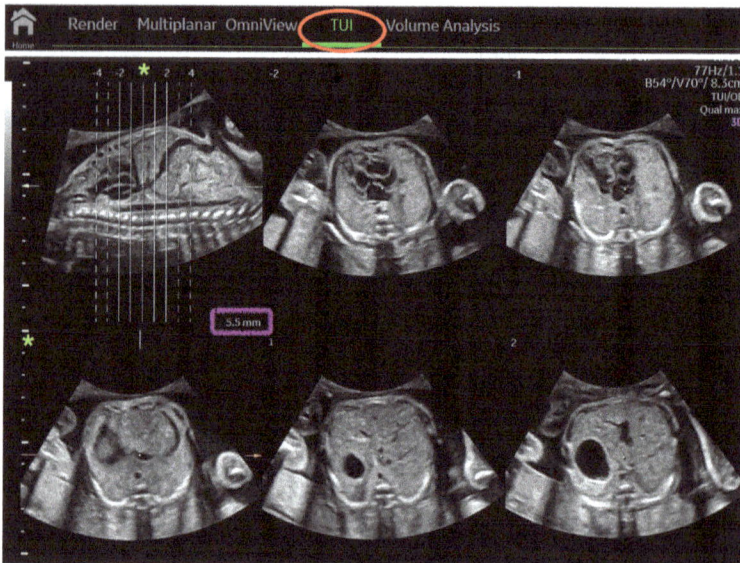

Fig. 6.2: In TUI, the upper left image is the orientation plane. The number of slices can be selected as needed. The green asterisk marks the reference plane; in this case, two planes are in front of the reference plane and two are behind it. The distance between the layers can be changed accordingly (purple box); in this case 5.5 mm was chosen. In Figure 6.3 the available functions are explained.

To improve the image quality, we recommend using either the V-SRI filter or the activation of the VCI mode (see Chapter 4) in order to reduce speckles and increase contrast (Fig. 6.3). The VCI thickness can be increased so that the result resembles a series of thickened slices. Figures 6.4 –6.9 show the different possibilities of the tomography mode. Figure 6.1 shows the original volume in orthogonal mode. With plane A being the reference plane (Fig. 6.6), the displayed images change when the number of slices or the distance between the slices is changed (Figs. 6.7–6.9). The number of slices displayed on the screen can be changed: 2x1, 2x2, 3x2, 3x3, 4x4, etc., as shown in Figures 6.4 to 6.9. Figures 6.8 and 6.9 show scrolling within a volume in tomography mode where the planes can be easily adjusted by selectively rotating the x, y or z-axis. The choice of the A, B or C plane on the touch panel results in a different display as shown in Figures 6.2, 6.4, and 6.5.

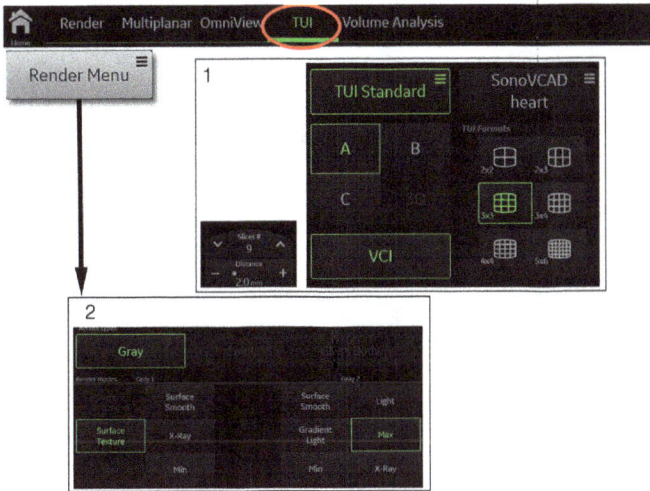

Fig. 6.3: Panel (1) shows the TUI submenu. In this menu, the selection of the parallel planes A, B or C can be made. In the lower left corner of the screen, the number of layers and the distance between layers can be selected. Tomography can be displayed on the screen in different formats, from 2x2 to 5x6 grids, as shown in figures 6.4 through 6.7. In addition, VCI can be enabled; when the Render submenu (panel 2) is opened, the gray mixture can be selected according to the purpose of the examination (tissue, bone, etc.). See Chapter 4 for VCI.

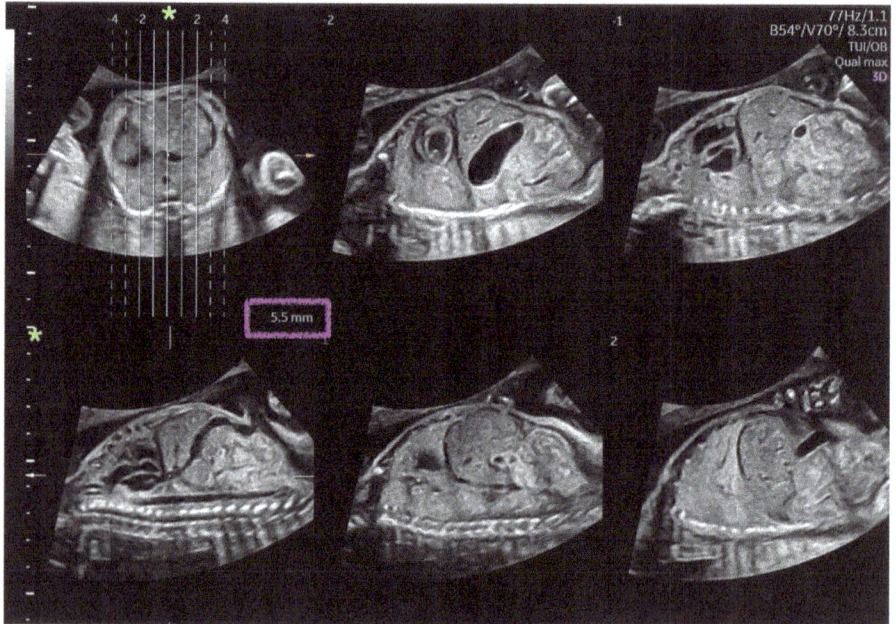

Fig. 6.4: The same display as in Figure 6.2, but plane B has been activated. In the upper left corner is the reference plane showing with the lines the planes from left to right, displayed in this figure.

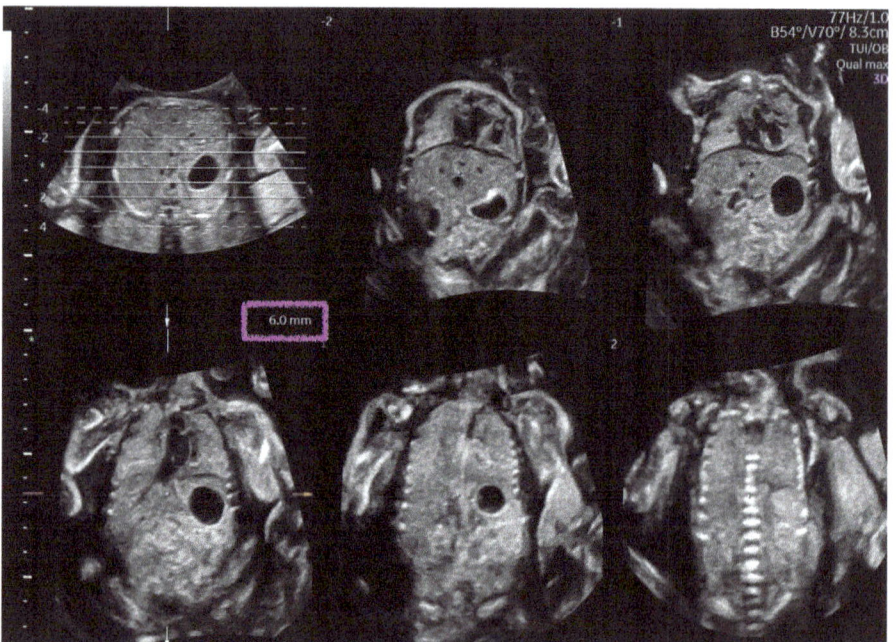

Fig. 6.5: The same display as in Figures 6.1 and 6.2, but in this case plane C has been activated with the display of the coronal planes from anterior to posterior.

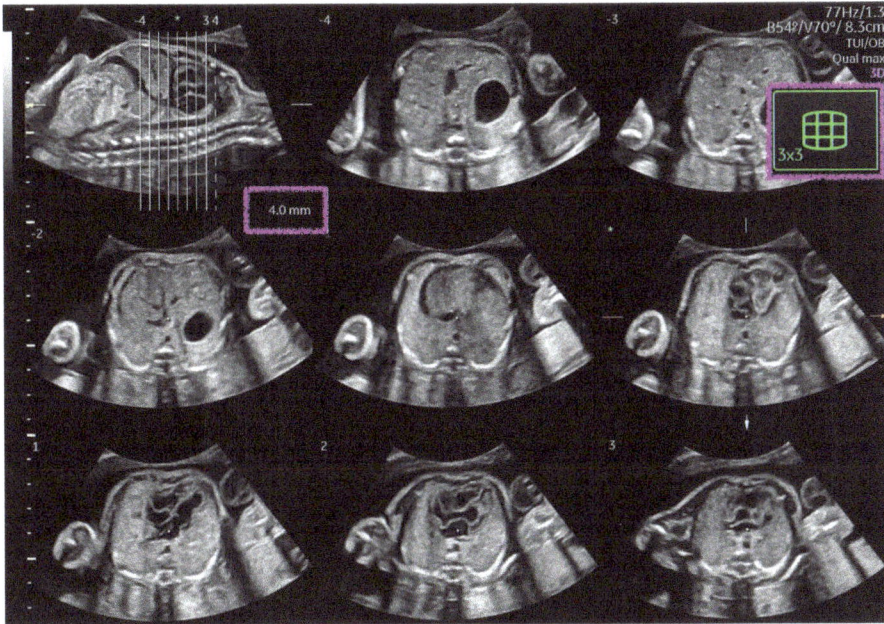

Fig. 6.6: The same display as in Figure 6.2, but here the number of shown layers has been changed from 2x3 in Figure 6.5 to 3x3. The distance between the slices is now 4 mm.

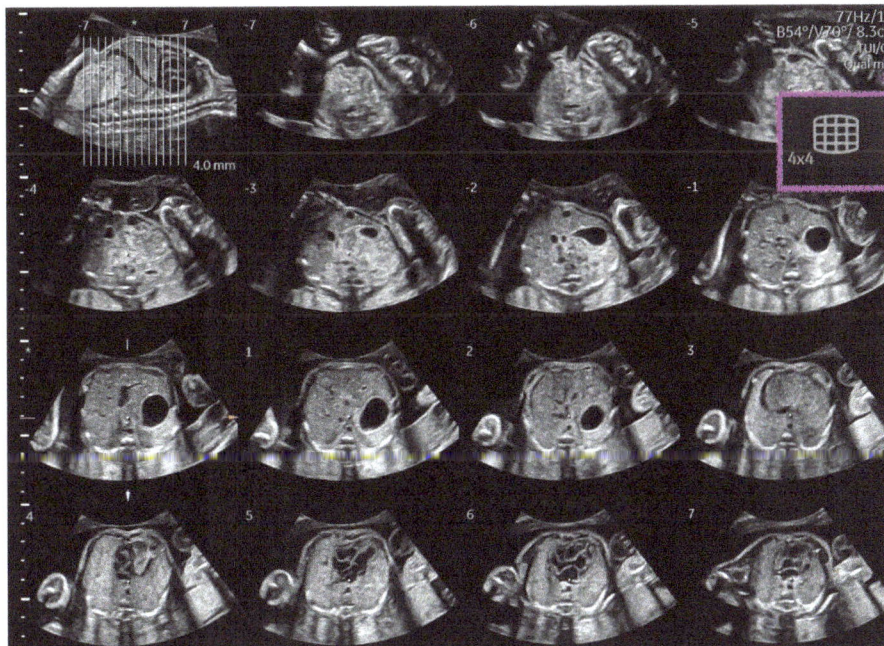

Fig. 6.7: The same representation as in Figure 6.6, but the number of images has been changed to 4x4 images.

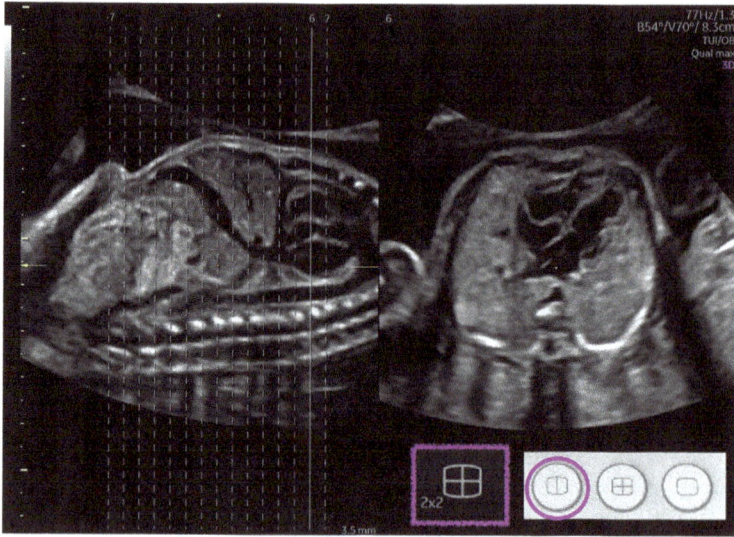

Fig. 6.8: In this example, 2x2 images were selected, but the display of two images was selected on the ultrasound panel, resulting in this duplicate view. What can be seen is the four-chamber view. On the orientation plane (left), the solid line shows the activated plane of interest; this approach can be used to move through the volume plane by plane, as shown in Figure 6.9.

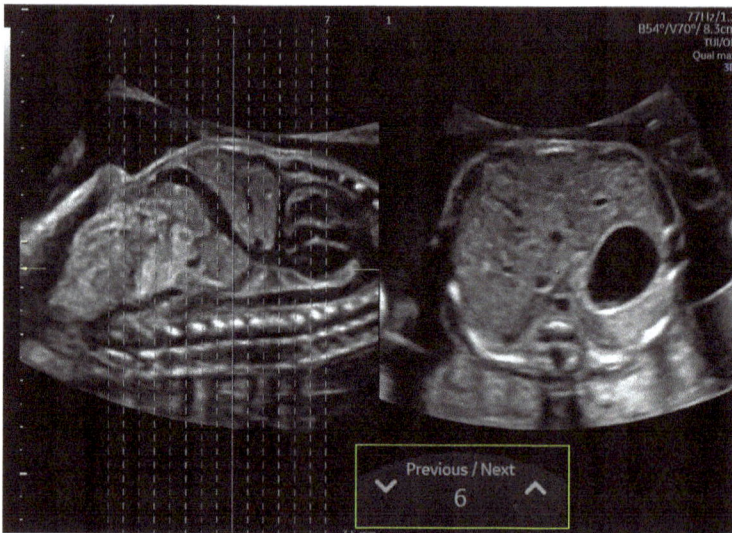

Fig. 6.9: Using the same presets as in Figure 6.8, the layer of the upper abdomen with the stomach can be seen here by scrolling through the images using the Previous/Next button.

6.3 Typical applications of the tomography mode

Tomography of the fetal head, face, and brain: Tomography can be ideally used to evaluate the fetal brain. For fetal neurosonography, volume acquisition can be performed either transabdominally (Figs. 6.10–6.14) or transvaginally (Fig. 6.15). Tomography provides an overview in which all intracerebral landmarks can be visualized at one glance (see also Chapter 16). The example in Figure 6.10 shows an overview of normal brain anatomy with 11 planes and Figure 6.11 the same volume with 29 planes. Figure 6.12 shows a midline acquisition across the fontanelle and Figure 6.13 shows a fetus with severe ventriculomegaly with following details: the normal cerebellum is seen along with a dilated third ventricle in another plane. Therefore, in this overview, diagnoses such as Chiari II malformation, Dandy-Walker malformation, or holoprosencephaly are excluded, and the probable diagnosis is aqueductal stenosis. The cavum septi pellucidi can be clearly seen and recognized in a coronal view in tomography mode; Figures 6.10 and 6.14 show normal and abnormal findings. Brain assessment is best performed transvaginally as shown in Figure 6.15, but see Chapter 16 for more information on fetal neurosonography.

Tomography of the thoracic and abdominal organs: Tomography is ideal for an overview of the thorax and abdomen, especially for clear delineation of structures, such as the lungs, diaphragm, heart, kidneys, liver, and other abdominal organs (Figs. 6.16–6.21). This allows accurate assessment of the extent of a lesion, such as a hyperechogenic lung (Fig. 6.16) or hydrothorax (Fig. 6.17). Tomography of the renal system (Figs. 6.18–6.20) is occasionally performed but can be of big value when an abnormality is identified (Fig. 6.20). Information about the various abdominal organs is best presented in tomography of axial cross-sectional planes showing the typical features of liver, stomach, bowel, bladder, abdominal wall, and kidneys (Fig. 6.7). This display mode is an ideal method in documenting a lesion, especially in fetal anomalies. Figures 6.20 and 6.21 show examples, such as multicystic kidneys in one fetus and the extent of ascites in another. Such image documentation can be of great clinical value for follow-up examinations.

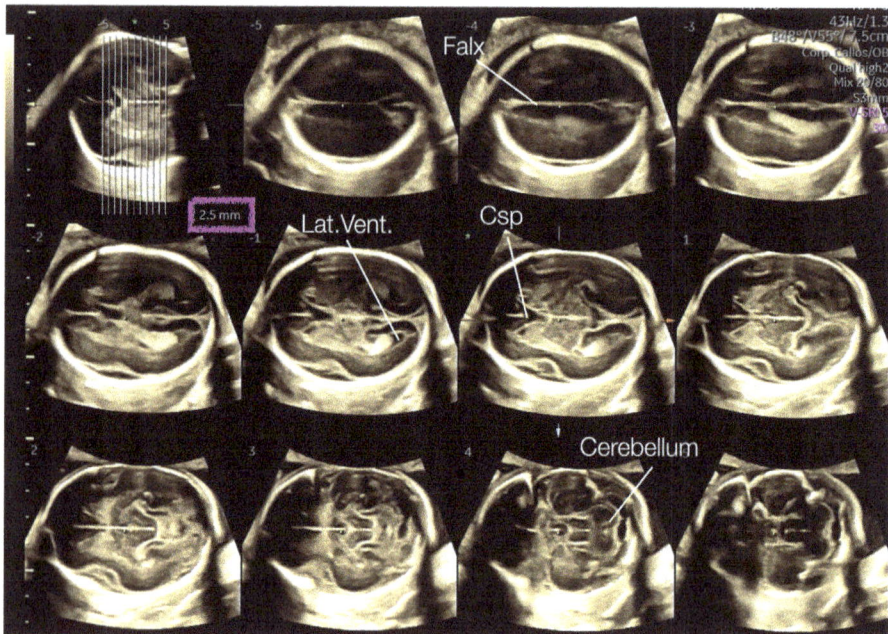

Fig. 6.10: 3D volume of a fetal brain shown in tomography mode in a 3x4 slice pattern with a slice spacing of 2.5 mm. The most important information needed is shown at one glance in these axial planes; cavum septi pellucidi (Csp), lateral ventricle (Lat. Vent.). See Figure 6.11.

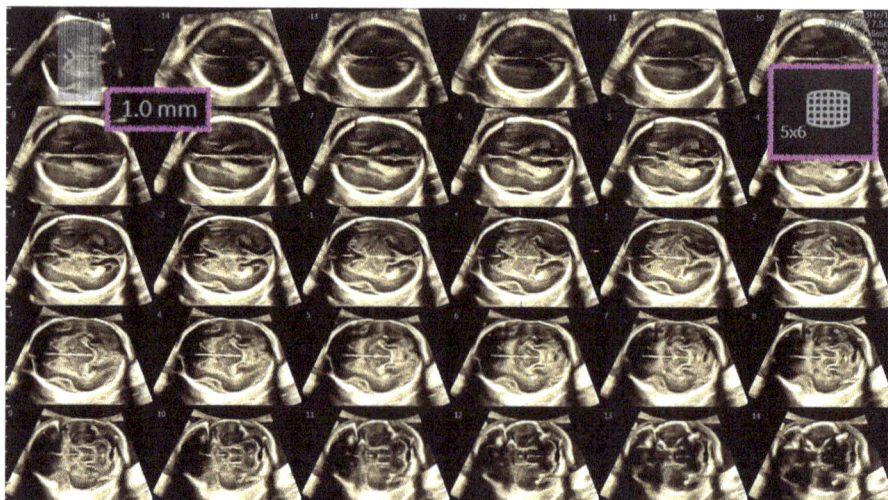

Fig. 6.11: The same volume as in Figure 6.10 was used here, changing the grid from 3x4 to 5x6 and adjusting the distance between layers from 2.5 mm to 1 mm.

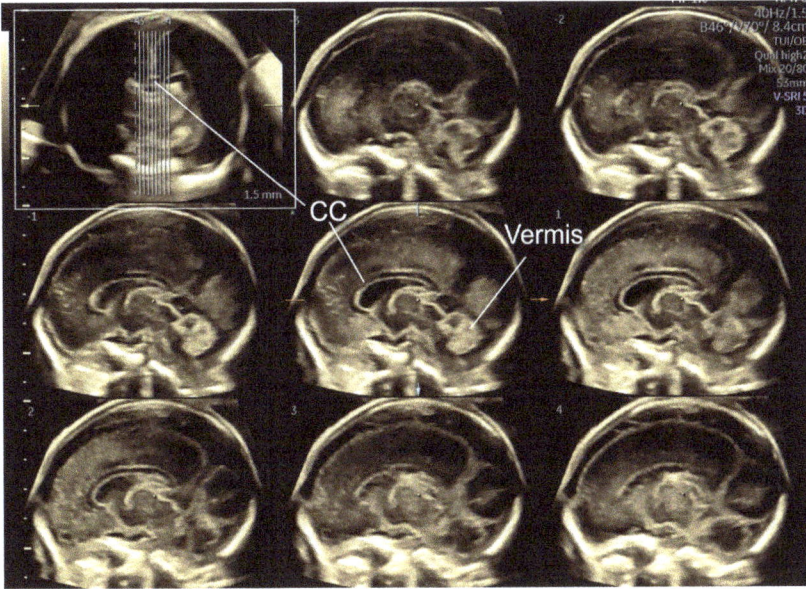

Fig. 6.12: 3D volume of a normal fetal brain at 22 weeks' gestation with insonation through the fontanelle, shown in tomography mode. Briefly, the overview required for a fetal neurosonogram in the midline as corpus callosum (CC) and vermis can be seen.

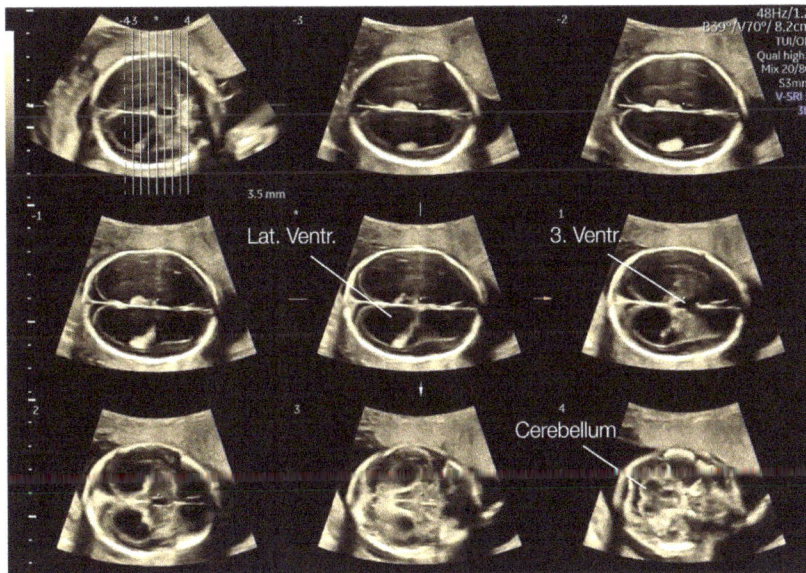

Fig. 6.13: Fetus at 19 weeks of gestation with ventriculomegaly, shown in tomography mode which provides a good overview. At one glance, the dilated lateral ventricles (Lat. Ventr.), the normal looking cerebellum (no Chiari II), and the dilated 3rd ventricle (3. Ventr.) can be easily seen. Presumably, there is an underlying aqueductal stenosis.

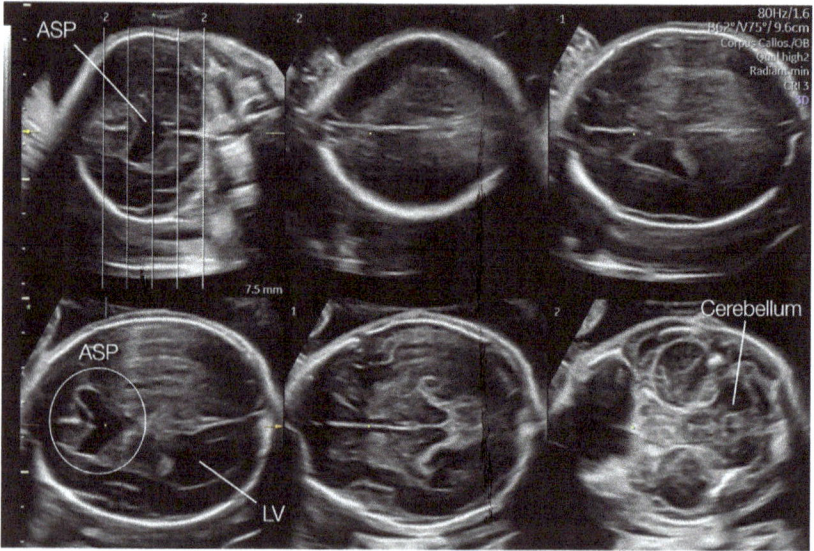

Fig. 6.14: Tomographic representation of the brain of a fetus with absent septum pellucidum (ASP) with communication of the anterior horns of the lateral ventricles.

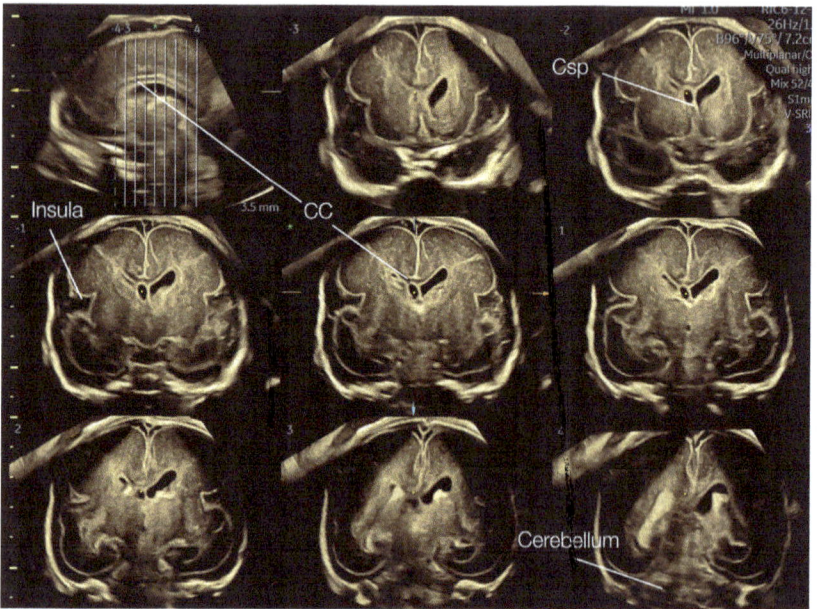

Fig. 6.15: Transvaginal neurosonography in tomography mode with coronal planes. Typical structures, such as the corpus callosum (CC), the cavum septi pellucidi (Csp), and the insula are clearly visible.

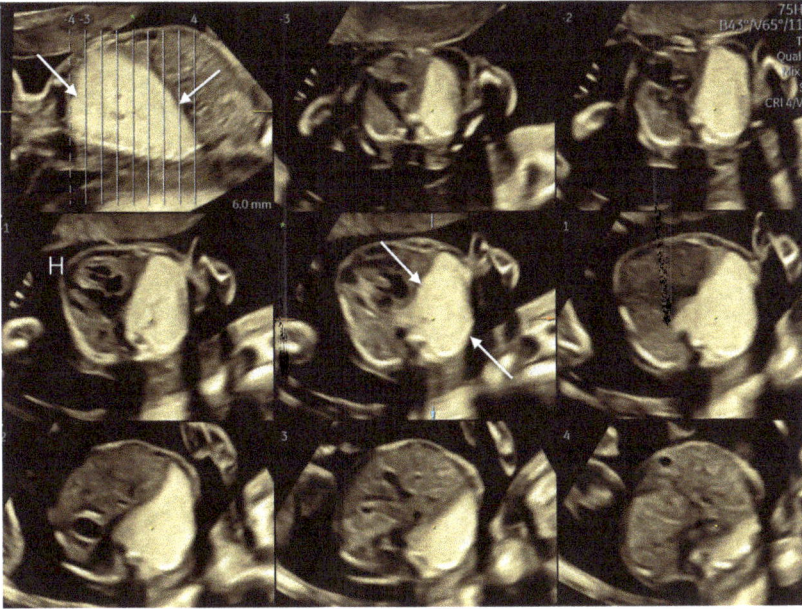

Fig. 6.16: This image shows a right hyperechogenic lung (arrows). The tomography mode shows the location and extent of the lesion as well as the difference in echogenicity compared to the contralateral lung. Note that the heart (H) has been shifted to the left.

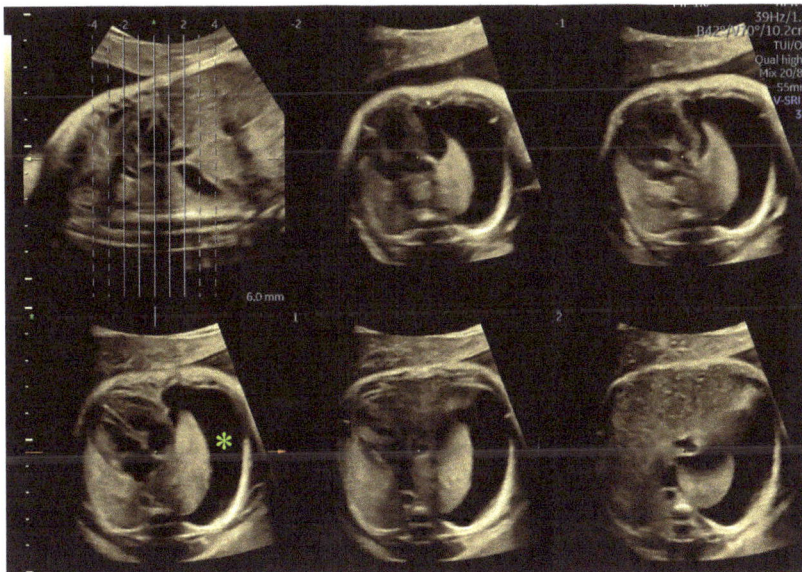

Fig. 6.17: Moderate right pleural effusion (*) shown in tomography mode.

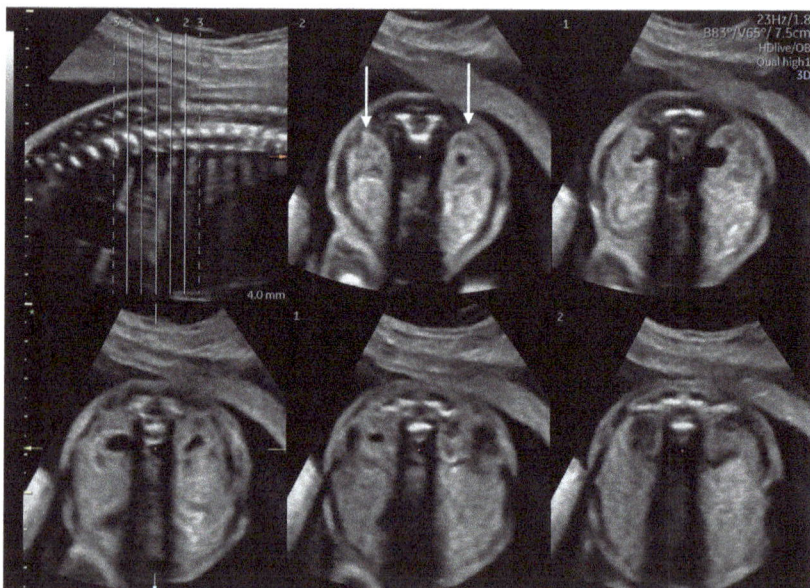

Fig. 6.18: This 3D volume acquisition shows the lumbar region with both kidneys (arrows), displayed here in tomography mode in transverse planes.

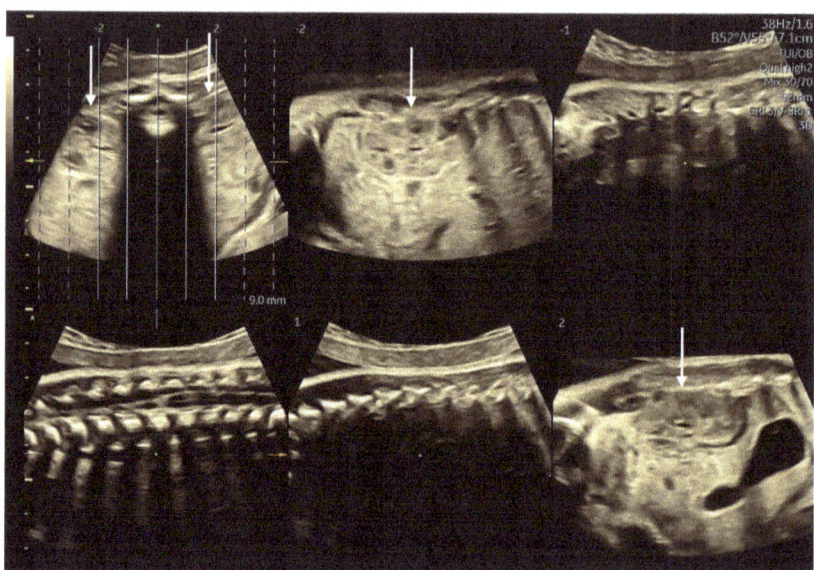

Fig. 6.19: This 3D volume acquisition in tomography mode shows the lumbar region with both kidneys (arrows) in sagittal and parasagittal planes.

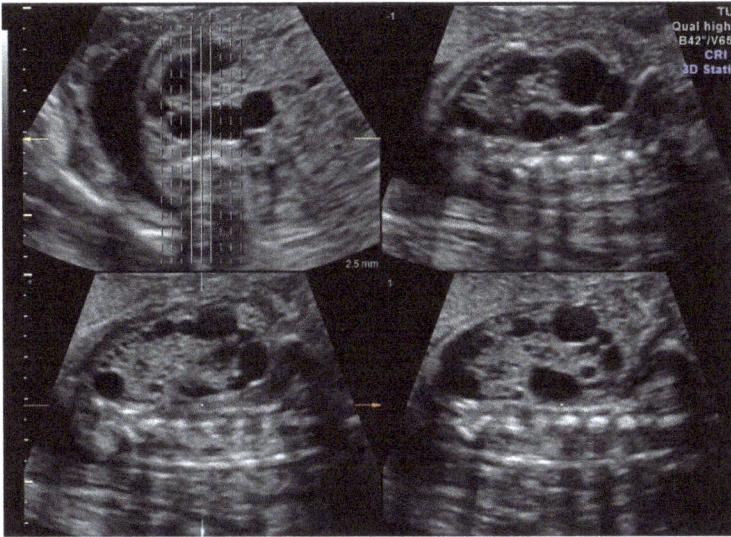

Fig. 6.20: Fetus with multicystic renal dysplasia shown in tomography mode. An overview of the lesion can be better visualized in tomography mode.

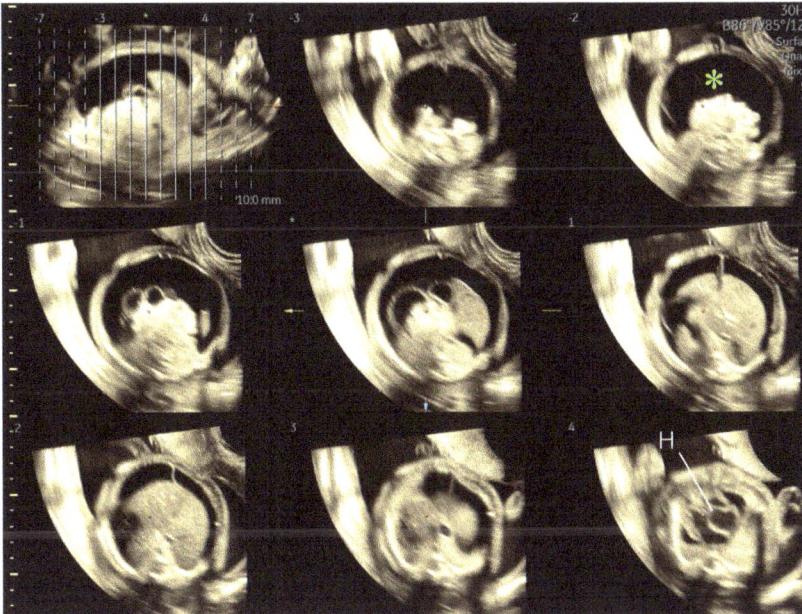

Fig. 6.21: Fetus with ascites (*) in heart failure with cardiac (H) dilation. The extent of ascites can be better assessed and documented in tomography mode compared to single images. These findings are more comparable, especially during follow-up examinations.

Tomography of the fetal heart: A comprehensive cardiac examination must be achieved in different planes, so tomography can be considered an ideal tool for obtaining the complete picture of a heart (Fig. 6.22). Tomography mode of the fetal heart can be performed with either grayscale (Figs. 6.22, 6.23) or color Doppler (Fig. 6.24) using static 3D or STIC volume acquisition. Typical adjacent planes, such as the upper abdomen, the four-chamber view, the five-chamber view, and the three-vessel and trachea view can be well and quickly visualized in one overview with this technique (Fig. 6.22). The Sono-VCAD software also enables the automatic generation of typical section planes out of a volume data set. Figure 6.23 shows an example of a fetus with a partial situs inversus where the opposite positions of stomach and heart can be recognized with one view. Compare to a normal fetus shown in Figure 6.22. For more examples on fetal cardiac tomography, see also Chapter 19 on the fetal heart.

Tomography in early pregnancy: In early gestation, the combination of transvaginal 3D ultrasound and tomography mode (Figs. 6.25–6.27) provides a high valuable information (see also Chapter 20). Because of the limitations of transvaginal probe manipulation, typical planes are more easily reconstructed from a volume than directly visualized on 2D. Acquisition of a 3D volume and its display in multiplanar mode, especially in tomography mode, provides a good overview. This is especially the case for regions such as the brain (Fig. 6.25), face (Fig. 6.26), thorax and abdomen (Fig. 6.27), and others.

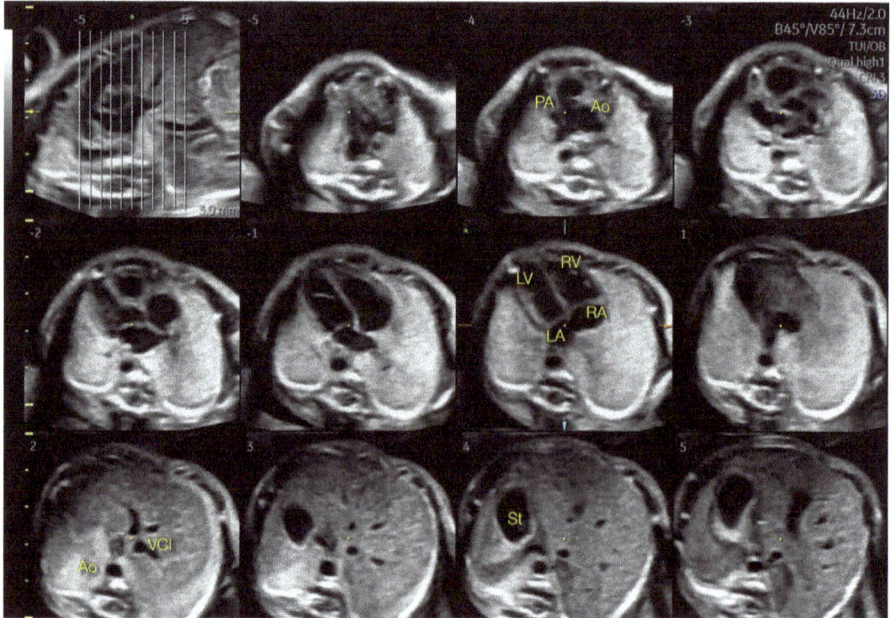

Fig. 6.22: Tomography mode of a 3D static volume of the heart. From the upper abdomen to the great vessels, the important structures can be visualized; aorta (Ao), pulmonary artery (PA), right and left ventricle (RV, LV), right and left atrium (RA, LA), stomach (St), inferior vena cava (VCI).

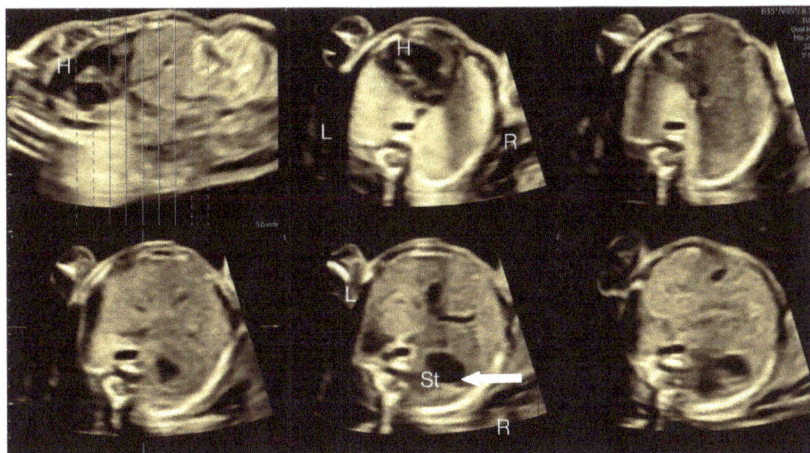

Fig. 6.23: Tomography mode in a fetus with partial situs inversus. Note that the stomach (St) is right-sided (arrow), while the heart (H) is left-sided. Tomography provides a good overview in such cases; left (L), right (R).

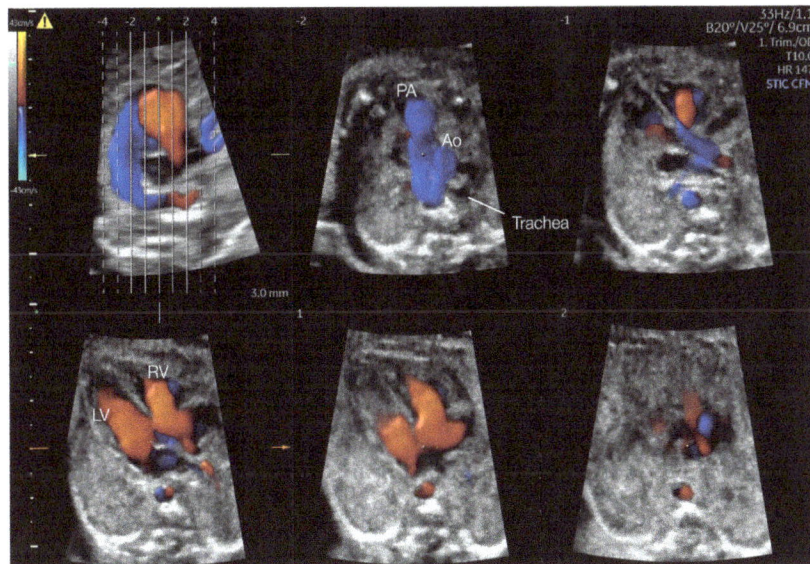

Fig. 6.24: Tomography mode of a STIC volume acquisition in color Doppler in the cardiac phase between diastole and systole. In diastole, the four-chamber view can be seen (bottom middle image) and systole can be seen in the three-vessel view. Aorta (Ao), left ventricle (LV), pulmonary artery (PA), right ventricle (RV).

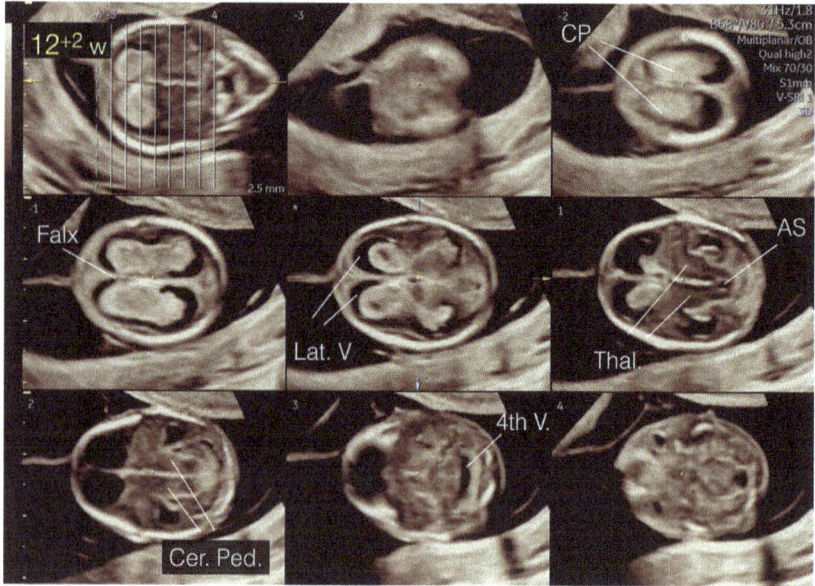

Fig. 6.25: Tomography mode of an axial view of the fetal brain at 12 weeks' gestation, providing an overview of the major landmarks of the brain at this stage of development. These include the greater choroid plexus (CP), the falx cerebri, the two lateral ventricles (Lat. V.), the thalami (Thal.), the Sylvian aqueduct (AS), the cerebral peduncles (Cer. Ped.), and the fourth ventricle (4th V.).

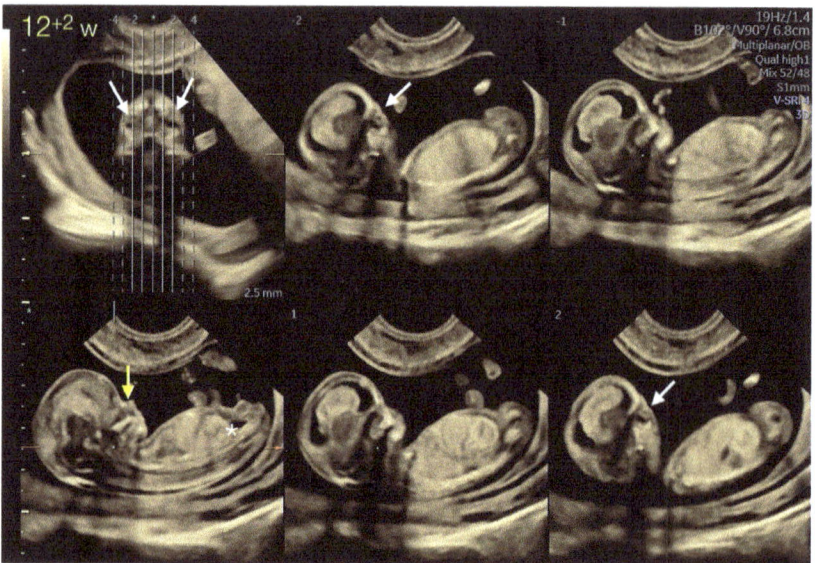

Fig. 6.26: 3D volume of a first trimester fetus in midsagittal view in tomography mode. The nasal bone (yellow arrow), maxilla, mandible, both eyes (white arrows), posterior fossa, thorax, abdomen, diaphragm, bladder (*) and abdominal wall can be seen in one plane.

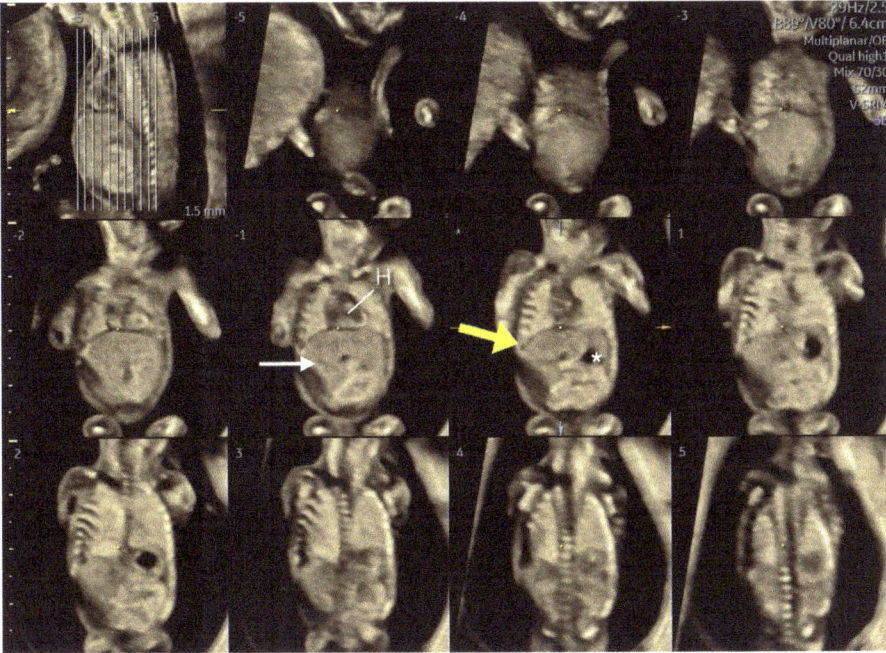

Fig. 6.27: Tomography of the body of a 13-week-old fetus showing the diaphragm (yellow arrow), lungs, liver, stomach (*), kidneys (arrows) and the left-sided heart position.

6.4 Conclusions

Tomography mode provides an optimal overview of the region of interest. The overall view of an organ with its neighboring structures enables a precise examination and is helpful in documenting a finding. The ability to display this region in two to 29 parallel successive planes simultaneously provides the flexibility to demonstrate the individual information needed. As experience is acquired, typical examination standards can be identified for the various body parts, and volume depth and interslice distance can be stored in specific presets. The fetal brain and heart are ideal regions to examine with this tool. Chapter 16 and Chapter 19 present some abnormal findings in these planes, and Chapter 18 presents some abnormal findings of the fetal thoracic, gastrointestinal, and renal organs.

7 The Surface Mode

7.1 Principle

Surface mode is the most often selected 3D and 4D rendering mode. It is used to visualize the surface of the region of interest; this is best demonstrated when covered by fluid, such as the face of the fetus or the limbs in the amniotic cavity. Within the render box, the surface mode displays the most superficial layer closest to the green render line (see Chapter 2). It is used to show the face, anterior or posterior body surface, limbs, or the entire fetus in early gestation. In addition, structures within the fetal body, such as cardiac chambers, the intracerebral ventricular system, intraabdominal organs, and others can also be visualized using the surface mode. This chapter presents the technical aspects of the surface mode and illustrates typical applications.

7.2 Practical approach

To obtain an appropriate 3D volume, the examiner should prepare the initial 2D image with good contrast between adjacent structures, e. g., between the echolucent amniotic fluid and the echogenic fetal skin. The preliminary settings for the 2D image were discussed in Chapter 1. Figures 7.1 and 7.2 show the effects of an a priori optimal grayscale gain enhancement on the acquisition result. As can be seen in these figures, a dark amniotic fluid in 2D is a prerequisite for a good surface mode image.

Positioning of the region of interest prior to 3D acquisition should be as perpendicular as possible to the surface to be imaged (Fig. 7.3 versus Figs.7.4–7.6). In Figure 7.3 the arm can be clearly seen on 2D, but the 3D result is not satisfactory. Only a perpendicular insonation of the arm, as shown in Figure 7.4, leads to an adequate 3D image; a similar case with legs and feet is shown in Figure 7.5. Ideally, the object of interest should be horizontal and parallel to the camera line (or rendering line) (Fig. 7.6).

For static 3D volume acquisition, it is also recommended to choose a wide box that covers a larger area than the selected region of interest (Figs. 7.6, 7.7B, 7.8B). This avoids missing parts of the fetus in the rendered 3D image, as shown in Figures 7.7A and 7.8A. Especially in early gestation, when the entire fetus is visible, a small volume box can cause parts of the fetus's arms and legs to be missing from the final 3D image. This is usually the case with static 3D images, whereas with 4D the examiner can adjust the resulting image in live mode accordingly.

https://doi.org/10.1515/9783111249513-007

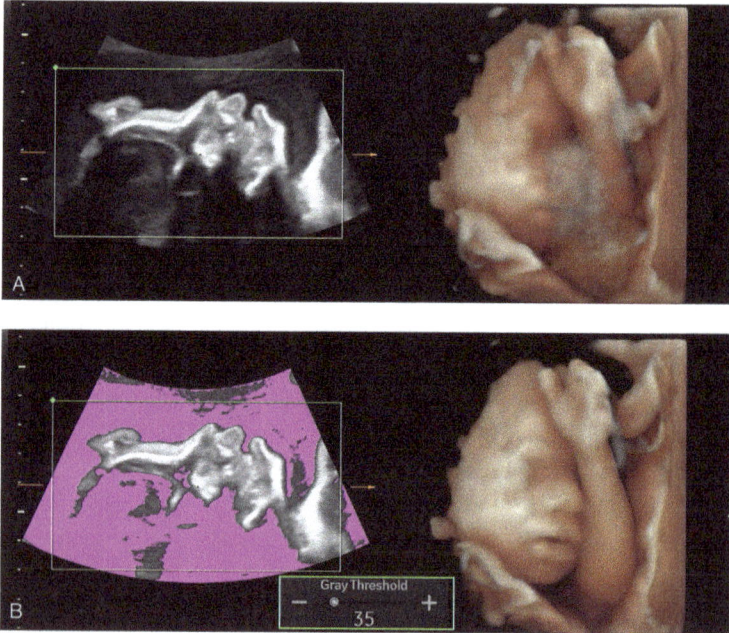

Fig. 7.1: 3D volume of the surface mode of a face. In (A), the preset of the grayscale image is not optimized and shows a low contrast with a gray-appearing amniotic fluid, resulting in an unsatisfactory 3D image. In (B), the gray threshold is increased, suppressing the gray amniotic fluid and showing the 3D image of the face. However, it is better to optimize the image before volume acquisition.

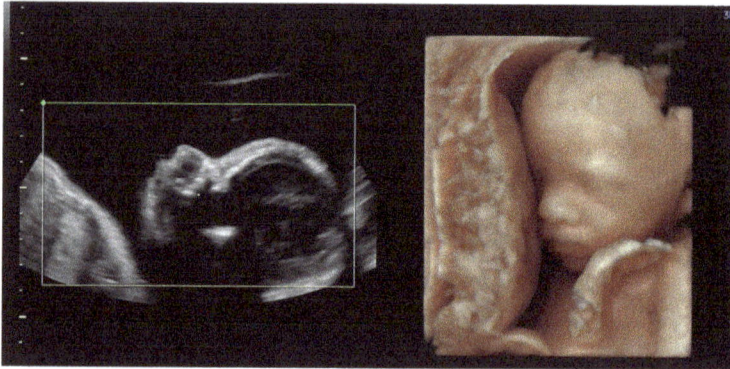

Fig. 7.2: In this fetus, the 2D image was optimized before volume acquisition and shows clear skin edges and black amniotic fluid. The result is an optimal 3D surface of the face.

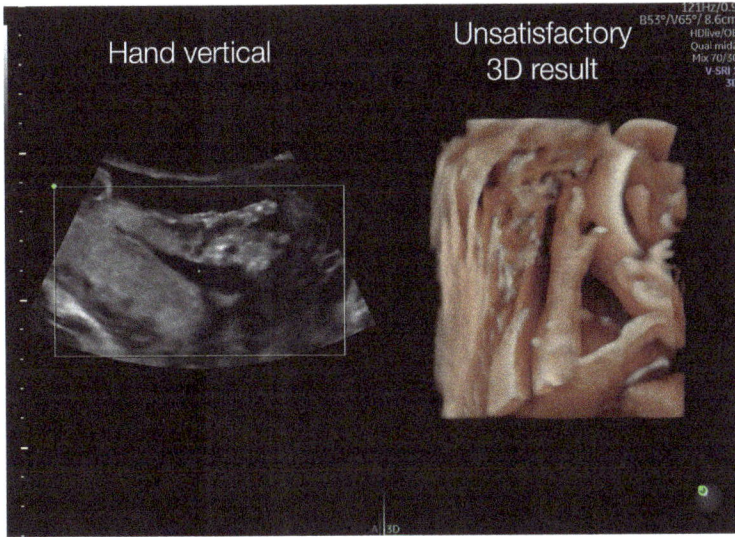

Fig. 7.3: For a good 3D image, the insonation angle during volume acquisition is important. In the left panel, the hand is well visible on the 2D image; in a 3D volume acquisition, however, the fingers are parallel to the ultrasound beam and not well visible on the 3D surface image. For best results, the hand should be horizontal. See Figure 7.4.

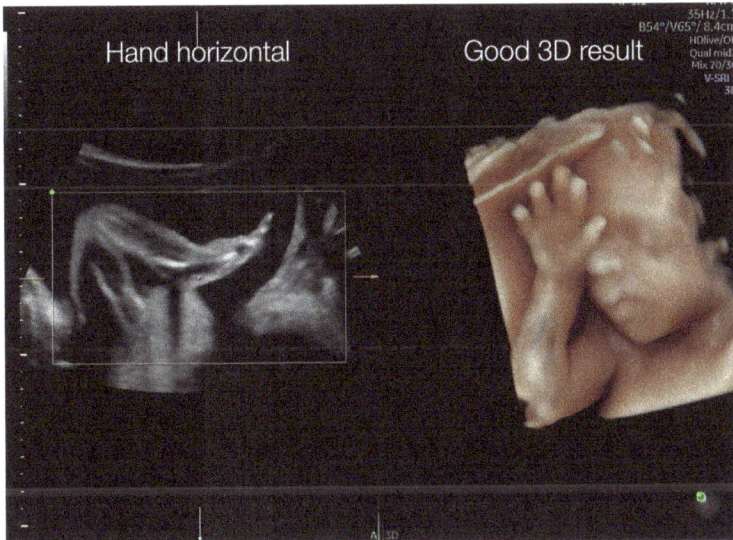

Fig. 7.4: Compared to Figure 7.3, the hand is horizontal and the ultrasound waves are perpendicular to it. This is ideal for 3D acquisition and the fingers are clearly visible.

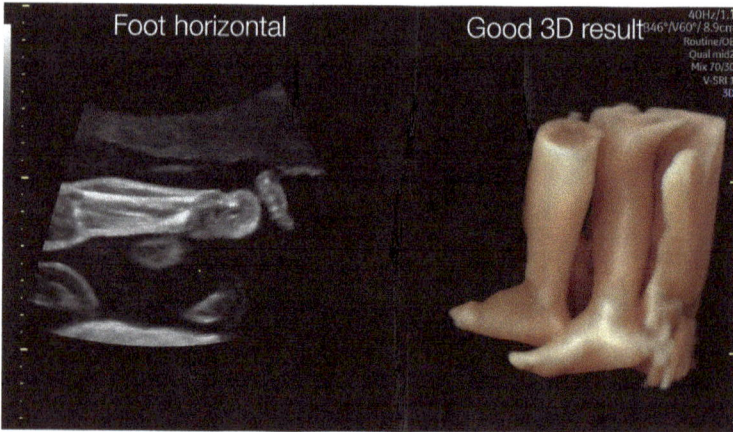

Fig. 7.5: Similar to imaging the hands is the 3D acquisition of the feet; the best insonation should be perpendicular, with the feet horizontal and viewed from the side, thus ideal for 3D acquisition.

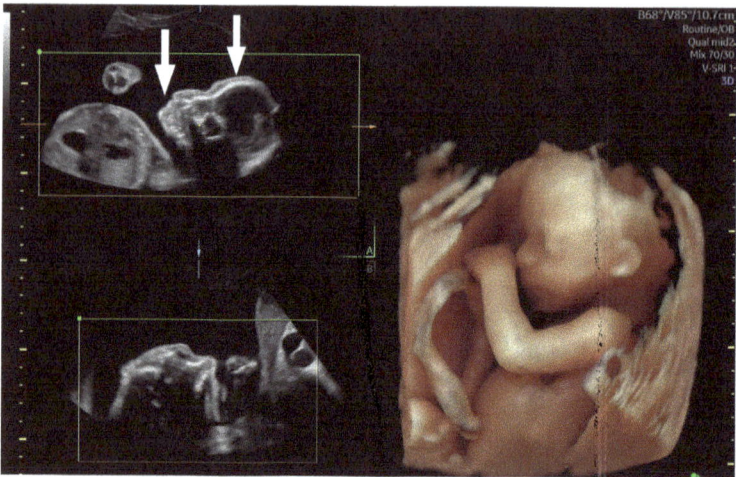

Fig. 7.6: 3D volume acquisition of a face in surface mode. Insonation is better from the side (arrows) with the forehead and face almost horizontal (arrows). This is easier to capture than a frontal view and gives a very good result.

After acquiring a volume, the examiner adjusts the rendering by resizing the box of the region of interest to include the structures to be displayed. The render box with the region of interest inside is then fixed (button "Fixed ROI") and one of the various surface mode functions is activated, as explained in Chapter 3. The quality of the rendering can vary and depends on the settings of the ultrasound system. The operator can switch between the different surface rendering modes and their combinations. The

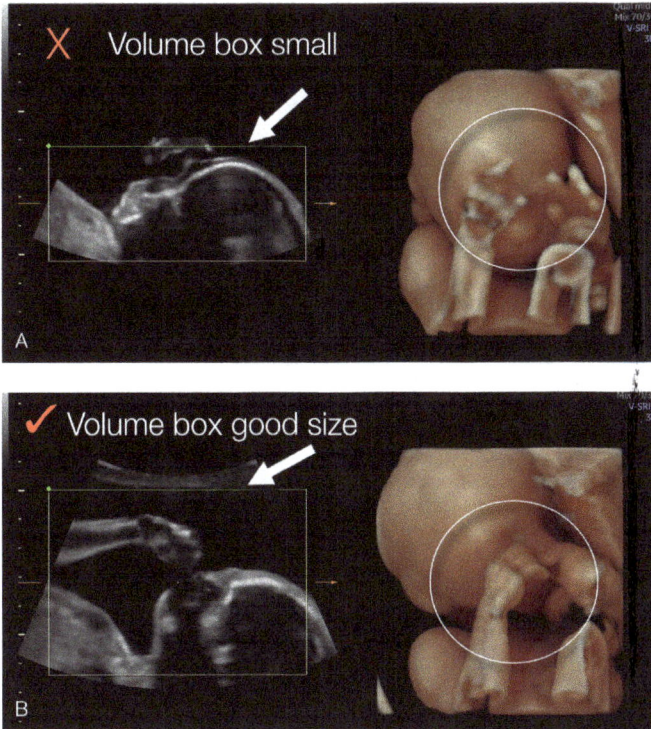

Fig. 7.7: 3D volume acquisition with a small volume box (A); the face can be seen, but part of the hand is missing. Acquisition of a larger box (B) is chosen for the static 3D acquisition; structures surrounding the region of interest can also be acquired. In the 4D examination, on the other hand, the examiner can adjust the size of the box during the live scan.

most often used mode currently is the combination of HDlive surface and HDlive smooth, giving the skin color appearance (Fig. 7.9) (see also Chapter 3). In recent years, the HDlive skin color has replaced the various sepia modes used in the past. There are no "best" presets, as a mix of different modes can also be a matter of aesthetic taste or preference. The softness of the image is defined not only by the resolution of acquisition but can also be slightly modified by using different levels of the filter called *Volume Speckle Reduction Imaging* (V-SRI). Figure 7.10 shows the same face with different V-SRI levels where the regions of mouth, nose, and eyes show the differences in softness. Image quality can also be improved by increasing image smoothness and shadowing. Magicut (see Chapter 3) can be used to remove structures in front of the region of interest provided the removed parts do not cast shadows on the background image. We often adapt the light source by changing its position to create an impression of depth and spatial effect. For the specific 3D rendering of the different organs, such as face or limbs, please refer to the corresponding chapters.

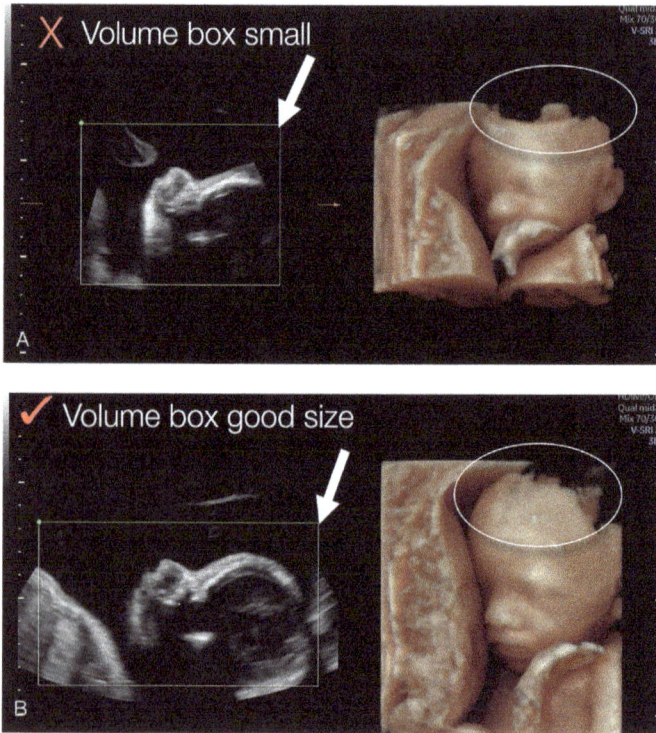

Fig. 7.8: 3D volume acquisition with a small volume box (A). The face can be seen, but part of the head is missing due to the small box. In (B), a larger box size was chosen to capture the entire head.

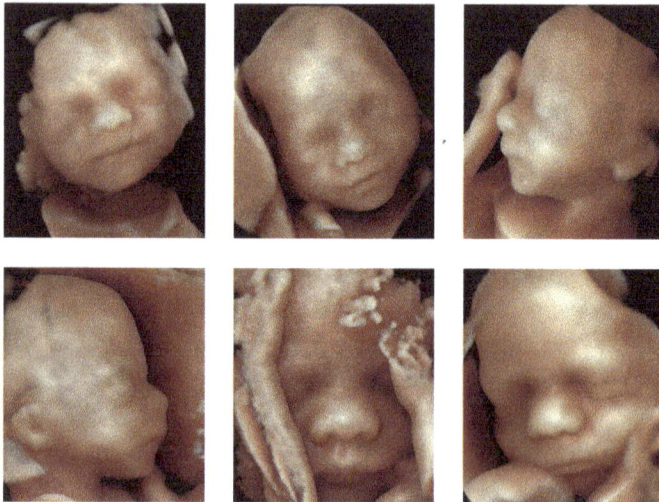

Fig. 7.9: 3D surface mode of different fetal faces in surface mode displays.

7.3 Typical applications of the surface mode

Head and face: The most common application of the surface mode is visualization of the fetal face, discussed separately in Chapter 15. The face can be visualized in 3D or 4D at different stages of gestation (Figs. 7.9–7.12). In addition to the frontal view, a lateral view allows visualization of the fetal profile and ear (Figs. 7.6, 7.9) which can be better assessed than with the conventional 2D view. In the first half of gestation, the fontanelles and sutures of the fetal skull are still large and can be easily visualized with the surface mode by decreasing the gain or increasing the transparency. With the real-time 4D, it is also possible to detect various fetal facial expressions and movements, including swallowing, yawning, eye opening, and others (Fig. 7.11). Figure 7.12 should be a warning to the operator to be careful when visualizing any 3D face image without using the electronic scalpel. The position of the umbilical cord around the neck or the umbilical knot in Figure 7.12 may be considered a variant by many operators, but in most cases, it is a concerning finding for the patient and her family. The goal of reassuring the parents by visualizing a cute fetal face in 3D will ultimately worry them for the entire pregnancy. The "how to visualize" approach for the face and the use of Magicut are discussed in Chapter 3 and Chapter 15.

Fetal limbs: Arms, legs, hands, and feet can also be well visualized from different perspectives and with different resolutions (Figs. 7.4, 7.5, 7.13). In many situations, the hands are near the face or covering it and are displayed together (Figs. 7.4–7.6, 7.13). Increasing the resolution in 3D acquisition often leads to a better representation of fingers and toes, even in early gestation (Figs. 7.13, 7.14C). Further improvement of the image is achieved by adjusting the softness of the image and the position of the light source. Further details can also be found in Chapter 17 on limbs.

Visualization of the body surface: The fetal body, either the back or the ventral side with the umbilical cord attachment, can be visualized well from early gestation (Figs. 7.14, 7.15). These can also be visualized at advanced gestational age if there is sufficient amniotic fluid to allow a surface view. Fetal anomalies such as gastroschisis, omphalocele (Fig. 7.16), spina bifida (Figs. 7.16, 7.17), sacrococcygeal teratoma (Fig. 7.18), and others that are present at the surface can be clearly observed in the surface mode. In gastroschisis, the intestinal loops can be visualized in detail in the early and late stages of pregnancy, as shown in Chapter 18. Identification and visualization of gender can also be done in surface mode (Fig. 7.19) where related anomalies can be well distinguished from normal external genitalia.

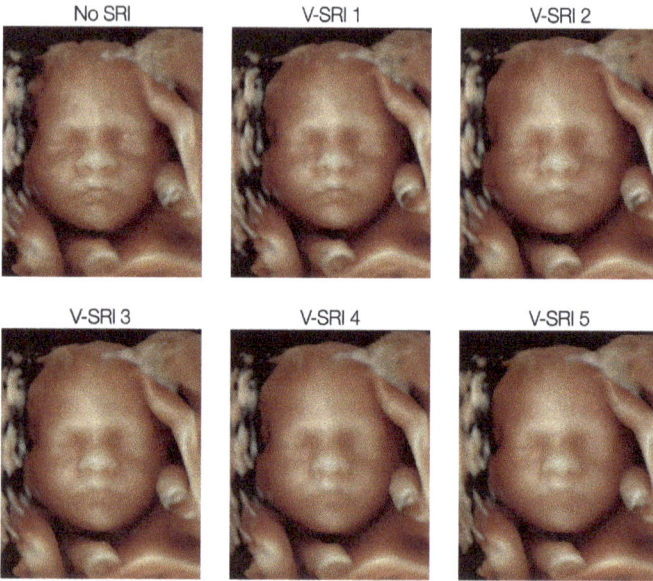

Fig. 7.10: Fetal face in 3D surface mode with HDlive. The result can be modified in its softness by using different levels of V-SRI, here from no V-SRI to level 5. The difference is most obvious in the region of the mouth and nose with nostrils. The authors prefer the use of a low V-SRI.

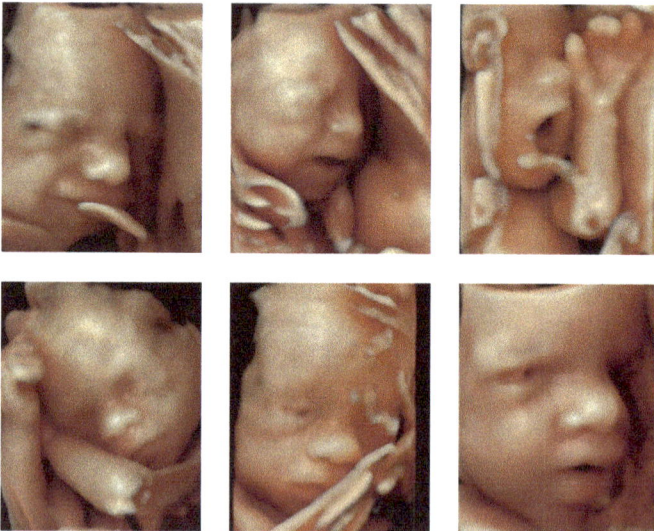

Fig. 7.11: During a real-time 4D examination, it is often possible to observe facial mimics as seen in these fetuses.

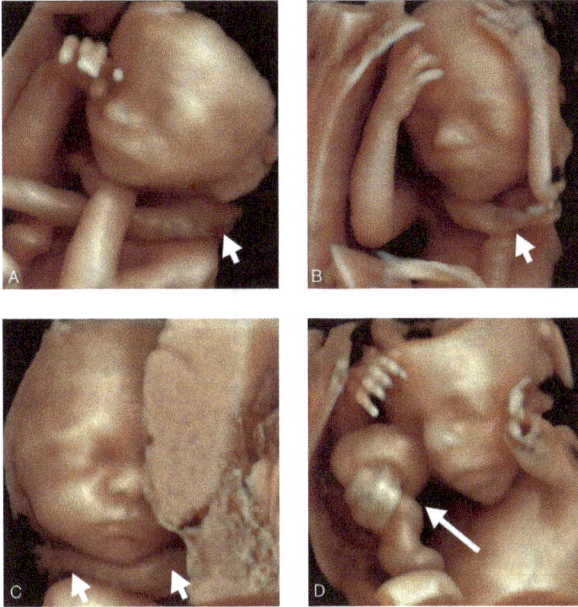

Fig. 7.12: When a face is rendered in 3D, additional adjacent structures, often not directly visible on the 2D image prior to volume acquisition, can be made visible. Here the umbilical cord (short arrows) can be seen around the neck; in image (D), a true umbilical cord node was even detected (long arrow). In such cases, consider removing the umbilical cord with Magicut (see Chapter 3).

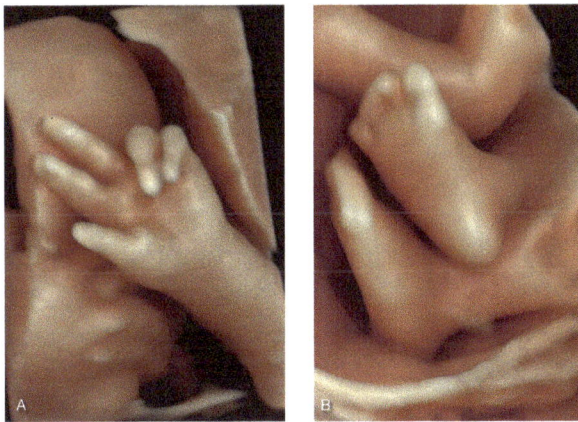

Fig. 7.13: With the 3D surface mode, hands with fingers and feet with toes can be seen clearly and their normal anatomy can be assessed. For this purpose, a perpendicular insonation angle and a higher resolution are recommended during acquisition.

Overview of the entire fetus: Rather than limiting the 3D view to the face, limbs, or other parts of the fetus by magnification, the examiner may also attempt to visualize the entire fetus. Ideally, a complete view of the fetus is possible between 8 and 18 weeks of gestation (Figs. 7.14, 7.15). Such a view is beneficial in delineating normal and abnormal findings, as shown in Figures 7.16, 7.18, and 7.20. At later stages of pregnancy, the fetus is too large to be fully visualized in one image.

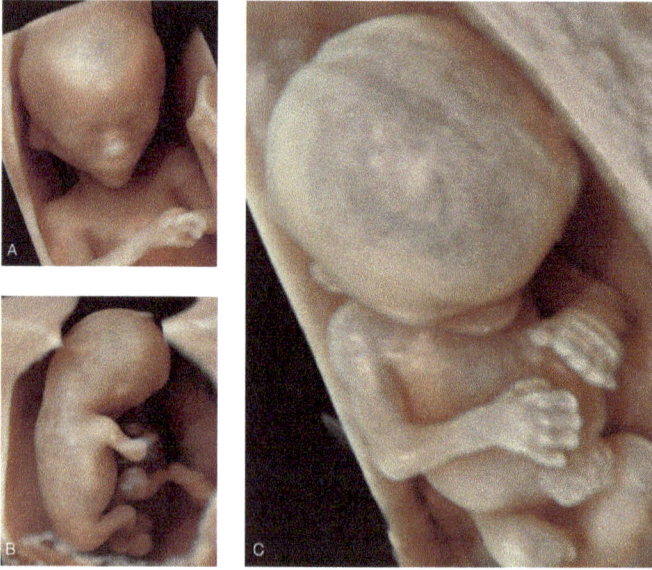

Fig. 7.14: Normal first trimester fetuses showing that 3D surface rendering can also be used to selectively represent some specific aspects such as the face (A), back (B) and hands with fingers (C).

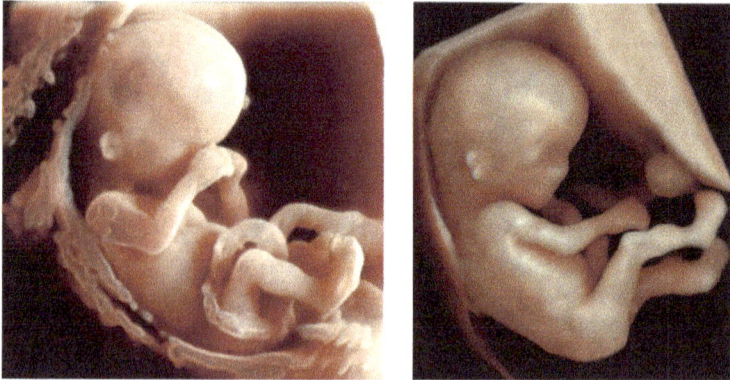

Fig. 7.15: Two normal fetuses at 12 weeks' gestation with transvaginal 3D volume acquisition and surface mode rendering to show the entire body with head, face, thorax, and limbs.

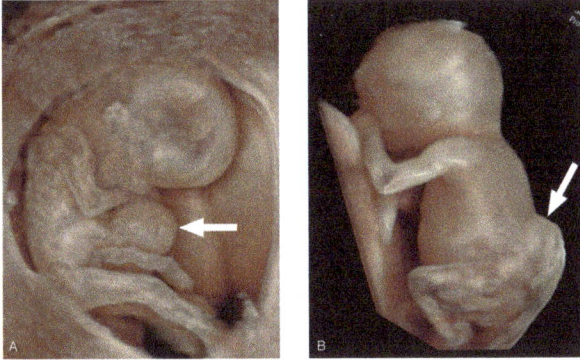

Fig. 7.16: 3D surface mode in two fetuses at 13 weeks of gestation with omphalocele (A) and with spina bifida (B). The surface mode can be used well to display such findings in overview.

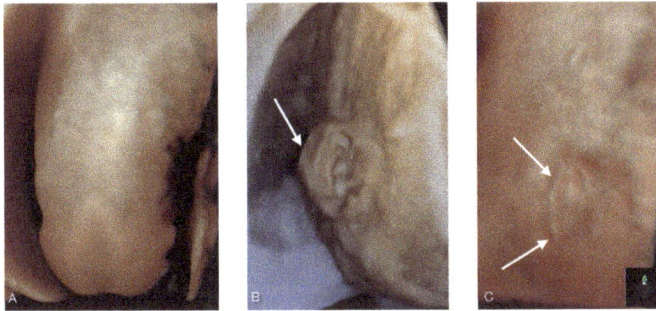

Fig. 7.17: 3D surface mode of the back of a normal fetus (A) and two fetuses with open spina bifida (B and C). In panel B the fetus has a myelomeningocele and in panel C a myeloschisis. While in (B) the finding is conspicuous and easy to recognize, the lesion is flat in (C) and can only be clearly recognized by increasing acquisition resolution and adjusting the light position (here from above).

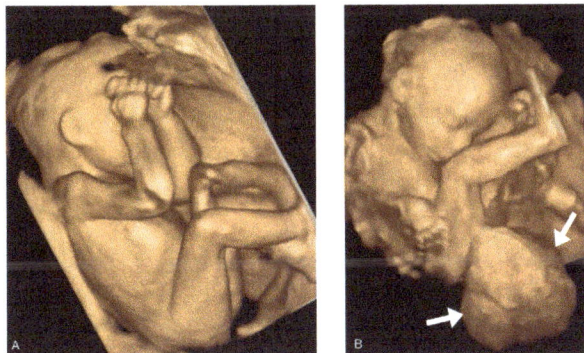

Fig. 7.18: 3D surface mode showing the complete fetus at 22 weeks of gestation (Panel A). In comparison, panel B shows a fetus with a sacrococcygeal teratoma (arrows).

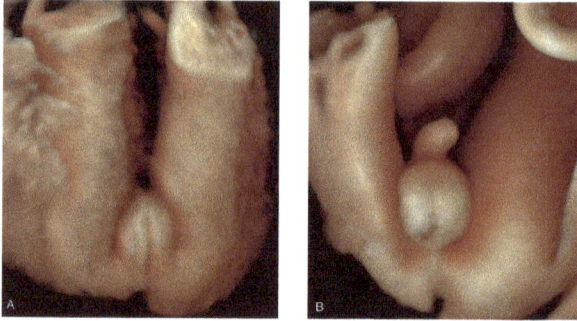

Fig. 7.19: The 3D surface mode can be used to visualize the gender, as can be seen in this girl (A) and this boy (B).

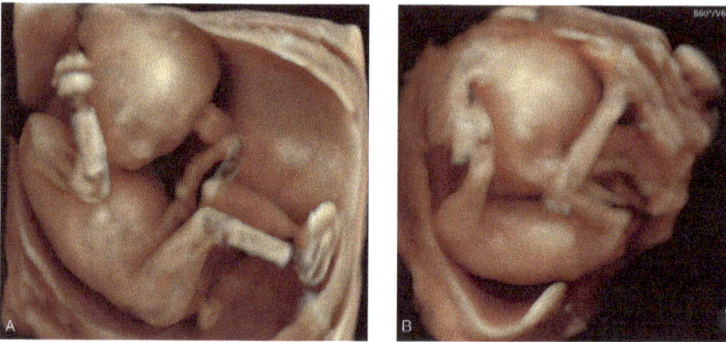

Fig. 7.20: Panel A: 3D surface mode showing a complete fetus at 22 weeks of gestation with normal head to body size ratio. Panel B, in comparison, shows a fetus with triploidy and severe growth restriction with a normal head compared to the small thorax and body.

Fetuses in multiple pregnancies: In multiple pregnancies, the surface mode is appropriate to obtain a complete view of the fetuses in the uterine cavity (Fig. 7.21). The amniotic membrane is often too thin to be visualized in monochorionic twins but, on the other hand, can be easily distinguished from a thick, separating chorion/amnion layer in dichorionic twins. The position and number of fetuses can be well visualized with the surface mode. A good effect can be reached by adding some silhouette mode (see Chapter 11).

Placenta, umbilical cord and amniotic membranes: The overview provided by the surface mode for visualizing the fetus may also show the surrounding structures, such as the placenta, the umbilical cord at its insertion and course, the amniotic bands, and various uterine anomalies.

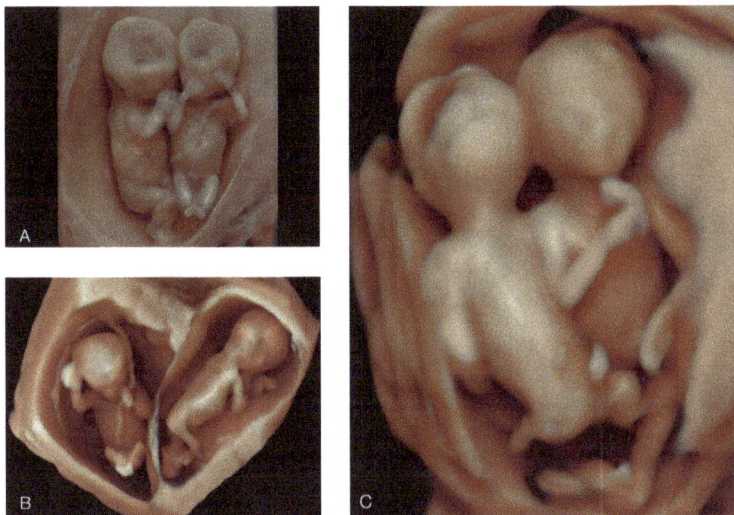

Fig. 7.21: The 3D surface mode can also be used in twin or multiple pregnancies to show the twins and their relationship to each other, as shown in these images. Even though the twins in (A) and (C) are very close, they are diamniotic twins, while the twins in (B) are dichorionic.

Visualization inside the body: Surface mode can be used to visualize internal body organs, such as the heart (Fig. 7.22), brain, thorax or abdomen, and others (Fig. 7.23). When applied to the heart, the heart cavities are well seen in the four-chamber view. The phases of the heart, diastole and systole, can also be demonstrated in a STIC acquisition (Fig. 7.22). When examining other organs, surface mode is rarely used under normal fetal conditions. However, it can be used well in anomalies, especially when there is increased fluid. These anomalies may include ascites (Fig. 7.24), pleural effusion (Fig. 7.25A), megacystis, cystic kidneys, hydronephrosis (Fig. 7.25B), hydrocephaly (Fig. 7.26), or brain anomalies in early gestation (Fig. 7.27).

Systole

Diastole

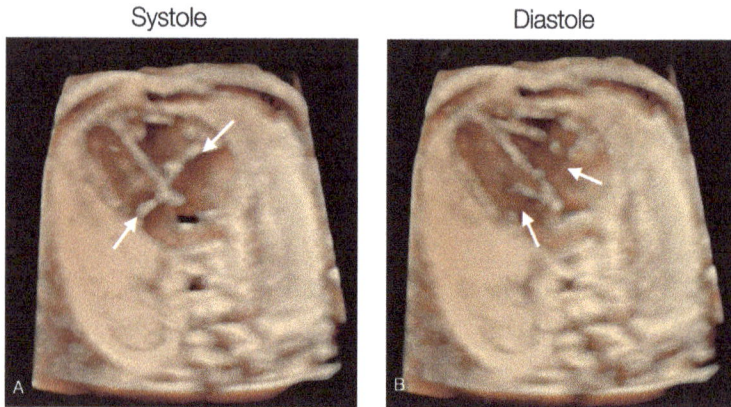

Fig. 7.22: STIC volume acquisition of a heart, looking into the ventricles in surface mode; in (A) during systole with atrioventricular valves closed (horizontal arrows) and in (B) during diastole with valves open (vertical arrows).

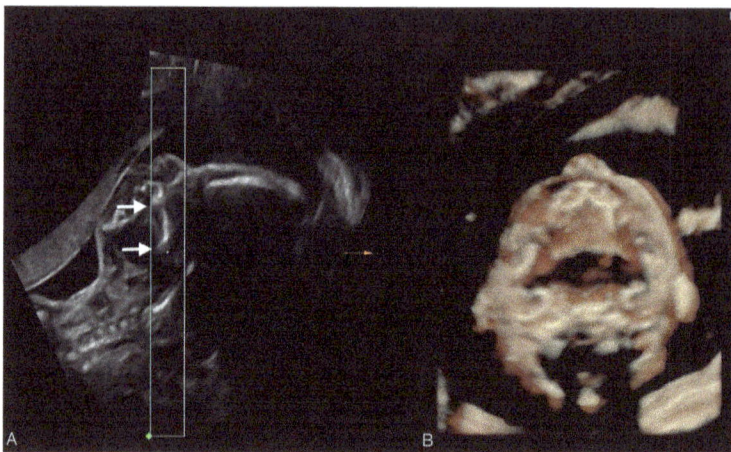

Fig. 7.23: The surface mode can be used to visualize structures hidden in the body, as shown here for the maxilla (B). The render line in (A) is in the mouth with a direct view of the upper jaw (arrows).

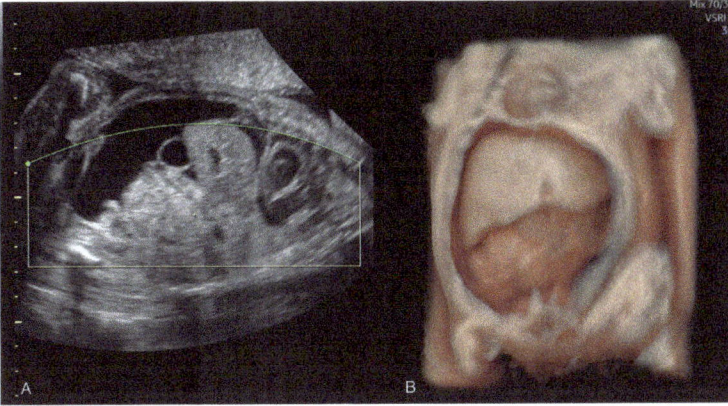

Fig. 7.24: Ascites shown in 3D surface mode, looking into the ascites at the liver and intestines. Note the position of the green projection line in the ascites in (A). Image B is reminiscent of a "virtual laparoscopy".

Pleural effusion   Hydronephrosis

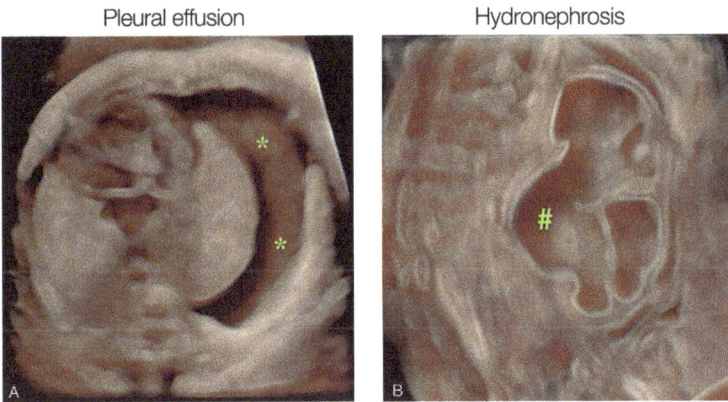

Fig. 7.25: Surface mode in two fetuses with malformations. (A) shows an axial view at the level of the thorax in a fetus with right pleural effusion (*); (B) shows a coronal view in a fetus with hydronephrosis (#).

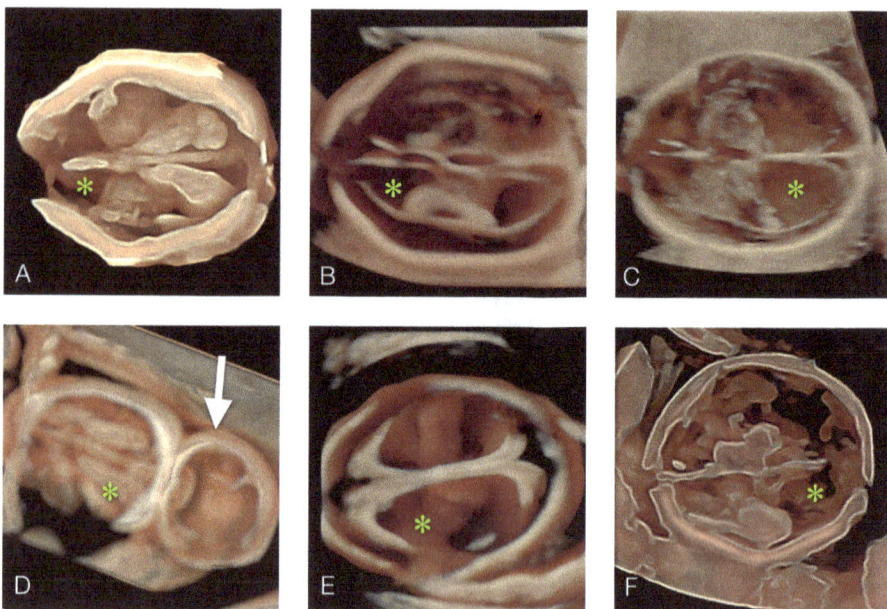

Fig. 7.26: Fetuses with ventriculomegaly of different etiologies between 16 and 22 weeks of gestation. The 3D surface mode is used to show the dilated lateral ventricles (*). Note how the surface mode is used here to see the interior of the brain and ventricular system. The fetus in (D) has a cephalocele (arrow).

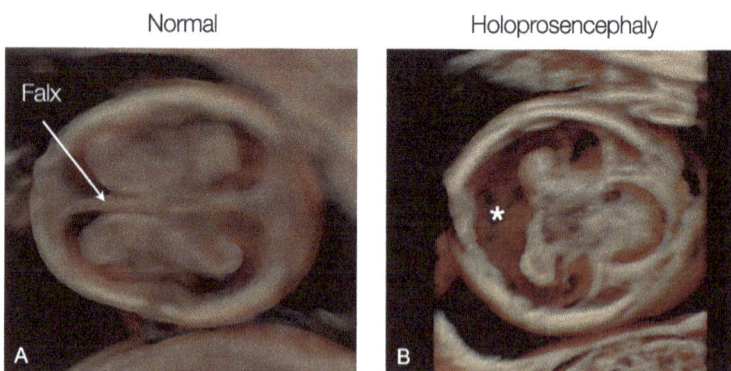

Fig. 7.27: Transvaginal 3D acquisition transventricular view in surface mode at 13 weeks' gestation, showing in (A) a fetus with normal anatomy in which the falx cerebri (arrow) separates both cerebral cavities, and in (B) a fetus with holoprosencephaly with fused lateral ventricles (*).

7.4 Conclusions

The 3D surface mode is the most used rendering mode in 3D ultrasound along with tomography display. Therefore, it is helpful for the examiner to learn how to use the various surface rendering tools. Documentation of normal body surface findings is becoming increasingly important to complete a 2D assessment of a fetus. In the case of fetal anomalies, surface mode can quickly provide a more complete picture of the findings, making them more understandable to patients and colleagues. In addition, combining it with some silhouette tools, as discussed in Chapter 11, can be very beneficial.

8 The Maximum Mode

8.1 Principle

Maximum mode has been introduced for the spatial visualization of hyperechogenic structures such as the fetal bones. In this transparency mode, all hyperechogenic structures within the render box are highlighted and displayed in a projection. In the upper panel of Figure 8.1A, we see the face of a fetus rendered with the surface mode; after activating the maximum mode (Fig. 8.1B), the skin is no longer visible and only the hyperechogenic signals of the facial bones are displayed. In recent years, the newly introduced silhouette mode has been combined with additional functions that now also en-

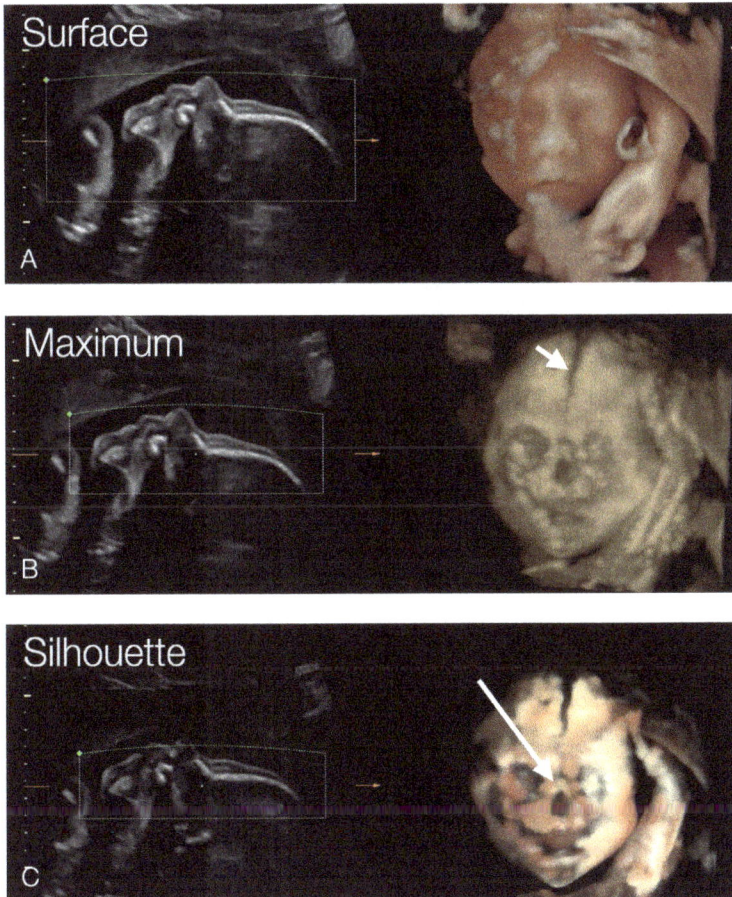

Fig. 8.1: 3D volume of a face in surface mode (A), after switching to maximum mode (B), or by selecting silhouette mode (C) with increased silhouette threshold. In panels B and C, the different facial bones can be seen, including the metopic suture (short arrow), the two orbits, the nasal bones (long arrow), the upper and lower jaw.

https://doi.org/10.1515/9783111249513-008

able the display of bony structures, as shown in Figure 8.1C. Many bones such as vertebrae, ribs, skull bones, and other curved bones cannot be properly visualized in a single 2D plane so that the main advantage of the maximum or silhouette modes is the ability to show a projection of the bones in a 3D volume data set. Figures 8.2 to 8.4 show examples of the use of surface mode in comparison with maximum and silhouette mode for bones.

Surface Mode   Maximum Mode

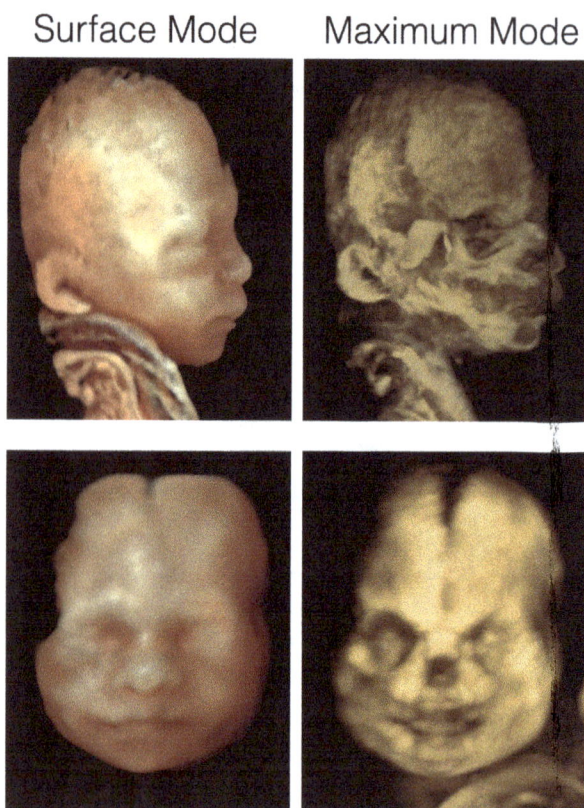

Fig. 8.2: 3D volume of two faces from the side (upper panel) and from the front (bottom panel). The images on the left are displayed in surface mode, while the images on the right were obtained after switching to maximum mode. When displayed in maximum mode, the different facial bones are well recognized.

Surface Mode Maximum Mode Silhouette Mode

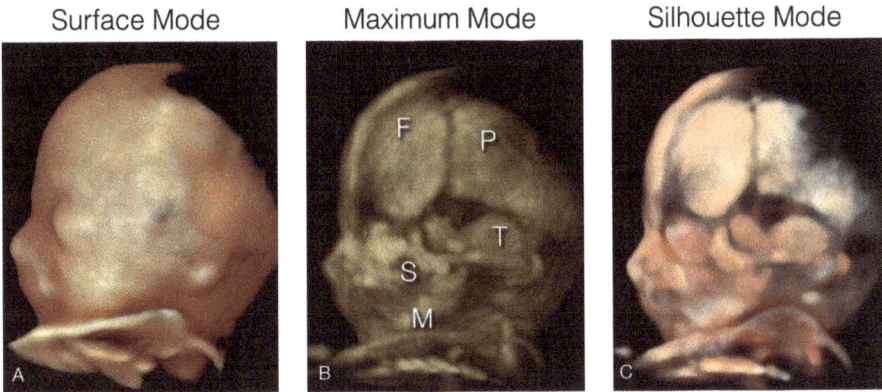

Fig. 8.3: Lateral view of head and face with 3D display in surface mode (A), maximum mode (B) and silhouette mode (C). Note that the skull bones are well recognized in this lateral insonation, such as the frontal bone (F), the parietal bone (P), the sphenoid bone (S), the temporal bone (T), and the mandible (M).

Surface Mode Maximum Mode Silhouette Mode

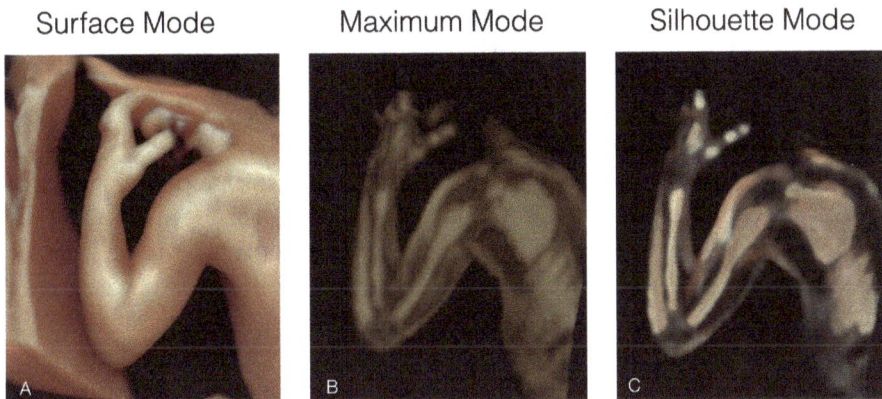

Fig. 8.4: Demonstration of an arm in surface mode (A), maximum mode (B) and silhouette mode (C). For this purpose, the box has been reduced in size to include only the arm with the result that the structures behind the arm cannot be seen.

8.2 Practical approach

When recording a volume, care should be taken to ensure that the volume is large enough to cover the entire area of interest. A better result is obtained if 2D image gain is reduced and contrast is increased during volume acquisition so that the bones appear "light" and the surrounding tissue appears "dark" (Fig. 8.5). In the third trimester, fetal skin shows an increased echogenicity and often overlays information from the bony structures. In our experience, therefore, the maximum mode is best performed between 15 and 25 weeks of gestation so that the bones are clearly visible.

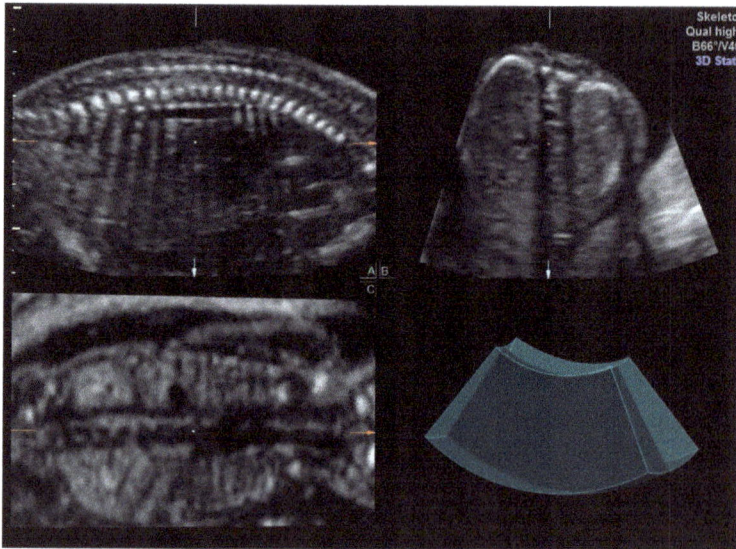

Fig. 8.5: Typical volume acquisition of a spine with ribs to be displayed in maximum mode, but here first in the orthogonal view. Note that the 2D image is rather dark with increased contrast to better highlight the bones and reduced signals from the skin and surrounding tissue.

Once the 2D image preset is adjusted, an acquisition box large enough to include the area of interest is selected (Fig. 8.5). In general, it is better to use a shallow box depth if only the superficial bones are included with very little information from the adjacent tissue or skin (Figs. 8.6 and 8.7). The resolution of the 3D volume ("low", "mid1" to "max") depends on the duration of the volume acquisition, as shown in Figure 8.8. The maximum mode is used not only in static 3D and 4D volume acquisition (Fig. 8.8), but also in VCI-Omniview (Figs. 8.9, 8.10); in all these cases a slice thickness of 15 to 20 mm is recommended. Generally, a maximum mode level of 100% is selected, but occasionally a mixture of maximum and surface modes (80%/20%) with an increased threshold may provide a better image. Figure 8.11 shows the use of VCI in maximum mode for highlighting the hard palate in orthogonal mode. Figure 8.12. shows demonstration of different regions of the skeleton by using silhouette mode for bones.

An interesting instrument is also the examination with VCI-A (see Chapter 4 and Chapter 14) in combination with the maximum mode: the 4D examination, which is ideally performed with a matrix probe, allows visualization of the bones of interest in a slice thickness of 10–20 mm (see Chapter 14).

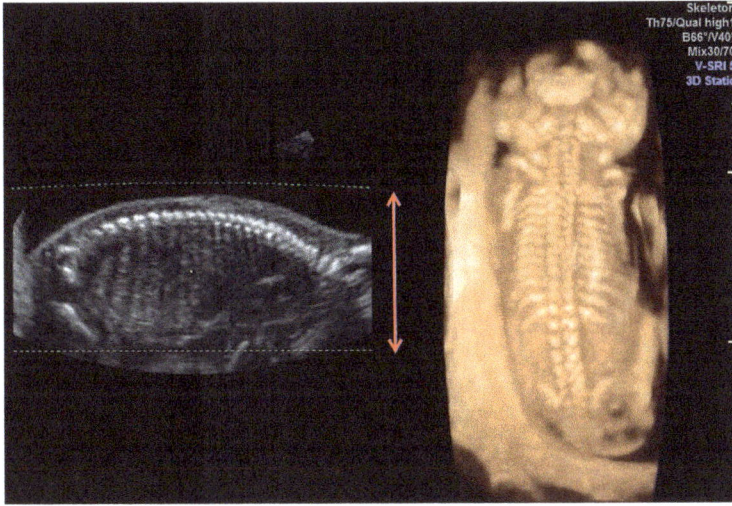

Fig. 8.6: In this example, the volume box is still very large (double arrow). In such a case, all signals inside the box are calculated, whereas only the information of the bone structures is needed. A better result can be achieved with a narrow box, as shown in Figure 8.7.

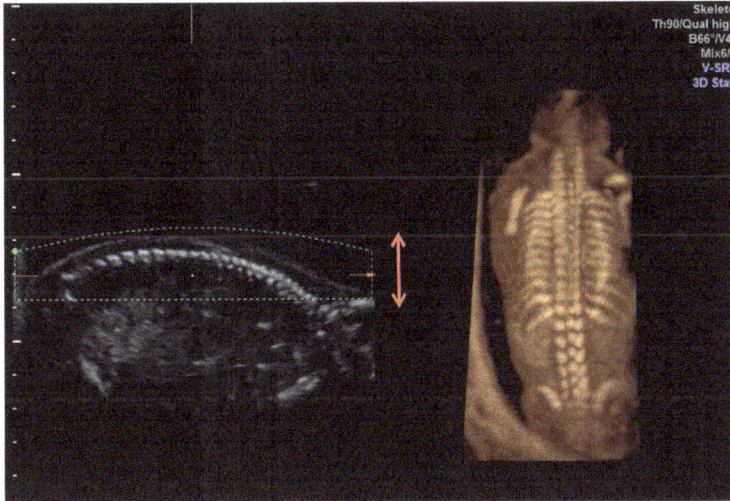

Fig. 8.7: Compared to Figure 8.6, the volume box has been reduced in depth (double arrow) to include mainly the bony structures. The 3D image then shows more details.

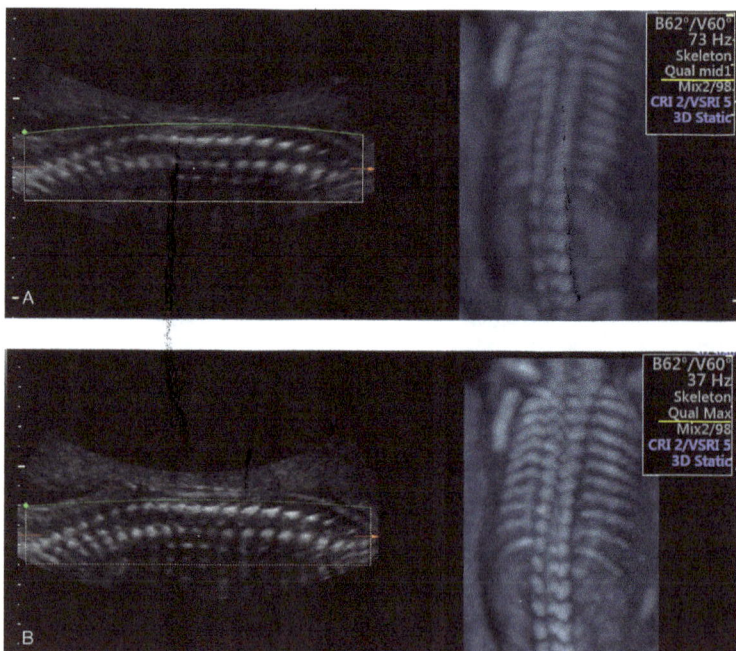

Fig. 8.8: 3D acquisition of a spine in two different resolutions with maximum mode rendering. In (A) the acquisition was taken with quality "mid1" and in (B) with quality "max". The difference in the resolutions is clearly visible in the 3D images.

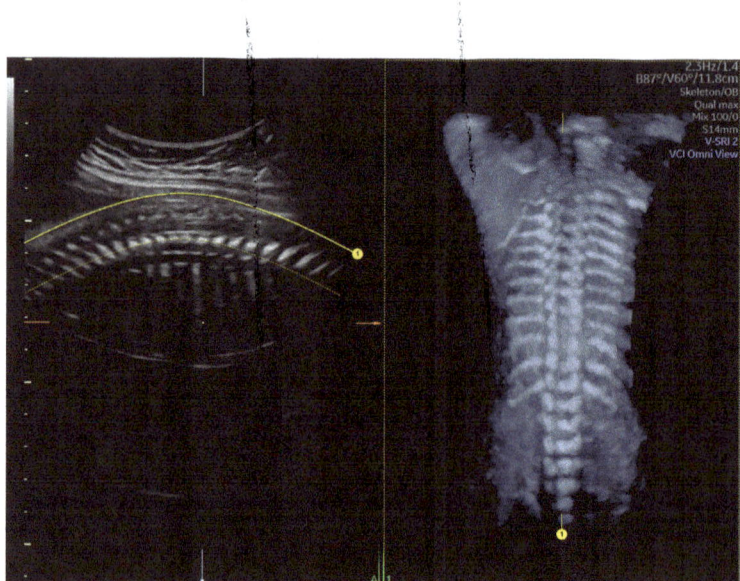

Fig. 8.9: Using VCI and the Omniview tool as VCI-Omniview during a 4D examination. The Omniview line was placed as a curved line along the spine with a slice thickness of 17 mm and the maximum mode was selected.

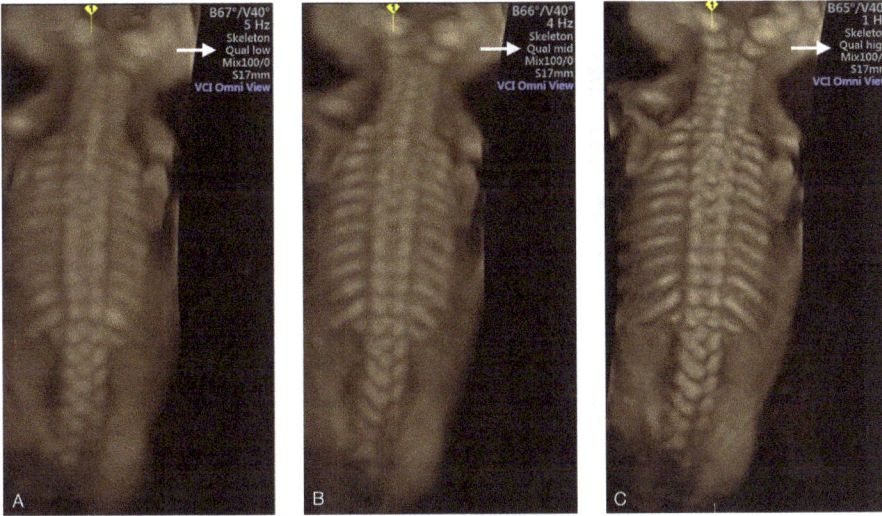

Fig. 8.10: During a 4D examination, the spine was displayed with VCI-Omniview as shown in Figure 8.9. Panels A, B and C show the difference in resolution depending on the acquisition quality. In (A) the volume acquisition quality was chosen "low", in (B) "medium" and in (C) "high".

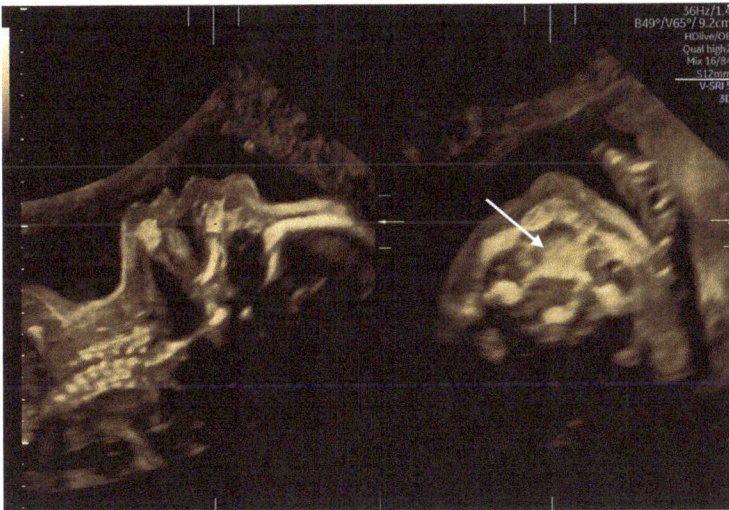

Fig. 8.11: Representation of the hard palate (arrow) in an orthogonal 3D view with a VCI thickness of 12 mm and maximum mode rendering to highlight the bones.

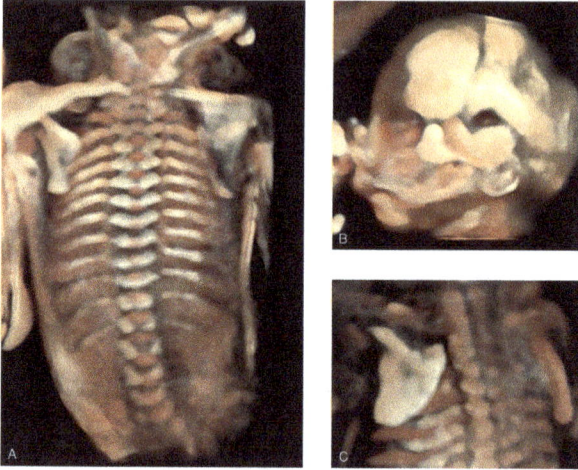

Fig. 8.12: Skeletal system with spine and ribs (A), cranial bones (B), and scapula (C) rendered with the surface mode and the silhouette tool with increased threshold. This approach can be used as a good alternative to the transparency maximum mode.

8.3 Typical applications for bones' visualization

In the following, some clinical aspects are briefly presented. Abnormal cases are demonstrated in Chapter 17 on the fetal skeleton and face.

Visualization of the spine and ribs: A dorsal view with a narrow 3D/4D box over the spine or with VCI-Omniview as a straight or curved line is ideal (Figs. 8.6–8.10, 8.12A). Figure 8.13 shows ribs at 13, 16, and 21 weeks of gestation, and Figure 8.14 shows a dorsal and lateral view of the spine. In this view, the shape of the spine and the symmetry of the vertebral bodies are easily seen, a view ideal for demonstrating spina bifida, hemivertebrae, kyphoscoliosis, rib count, and others (Fig. 8.15). See also Chapter 17.

Frontal view of the face: Acquiring a facial volume from the front allows visualization of the bony face (Figs. 8.1, 8.16, 8.17) showing frontal bones with the metopic suture, orbits with the nasal bones, maxilla, and mandible. Absent nasal bones (Fig. 8.17), abnormal metopic suture, facial clefts, and abnormal orbital sizes are the main areas of interest (see Chapter 17).

Cranial bones and sutures: The maximal mode is ideal for visualizing the curved shape of the cranial bones with sutures and fontanelles (Figs. 8.18, 8.19). This approach is also excellent for visualizing wide sutures, abnormal ossifications, and prematurely closed sutures in craniosynostosis. A special examination technique is real-time 4D with VCI-A for bones, which is ideal for cranial sutures (see Chapter 14).

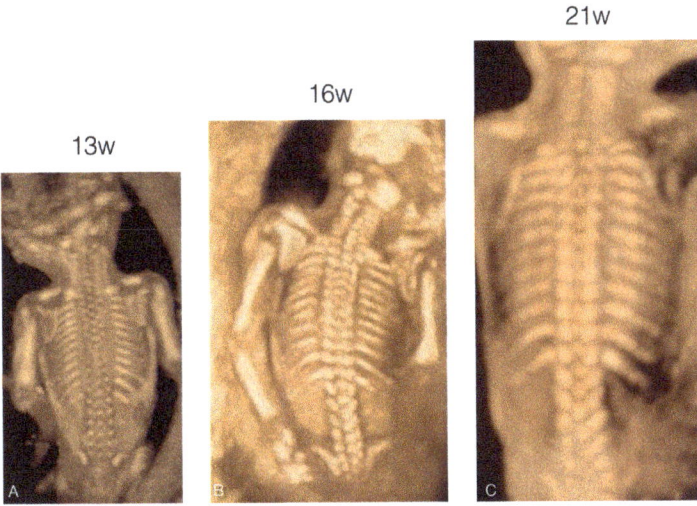

Fig. 8.13: Fetal spine and ribs in a fetus at 13 weeks (A), 16 weeks (B) and 21 weeks (C). Note the increasing ossification of the spine and ribs as gestation progresses.

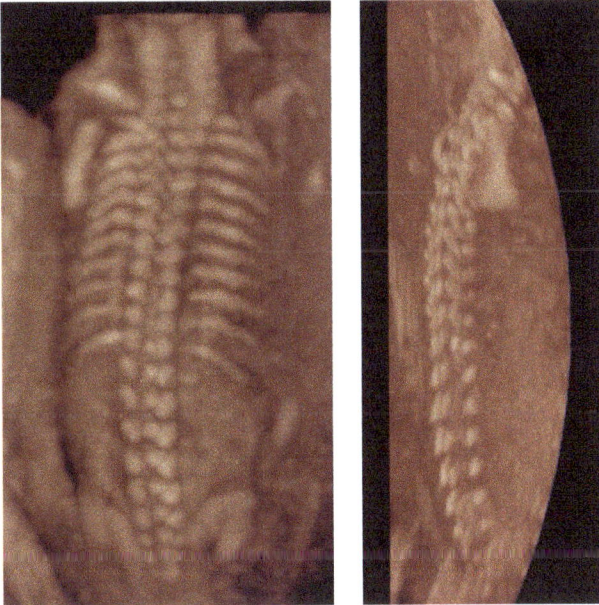

Fig. 8.14: Spine viewed from dorsal (left) and lateral (right) in maximum mode.

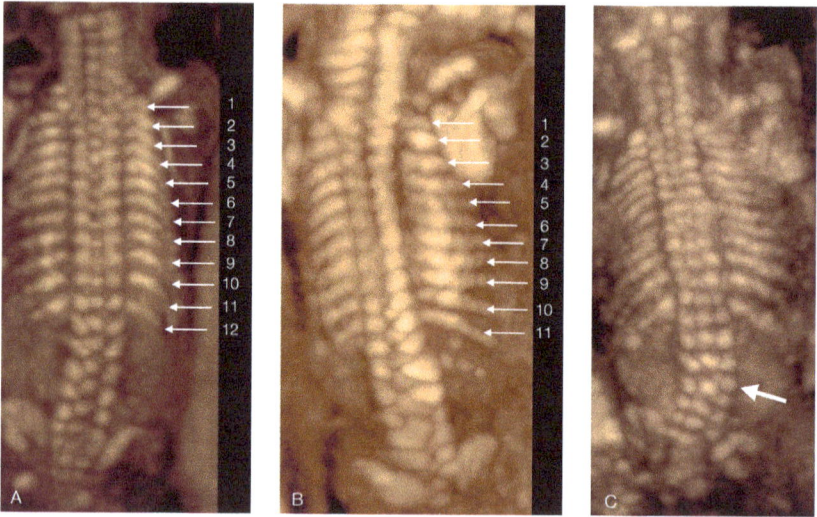

Fig. 8.15: Rib number and vertebral bodies under normal and abnormal conditions. In (A), 12 pairs of ribs are typically clearly visible, while the fetus in (B) has only 11 pairs of ribs and the fetus in (C) has a hemivertebra (arrow) with a kink in the lumbar spine.

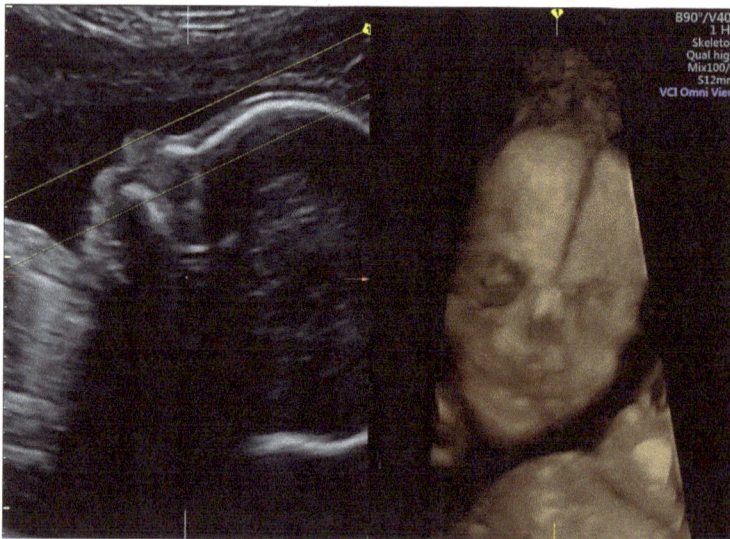

Fig. 8.16: During a 4D examination, the face was imaged using VCI-Omniview with a slice thickness of 16 mm and maximum imaging. The fetal face shows the details already shown in Figure 8.1.

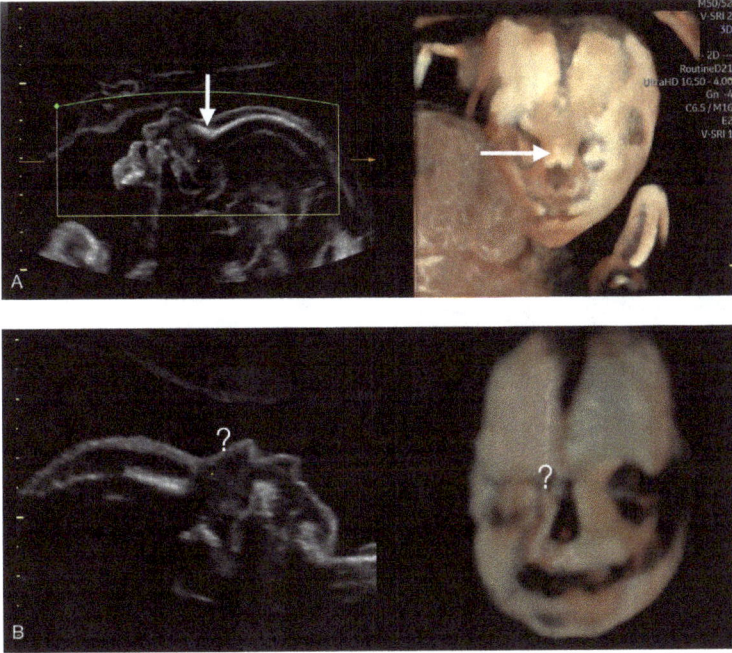

Fig. 8.17: Two fetuses with present ossification (A) and absent ossification (B) of the nasal bone shown in 2D (left images) and in 3D silhouette mode (right images). The nasal bone is clearly visible in (A) (arrow) and absent in (B) (?).

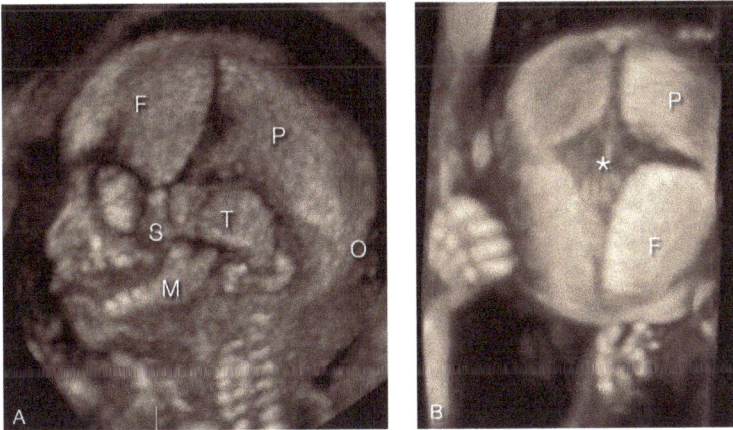

Fig. 8.18: In panel A, the skull bones are well visualized with a lateral insonation in maximum mode, recognizing the following bones: Frontal bone (F), Parietal bone (P), Sphenoid bone (S), Temporal bone (T) and Occipital bone (O), and the Mandible (M). In panel B, the 3D volume with maximum mode shows a top view of the head with the anterior fontanel (*).

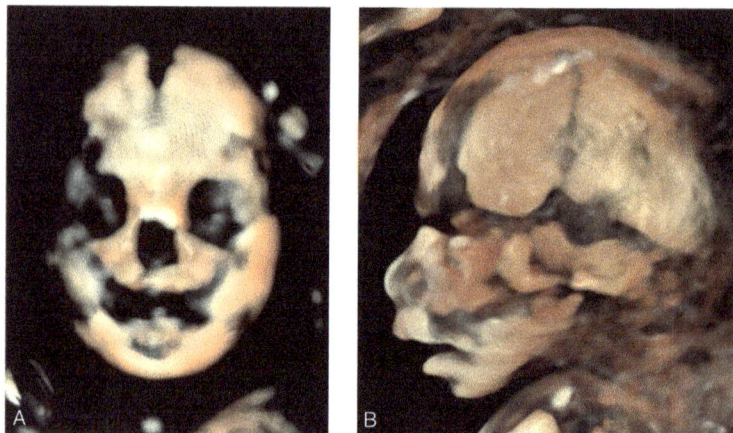

Fig. 8.19: In these two fetuses, the face (A) and the cranial bones (B) are well visualized with the silhouette mode, showing that this can be a good alternative to using the maximum mode.

Visualization of the long bones and limbs: The long bones of arms and legs as well as hands and feet can be clearly seen in maximum and silhouette modes (Fig. 8.4) (see Chapter 17). The 3D visualization is ideal when the long bones are horizontal with an almost vertical insonation. Bones' size, shape and proportions, skeletal anomalies, club-feet, and anomalies of the hands and feet are important regions of interest.

Visualization of the fetus in the first trimester: Interest in fetal skeletal anatomy in early pregnancy has increased in recent years along with the increase in image resolution. In addition to visualizing the developing spine and ribs, the limbs and the cranial bones can also be examined well, depending on the question of interest. For this purpose we use more often the silhouette mode (Figs. 8.20, 8.21).

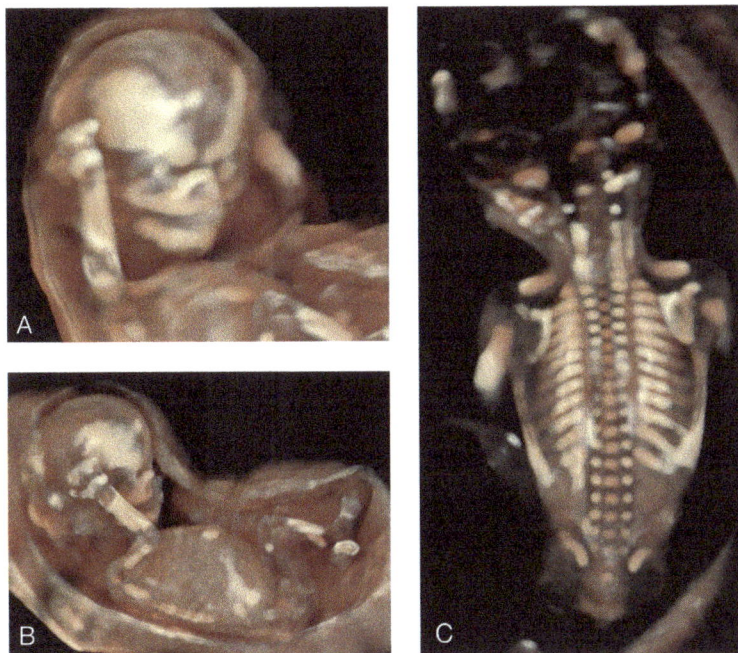

Fig. 8.20: Visualization of the bones of the fetus in the first trimester, shown here at 12 weeks (A and B) and 13 weeks of gestation (C); they may include the spine, ribs, limbs, facial and cranial bones. Note that ossification progresses rapidly between the first and second trimester.

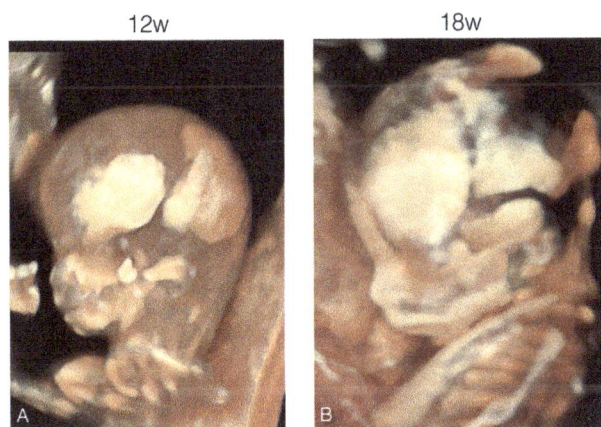

Fig. 8.21: Development of the skull bones between 12 weeks (A) and 18 weeks of gestation (B), visualized with silhouette mode for bones.

8.4 Conclusions

Maximum mode and silhouette mode for bones are the ideal 3D tools for visualizing the different parts of the fetal skeleton. It is easiest to start with a static 3D visualization of the fetal spine and long bones. The best results are obtained with a vertical insonation of the horizontal bones. A thin slice in the static 3D view or in the VCI-Omniview view allows selection of the region of interest. Chapter 17 discusses some 3D skeletal anomalies in more detail.

9 The Minimum Mode

9.1 Principle

Fluid-filled structures are easily seen on ultrasound because they are echolucent and have a clear delineation from adjacent organs. Minimum mode is a transparency mode with the ability to display information within the volume box by highlighting hypo- or anechoic structures. However, this advantage is limited when amniotic fluid or bone shadows are selected in the volume box. In recent years, the use of minimum mode has decreased and has been replaced first by other tools, such as inversion mode (see Chapter 10), and more recently by the various features of silhouette mode (Chapter 11).

From a clinical point of view, the most important aspects for which we use the minimum mode are the increased fluid accumulation in the thoracic and abdominal organs, especially the kidneys and urinary tract, but also the visualization of cerebral vesicles, cerebral ventricles, and the nuchal translucency in early stages of pregnancy. In addition, the heart, great vessels, and vasculature provide good structures to use with the minimum mode.

9.2 Practical approach

Prior to volume acquisition, the 2D image should be carefully prepared by optimizing the contrast so that the fluid is seen as "smooth black" without artifacts or speckles (Fig. 9.1). Ideally, the volume is acquired from a perspective with as little shadowing by the bones as possible since the shadows will affect the rendered image in the same way as the fluid. When rendering a volume with the minimum mode, the examiner should choose a flat volume box that primarily contains only the organs of interest and very little information from the adjacent tissue (compare Figures 9.1 and 9.2). Within the box, the presence of amniotic fluid should be avoided because it casts a large black shadow (Fig. 9.1). In other words, the anterior and posterior lines of the volume box should be ideally placed in the tissue and not in the amniotic fluid (Fig. 9.2).

A good result is often obtained with a "minimum mode" in combination with an "X-Ray mode" (80%/20% mix). However, the "gray threshold" should be increased and, in some cases, post-processing by changing contrast and gain can improve the image result. Rotation along the vertical Y-axis often leads to a better 3D effect in the region of interest (Figs. 9.3A, 9.3B).

https://doi.org/10.1515/9783111249513-009

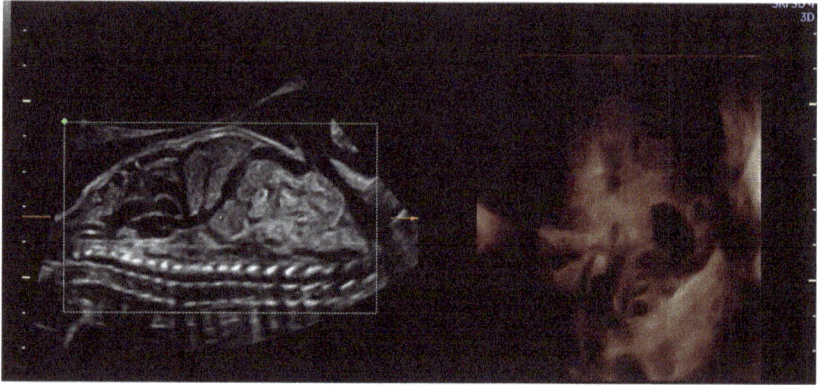

Fig. 9.1: The render box was placed over the fetal abdomen and minimum mode was activated. The box is deep and contains amniotic fluid, which is why the result appears almost black and no structures can be seen (see Fig. 9.2).

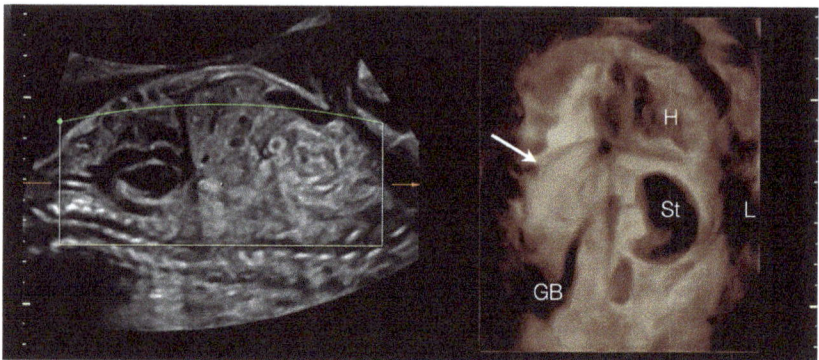

Fig. 9.2: The render box shown in Figure 9.1 is now less deep and no longer contains amniotic fluid in the volume field. The contours of the thorax and abdomen can be seen better and the hypoechoic organs such as the heart (H), stomach (St) and gallbladder (GB) can be identified clearly.

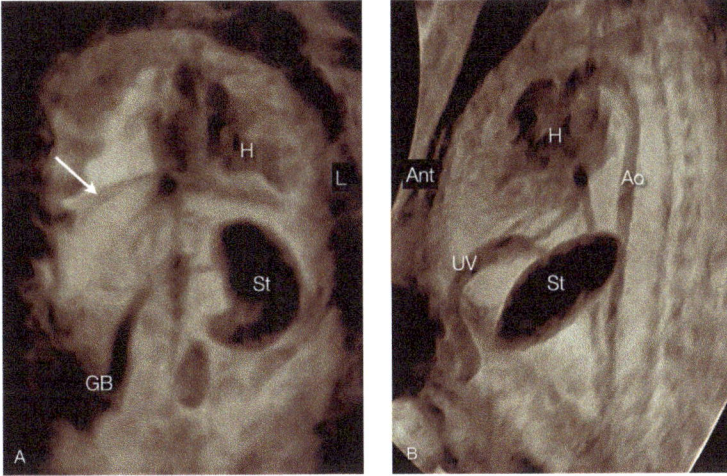

Fig. 9.3: Thorax and abdomen in 3D minimum mode in antero-posterior (A) and lateral projection (B). In both views, typical structures such as the stomach (St), gallbladder (GB), heart position (H), diaphragm (arrow), umbilical vein (UV) and descending aorta (Ao) are well identified. Note the use of this 3D tool to visualize the normal situs with stomach and heart on the left side of the body. Compare with Figure 9.4; left (L), anterior (Ant).

9.3 Typical applications of the minimum mode

Typical structures that are rendered with minimum mode in the normal fetus are the echolucent organs such as the urinary bladder, stomach, gallbladder (Fig. 9.4), umbilical and portal veins, the heart with the great vessels, and the intracerebral ventricular system. Because some fetal anomalies are often associated with increased fluid accumulation, these can be clearly visualized with minimum mode. However, we must admit that border and shape discrimination is better provided by the other tools, especially inversion or silhouette modes (see Chapter 10 and Chapter 11).

Intra-abdominal organs with blood vessels: One of the typical approaches that can be easily combined with the minimum mode is to image the abdomen and thorax from the front (Fig. 9.3). The 3D view is then either a frontal or lateral insonation with the projection of the situs with stomach, heart, diaphragm, but also the umbilical vein with gallbladder, inferior vena cava, and descending aorta. In this view, the situs inversus or ambiguous is clearly visible (Figs. 9.5A, 9.5B). In the lateral view, an abnormal course of the umbilical vein in agenesis or an atypical course of the ductus venosus can be easily distinguished from a normal finding. The absence of stomach filling or, better, a dilated stomach, as observed in the double bubble sign (Fig. 9.6), can be well documented.

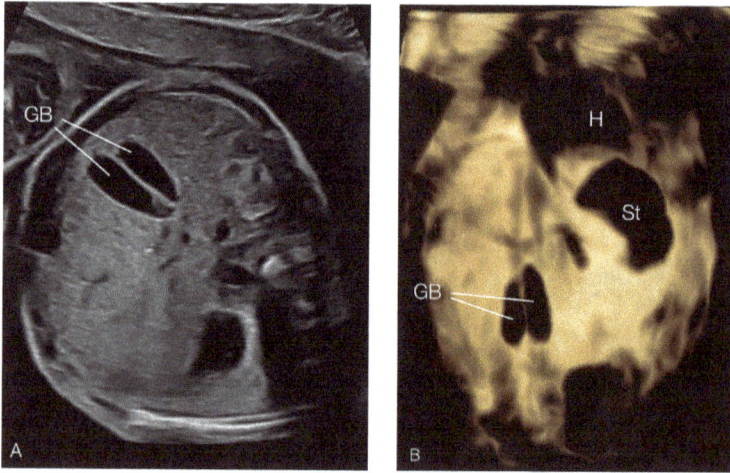

Fig. 9.4: Fetus with a gallbladder duplication (GB) in 2D (A) and in 3D minimum mode projection (B). Heart (H), stomach (St).

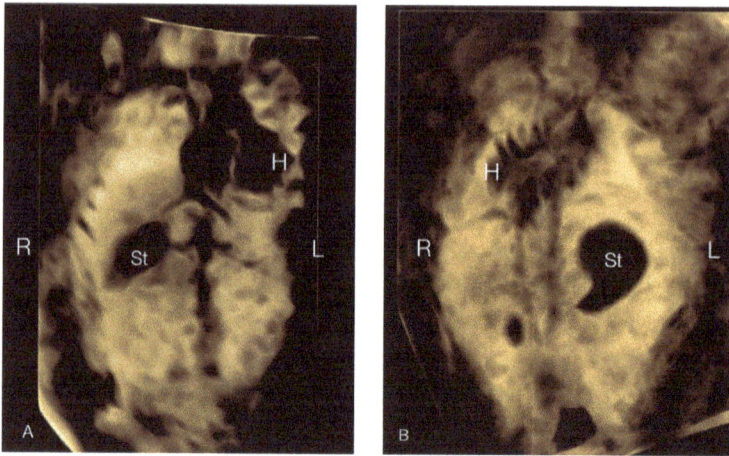

Fig. 9.5: Thorax and abdomen in 3D minimum mode in antero-posterior projection in two fetuses with partial situs inversus. In (A), the stomach (St) is on the right side of the body (R) and the heart (H) is on the left side (L). In (B), the heart is on the right side and the stomach is on the left side.

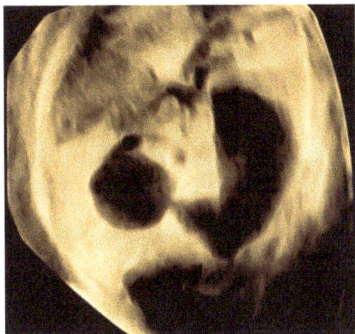

Fig. 9.6: Stomach in duodenal atresia with double bubble sign in 3D minimum mode.

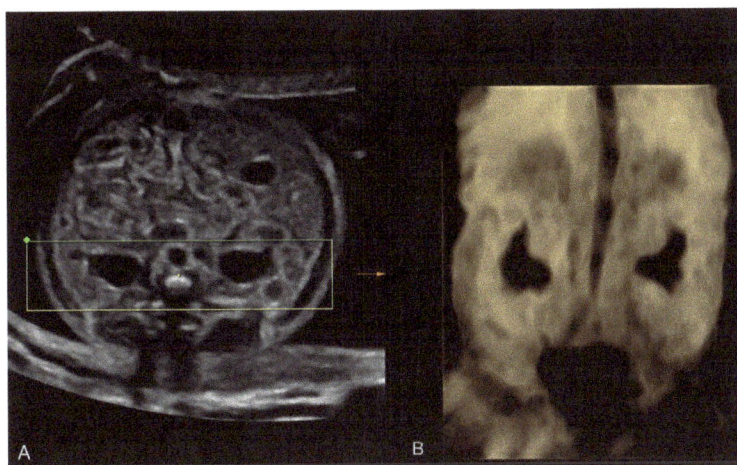

Fig. 9.7: Bilateral mild pyelectasia in axial view in 2D (left) and in minimum mode in coronal projection (right).

Other abnormal conditions in the abdomen with increased fluid volume include the presence of megacystis, pyelectasia (Fig. 9.7), hydronephrosis (Fig. 9.8) with or without dilated ureter (see Chapter 18), multicystic renal dysplasia (Fig. 9.9), and others. However, fetal ascites is better visualized in surface mode or in combination with silhouette mode.

Thorax with heart and great vessels: A frontal acquisition of the thoracic cavity with minimum mode display shows the shape of the heart with the crossing of the vessels as well as the two slightly echogenic lungs and the dark border of the diaphragm (Fig. 9.3). A lateral view allows visualization of the crossing of the great vessels with the aortic arch (Fig. 9.10A).

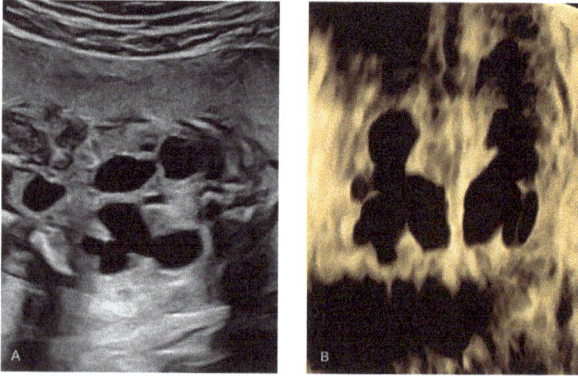

Fig. 9.8: Fetus with moderate bilateral hydronephrosis in 2D (A) and in 3D minimum mode (B).

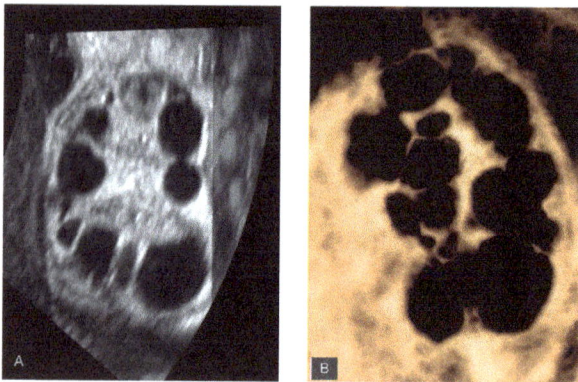

Fig. 9.9: Multicystic kidney dysplasia with multiple cysts of different sizes in 2D (A) and in 3D minimum mode (B).

Normal   TGA

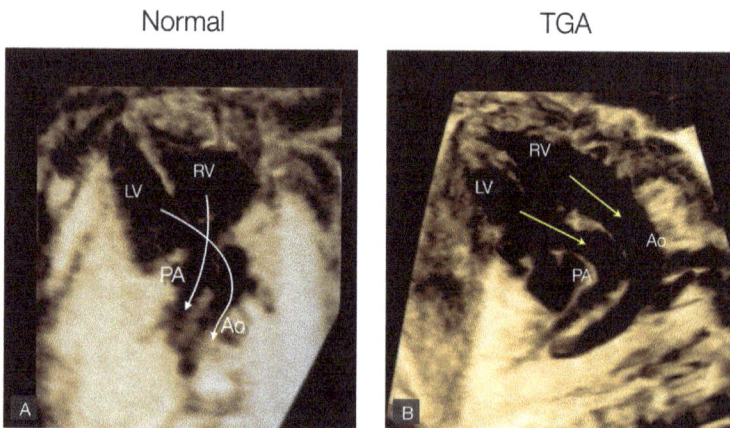

Fig. 9.10: STIC volumes in minimum-transparent mode in two fetuses: one with a normal heart (A) and the other with a transposition of the great arteries (TGA) (B). Note the crossing of the great vessels in (A) compared with the parallel course of the vessels in (B). Aorta (Ao), left ventricle (LV), pulmonary artery (PA), right ventricle (RV).

Abnormal findings, such as lung cysts, hydrothorax (Fig. 9.11), and the location of the stomach in diaphragmatic hernia can be clearly observed and identified with this rendering mode. Cardiac defects, however, are more difficult to visualize unless the size or course of the great vessels is involved (Fig. 9.10). For this purpose, we generally prefer to use the inversion mode or glass-body mode.

Intracerebral ventricular system: The fluid-filled ventricular system can also be visualized well with the minimum mode (Fig. 9.12). However, a major limitation of this

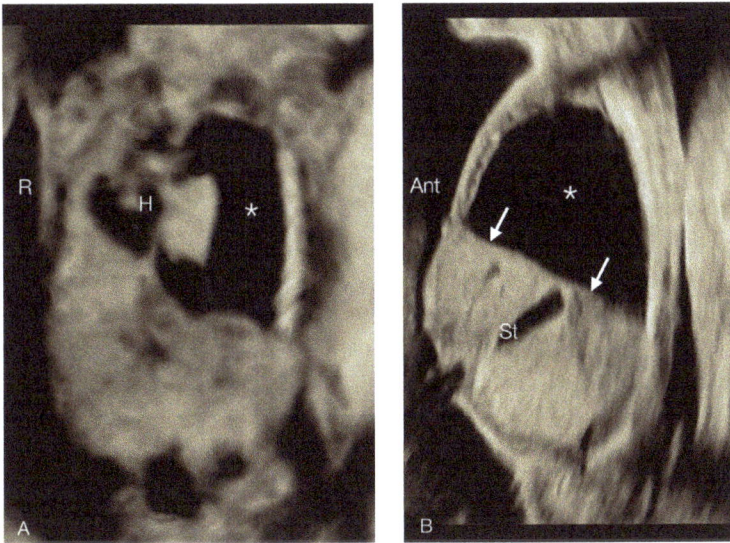

Fig. 9.11: Fetus with unilateral pleural effusion (*) in minimum mode. (A) shows the antero-posterior projection with the heart (H) displaced to the right (R). (B) shows a lateral projection at the level of the effusion, with the diaphragm (arrows) and stomach (St) clearly visible; anterior (Ant).

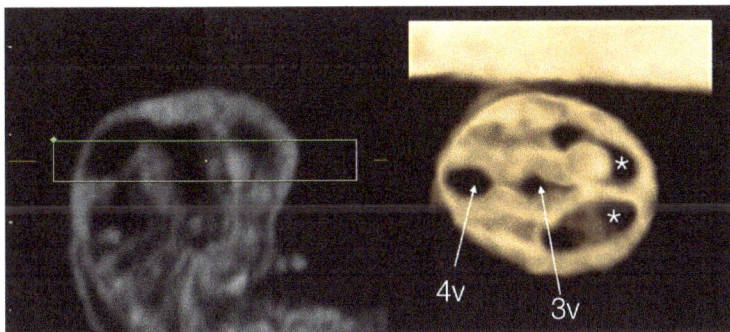

Fig. 9.12: Projection of the intracerebral ventricular system at 9 weeks' gestation. In minimum mode, both lateral ventricles (*) and the developing third ventricle (3v) and fourth ventricle (4v) can be readily identified.

application in the second and third trimesters is bone shadowing, so we recommend that the volume ideally be imaged through the fontanelle. Minimum mode can also be used in anomalies with increased fluid accumulation, as seen in ventriculomegaly, hydrocephaly, holoprosencephaly, absent septum pellucidum, and others. An interesting application is the visualization of the cerebral ventricles in early gestation (Fig. 9.12) before ten weeks of pregnancy. At this stage, the cranial bones are minimally ossified and the ventricles are adequately filled with fluid. A combination of minimum mode and X-Ray mode is appropriate to obtain a high-contrast image, as shown in Figure 9.12 This approach has also been replaced by the silhouette mode in recent years (see Chapter 11).

9.4 Conclusions

Minimum mode can be used as a projection that highlights the anechoic structures in a volume, like an X-Ray examination in radiology. Transparent structures and their neighboring organs can be clearly observed and identified, and abnormally increased fluid in the fetal body can be well visualized. Diagnoses such as hydronephrosis, hydrothorax, double bubble, cystic lesions, and hydrocephaly can be visualized with the minimum mode. Interestingly, hyperechoic lesions, as seen in hyperechogenic lungs or kidneys, can also be well highlighted compared to adjacent tissues. The two prerequisites for a good result are, first, the avoidance of bone shadows during acquisition and, second, the use of a narrow display field, especially to avoid the presence of amniotic fluid. In recent years, however, the minimum mode has been used less and less as a single mode as other transparent modes have been preferred.

10 The Inversion Mode

10.1 Principle

The inversion mode rendering discussed in this chapter is simply the inversion of the information provided by the echolucent (anechoic) structures so that they are represented echogenic instead of anechoic (Fig. 10.1). The term was introduced so as to differentiate it from the minimum mode (see Chapter 9) since this mode inverts areas with absent echo signals to solid structures (Fig. 10.1). The image resembles a 3D digital cast of the structures of interest, and spatial depth is better perceived in comparison to the minimum mode. In addition, most of the information about the surrounding tissue is blacked out. Unlike minimum mode, Magicut (see Chapter 3) can be applied to an inversion mode volume to remove artifacts around the region of interest. Previously, the color of inversion mode was primarily displayed in sepia, with limited post-processing light options, but the advent of HDlive has enabled the use of new tools such as surface softness, light source, and others. These are also presented and discussed in this chapter.

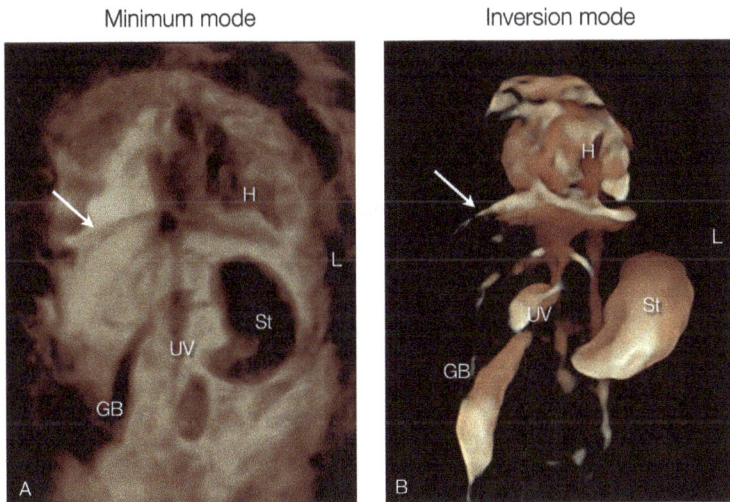

Fig. 10.1: Thorax and abdomen in 3D minimum mode in antero-posterior projection (A) and the same volume after activating and adjusting the inversion mode tool (B). In both views, typical structures, such as the stomach (St), gallbladder (GB), heart position (H), diaphragm (arrow), and umbilical vein (UV) are clearly visible.

https://doi.org/10.1515/9783111249513-010

10.2 Practical approach

During 3D volume acquisition, care should be taken to minimize ultrasound shadows (e. g., bone shadows), as shadows are falsely represented as echogenic information in inversion mode. Prior to volume acquisition, image contrast should be adjusted to allow for clear black/gray discrimination and better edge detection. The box size in inversion mode should ideally include the entire region to be imaged. For successful 3D image display, it is recommended to either know the different steps towards the result, or even better, to have a special pre-programmed preset for the inversion mode. The step by step procedure is explained below and in Figures 10.2 to 10.4.

After capturing a volume and selecting inversion mode, the image turns black and little information is displayed in inversion mode (Fig. 10.1). The size of the box must be adjusted to include the area of interest, and then the "gray threshold" level must be increased (level 70 or more) until the result of the inversion appears on the screen (Fig. 10.2). For some systems, the default inversion setting is "light" color, but the authors prefer to use "gradient light" or HDlive, which combines well with a surface mode. Magicut can be used to remove additional neighboring artifacts (see Chapter 3, Fig. 10.3), and the "Gain" and "Threshold" buttons can be used to enhance the image. A soft HDlive image is achieved by increasing the shadow value from 50 to 100 or more.

Step 1: Activate Inversion mode and choose HD-live smooth

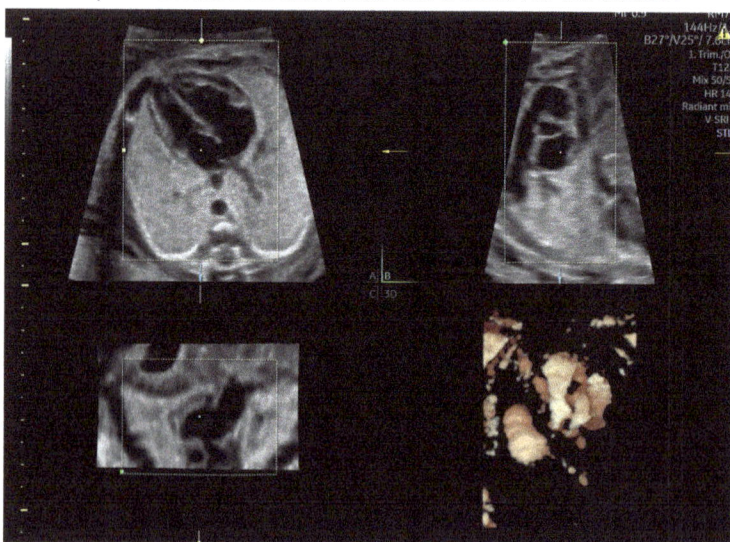

Fig. 10.2: The main steps for a 3D rendering in inversion mode using the example of a STIC volume of a heart. The render box is placed to cover the heart, the inversion mode is activated and HDlive smooth is selected (continued in Figure 10.3).

Step 2: Increase gray threshold

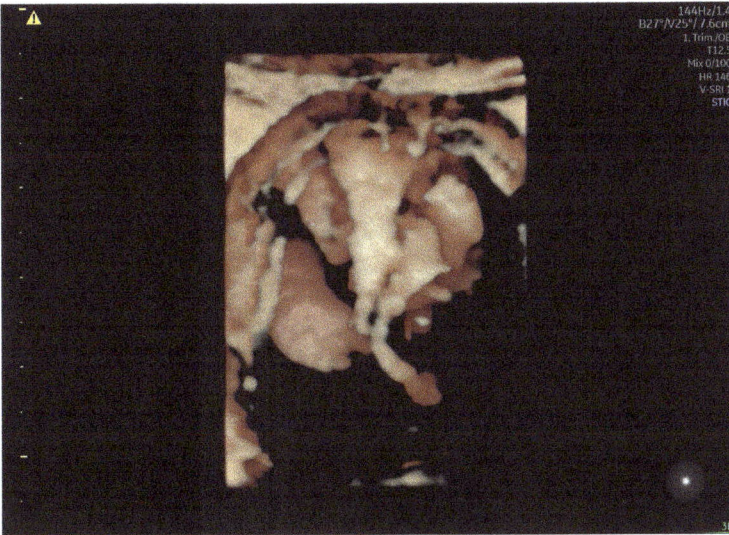

Fig. 10.3: In a second step, the gray threshold is increased from e. g., 20 to 60 and the gain is adjusted until the desired anatomical details are visible.

10.3 Typical applications of the inversion mode

There are many similarities between the use of the minimum mode and inversion mode in terms of the organs of interest.

Thorax and abdomen: In inversion mode, echolucent structures in the thorax and abdomen can be visualized under normal and abnormal conditions. Typical structures include the stomach (Fig. 10.5), urinary bladder, gallbladder (Fig. 10.6), and various large vessels in the thorax and abdomen (Figs. 10.4, 10.7).

Intracerebral structures: the fluid-filled intracerebral ventricular system can be visualized with the inversion mode, especially in the early embryonic period (Fig. 10.8). One of the major limitations of the inversion mode is that the surrounding structures cannot be visualized. However, the inversion mode is used clinically to study the embryology of brain development, particularly the ventricular system between 8 and 13 weeks of gestation (Fig. 10.8), and to demonstrate conditions such as holoprosencephaly in first and second trimester (Fig. 10.9). Later in pregnancy, the inversion mode can be used for conditions with increased fluid accumulation, such as ventriculomegaly and others which are best detected after transvaginal volume acquisition (Figs. 10.10, 10.11). In a recent study on the use of inversion mode on the fetal brain the scientists Chen and Li from China showed how to visualize the Sylvian fissure and gyrations in the distal hemisphere, an interesting approach with promising potential (Fig. 10.12).

Step 3: Remove artifacts with Magicut   Step 4: Adjust for your purpose

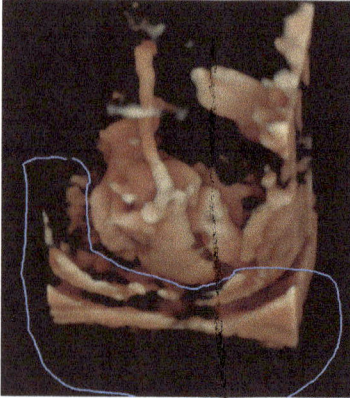

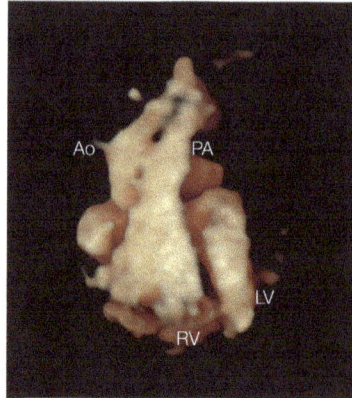

Fig. 10.4: In a third step, artifacts caused by ribs shadows and other disturbing structures are removed with the Magicut electronic scalpel. In step 4, the image is finalized by adjusting the threshold and gain and blurring the image by increasing the value of shadow function. Aorta (Ao), left ventricle (LV), pulmonary artery (PA), right ventricle (RV).

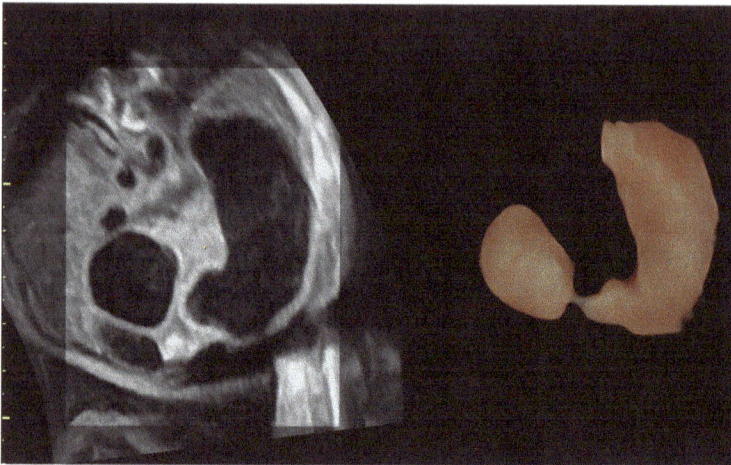

Fig. 10.5: Dilated stomach and duodenum in a fetus with duodenal atresia with the double bubble in 2D (left) and in inversion mode (right).

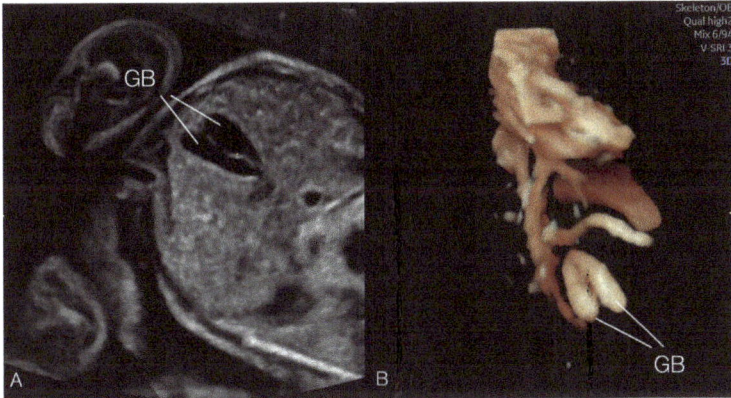

Fig. 10.6: Axial view of the abdomen with gallbladder (GB) duplication in 2D (A) and in inversion mode (B).

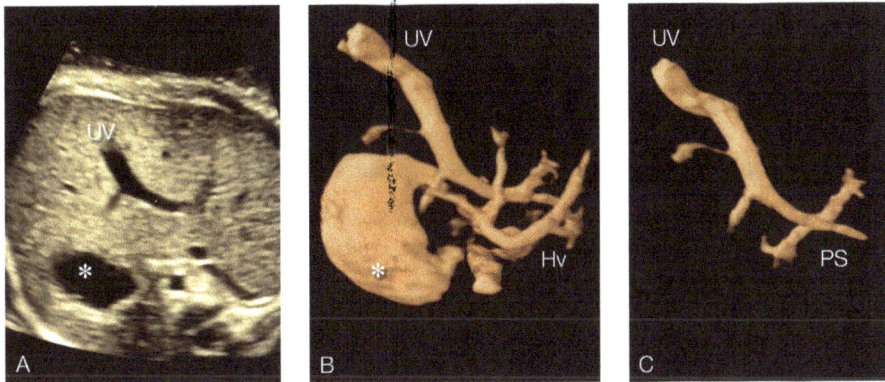

Fig. 10.7: Image A: 3D volume acquisition of an axial cross-section of the fetal abdomen at the level of the stomach (*) and liver in the 33rd week of gestation. Image B: the inversion mode view allows demonstration of the stomach (*), hepatic veins (Hv), and umbilical vein (UV) with the portal system. Image C: here, stomach and hepatic veins have been digitally removed and the umbilical vein can be seen with its connection to the portal sinus (PS).

Urogenital system: Abnormal renal findings associated with fluid accumulation can be clearly visualized with the inversion mode. Typical conditions include multicystic renal dysplasia (Fig. 10.12), hydronephrosis (Fig. 10.13), megacystis, and others. Further examples are shown in Chapter 18.

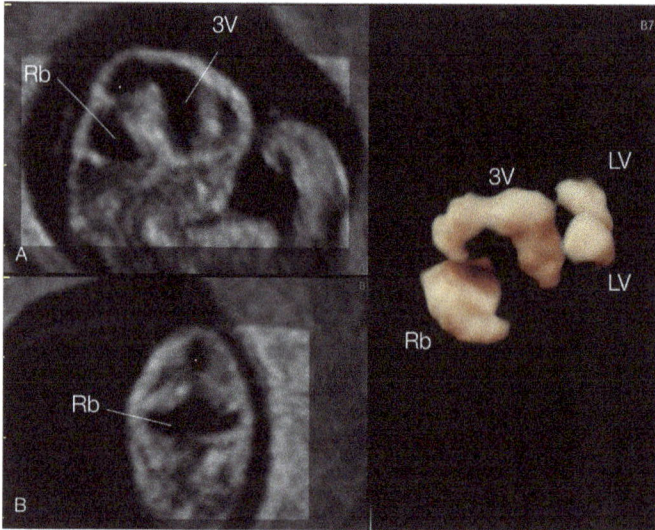

Fig. 10.8: The intracerebral ventricular system of a 9-week-old embryo shown in orthogonal mode (A and B) and inversion mode (C); lateral ventricle (LV), rhombencephalon (Rb), third ventricle (3V).

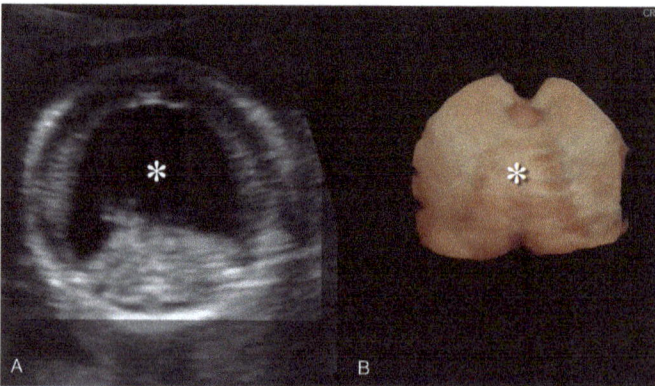

Fig. 10.9: Fetus with holoprosencephaly at 18 weeks of gestation in 2D (A) and in 3D inversion mode (B) showing the monoventricle (*).

Heart and great vessels: one of the main applications of the inversion mode is the heart and adjacent vessels, where spatial orientation can be clearly visualized (see Figs. 10.2–10.4). Inversion mode can be used in both static 3D and STIC (Fig. 10.14). In frontal view, a STIC volume can be displayed with good contrast to show the atria, ventricles and the crossing or the abnormal parallel course of the great vessels (Fig. 10.14).

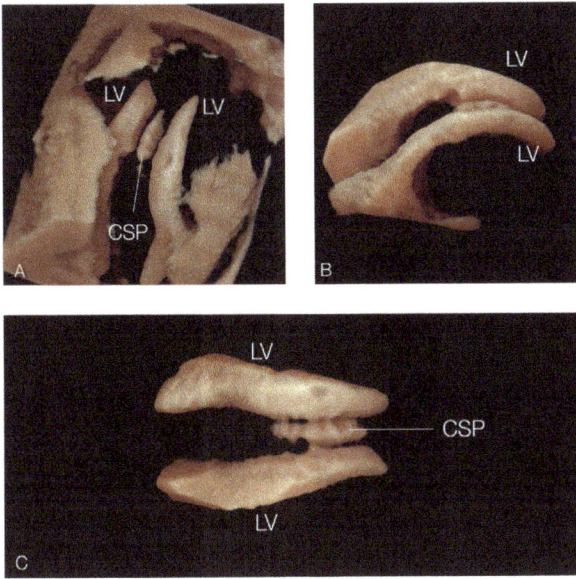

Fig. 10.10: Ventriculomegaly in a fetus at 25 weeks' gestation after transvaginal 3D volume acquisition and rendering in inversion mode. Image A: ventricular system is rendered with other adjacent information, mainly due to shadowing. Image B: after removal of artifacts with Magicut, only the two lateral ventricles (LV) are shown from lateral view. The cavum septi pellucidi (CSP) is shown from cranial view in (C).

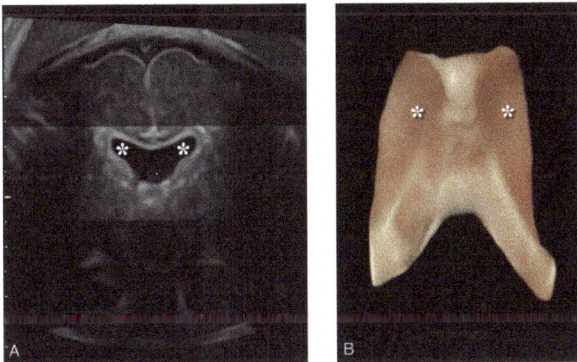

Fig. 10.11: Ventricular system of a fetus at 20 weeks with absent septum pellucidum after transvaginal 3D volume acquisition. Image A: in 2D, the two anterior horns (*) of the lateral ventricles are communicating due to the absence of the laminae of the septum pellucidum. Image B: after rendering in inversion mode and manipulation with Magicut, the ventricles communicating along the midline are clearly visible in the view from below.

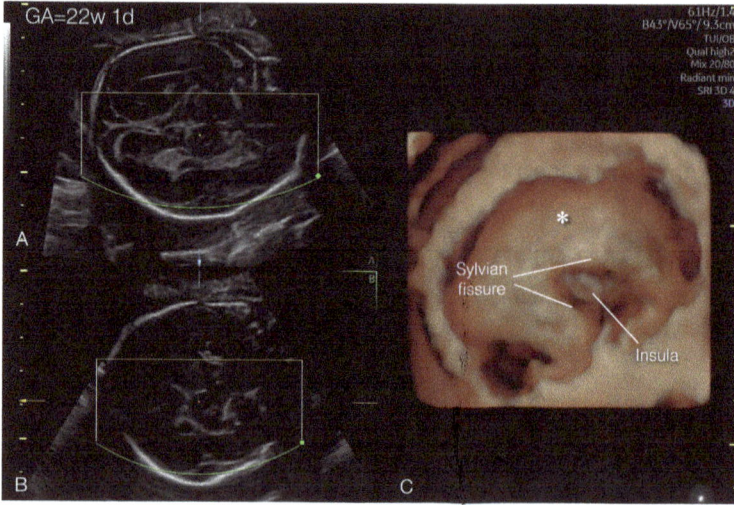

Fig. 10.12: Inversion mode of the convex surface of the distal cerebral hemispheres showing the cortex (*) smooth and the Sylvian fissure and insula. Compare also with Figure 16.26.

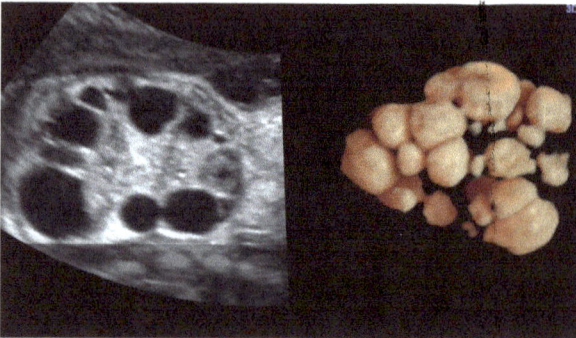

Fig. 10.13: Multicystic renal dysplasia in 2D (left) and in inversion mode (right). The individual cysts are easily seen in 2D but are spatially better visualized in 3D inversion mode with HDlive.

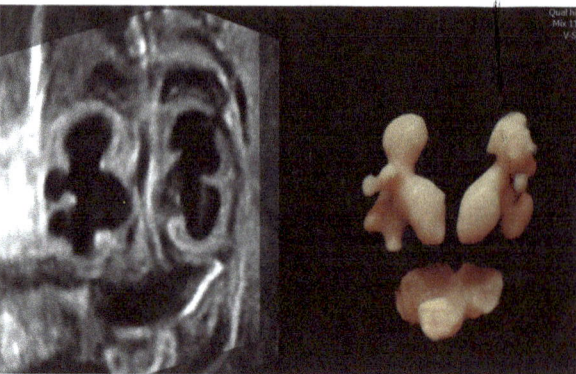

Fig. 10.14: Bilateral hydronephrosis in a fetus with vesicoureteral reflux in 2D (left) and in inversion mode (right).

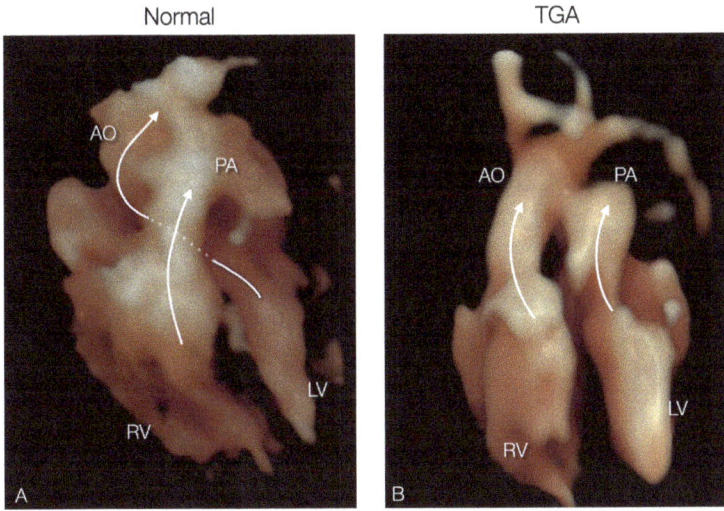

Fig. 10.15: STIC acquisition of two hearts shown with the inversion mode. Image A: normal heart with right (RV) and left ventricles (LV) and normal crossing of aorta (Ao) and pulmonary artery (PA). Image B: fetus with transposition of the great arteries (TGA) with the wrong origin of the Ao from the RV and PA from LV and the parallel course of the vessels.

10.4 Conclusions

Fluid in the fetal body that contrasts well with adjacent tissues and is not shadowed by bones is the ideal region for imaging in inversion mode. The image is similar to a digital cast and can be enhanced by using HDlive and changing the position of the light source. A prerequisite for a good image is a contrast optimized 2D image prior to acquisition and a good balance when using the threshold and gain buttons. Often Magicut is required to remove additional artifact information. Recently, with the significant improvement of the silhouette mode software (see Chapter 11), inversion mode has been less used in favor of the newer one, which will be discussed in the next chapter.

11 The Silhouette Mode

11.1 Principle

When selecting the mode of a 3D volume rendering for a region of interest, the operator generally chooses between either the surface mode and a transparent mode or a mixture of both (see Chapter 3, Chapter 7 and Fig. 3.28). The new software named *silhouette mode* has changed this rigid differentiation between surface and transparency modes as it combines both. It enables the demonstration of contours of the structures to be visualized within the selected region of the volume (Fig. 11.1). At the time of its introduction, it was an extension of HDlive rendering mode, but since then it has become a more independent mode with a variety of transparency functions. Some of the potential of the silhouette mode is shown in Figure 11.2 and will be discussed in this chapter. We believe that the potential of this new method has not been yet fully exploited and we encourage the user to try different combinations. Color Doppler silhouette mode is shortly discussed in Chapter 12.

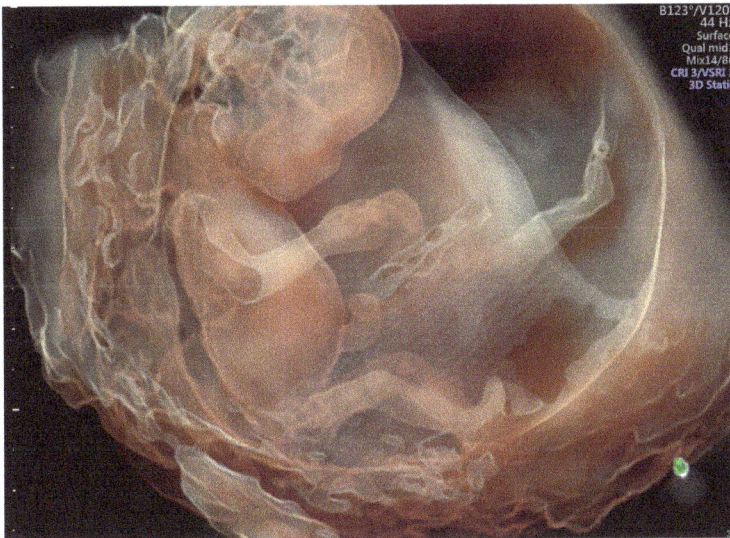

Fig. 11.1: Transvaginal 3D acquisition of a 12 weeks of gestation with surface rendering and display with silhouette mode. The placenta in front of the fetus was only partially removed with Magicut, but the silhouette mode allows the placenta to be transparent.

https://doi.org/10.1515/9783111249513-011

11.2 Practical approach

The silhouette mode software algorithm creates a gradient at organ boundaries, or even within the same tissue, when a significant change in acoustic impedance is detected. Using this algorithm, this mode allows separate highlighting of the structures of interest. As shown in Figure 11.2, organ boundaries can be found between bone and tissue, between fluid-filled structures (e. g., cavities or vessels) and tissue walls, or even within the same tissue if different acoustic information is present. Hyperechogenic or slightly echogenic structures can be seen at their clear borders, such as bone (Fig. 11.2B), liver (Fig. 11.2E), myocardium (Fig. 11.2G), or brain tissue (Fig. 11.2H). Echolucent structures, on the other hand, can be clearly visualized with their boundaries in the transparent view, such as cardiac cavities, cardiac and extracardiac vessels, intracerebral ventricles in early gestation, and other fluid-filled structures. This view across all layers highlighting structures with fluid collection, let Dr. Ritsuko Pooh (Japan) call this rendering a "see-through fashion" tool.

Variations of Silhouette Mode

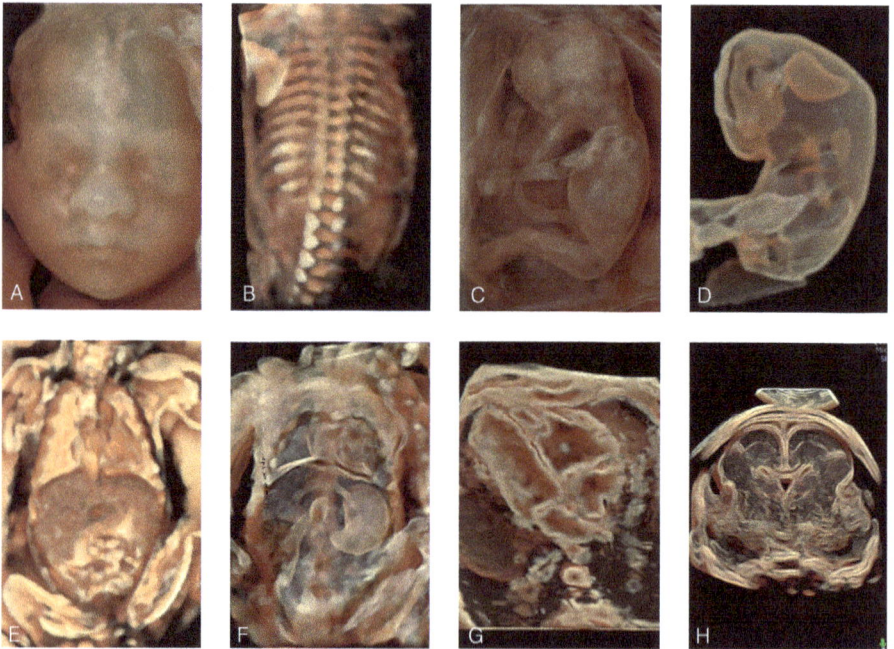

Fig. 11.2: Silhouette mode should not be considered as a single rendering tool. These eight examples show different applications of silhouette, from softening the image (A) to visualizing the skeletal system (B) to highlighting boundaries (E, G) or making structures transparent (C, D, F, H), among others. The combination of the different sub-functions of the silhouette mode and the choice of the appropriate volume depth provides the different rendering results.

All these details cannot be presented with one single preset but require some changes in the presets, depending on what information is to be extracted from the volume. The following sections attempt to explain the different presets by illustrating them with the figures in this chapter.

To make the best use of the silhouette mode, the operator must combine the three silhouette sub-functions gray-silhouette, silhouette-threshold, and silhouette-radius, each of which can be incrementally increased or decreased. Since the silhouette mode focuses on 3D visualization of the grayscale contours, additional functions that modify the post-processing of the grayscale information should also be adjusted accordingly. These functions include "gain", "gray-threshold" and "gray-transparency".

The final image can be optimized by adjusting the "shadow" of HDlive, the "volume SRI" and the "light source". For this reason, it is impossible to remember the combination of all nine components for each view, and we recommend using some presets preselected in the system and modifying them slightly to achieve the desired result. Nevertheless, it may be important to know the key functions of the silhouette tools, which are explained below and illustrated with several examples in this chapter. The following suggestions are based on the authors' experience, and each operator can use his or her own combination as desired.

Gray silhouette: The term *gray silhouette* is used to distinguish it from the color Doppler and HD Flow silhouette (see Chapter 12). At level 0, the silhouette mode and the other silhouette sub-functions are disabled. The silhouette mode is active from level 1 to 100. The transparency of the silhouette increases with the selected level. At low levels, the images of the skin appear waxy (levels 1–10) (Figs. 11.2A, 11.3). The skin becomes transparent at levels around 25, whereas the use of levels between 35–45 makes not only bones visible but also internal body organs in the first trimester. Almost all other silhouette presets use levels from 70–100. Figure 11.3 shows the difference in increasing the silhouette level when the other silhouette features are kept low.

Silhouette threshold: Changing the threshold changes the gray value around which a silhouette is displayed. Values range from 0 to 250, and we choose values between 30 and 50 for tissues, vessels, and fluid organs, increasing the value for brain vesicles and to highlight the borders of fluid-filled organs. On the other hand, high values of 120 to over 200 can be chosen to visualize bones along with a low gray silhouette of 30. It should be kept in mind that this threshold should also be considered as a complement to the gray-threshold used in the 3D surface mode, and both should ideally be changed together to achieve a good result.

Silhouette radius: The radius function specifies the thickness of the displayed silhouette with a range between 0 and 100. The value is a relative number between a minimum of 0 and a maximum of 100 thickness. In most cases we use values between 60 and 100.

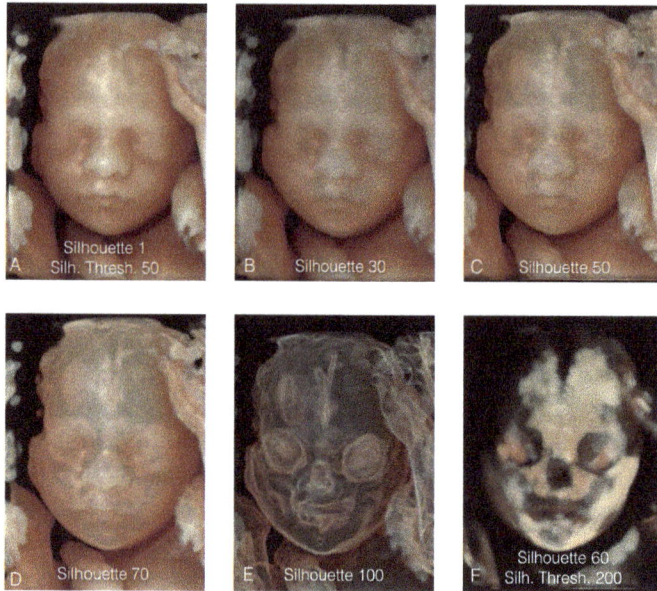

Fig. 11.3: The same face rendered in surface mode without activating the silhouette (A) and gradually adding the silhouette with different levels. Notice that images B through E become more transparent. In image F, the silhouette was selected at level 60, but the silhouette threshold was increased to 200.

Even if the combination of values can be copied to new volumes, the operator should keep in mind that the thickness of the 3D layer chosen as the region of interest can change the result. The result essentially depends not only on the previously described selected features, but also on the size and amount of information within the render box. Therefore, it is advised to always choose the smallest possible size with the maximum amount of information. Another helpful tip is to increase the contrast of the 2D image before capturing a volume if vessels or fluid-filled organs are to be displayed.

11.3 Typical applications of the silhouette mode

In their initial experience, the authors have obtained good results in the conditions presented below. The user is encouraged to explore new applications with the silhouette mode.

Embryo and early fetus: From visualization of the 5 mm embryo to the fetus at the 14 gestational week, silhouette mode can be applied throughout the first trimester and provide surprisingly interesting images (Figs. 11.4–11.11). However, this requires excellent 3D volume quality which is usually achieved with a transvaginal transducer. Ideally, the volume size is chosen to be as large as possible, which in turn allows better

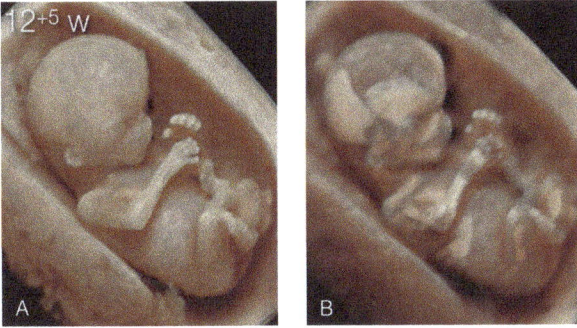

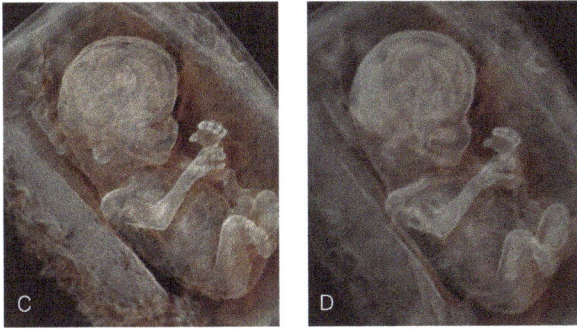

Fig. 11.4: Fetus at 12 weeks' gestation visualized with different levels of silhouette mode highlighting the skin (A), bones (B), or surface and internal structures (C and D).

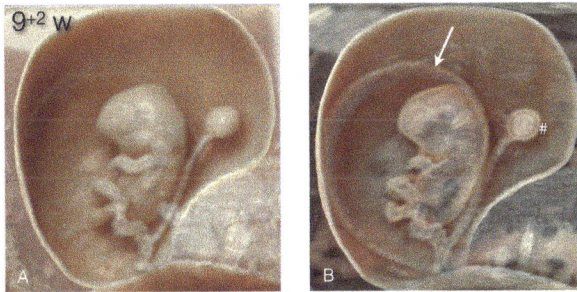

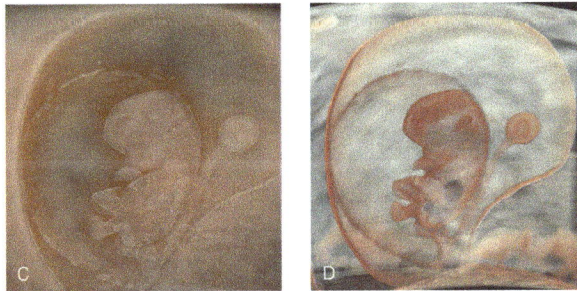

Fig. 11.5: Embryo at 9 weeks' gestation shown with different levels of silhouette mode. In (A), the gray threshold is high and the amniotic membrane is not clearly visible, while in (B), (C) and (D) a decrease in the threshold makes the membrane (arrow) visible. In (D), the light source comes from behind. The yolk sac is well visible in all four images (#).

visualization of the embryo/fetus and its surroundings. The amniotic cavity can be well visualized with this tool, which contributes to a good differentiation of the chorionicity in multiple pregnancy. The intracranial structures are discussed below. A simple application of the silhouette mode in early pregnancy may be to make the placenta and uterus transparent in order to visualize the shape of the fetus or embryo, as shown in Figures 11.1 and 11.6 to 11.8. For multiple pregnancies, a complete overview is better displayed using the silhouette mode, as shown in Figures 11.8 and 11.9. Figure 11.10 shows the use of 3D to visualize the fetal body in the first trimester with tomographic mode and then with different levels of silhouette mode. The view of the fetal brain at week 12 in a normal and an abnormal case is shown in Figure 11.11.

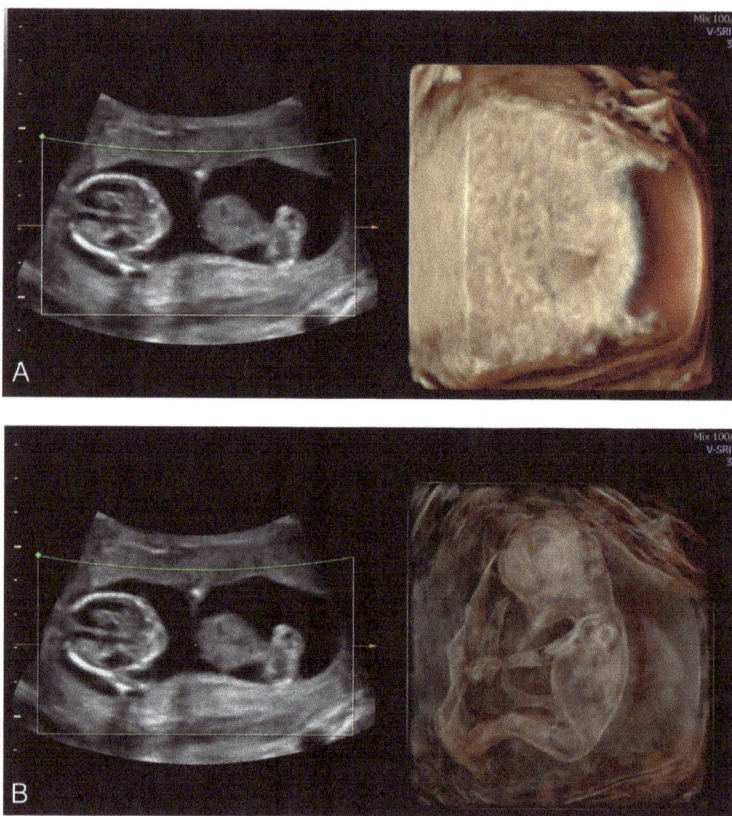

Fig. 11.6: One of the typical advantages of the silhouette mode is that some tissues are made transparent. Panel A shows a lateral view of a first trimester fetus partially covered by the placenta. In panel B, after activating the silhouette mode, the silhouette of the fetus appears with head, body, and limbs. See Figures 11.7–11.11 for similar examples.

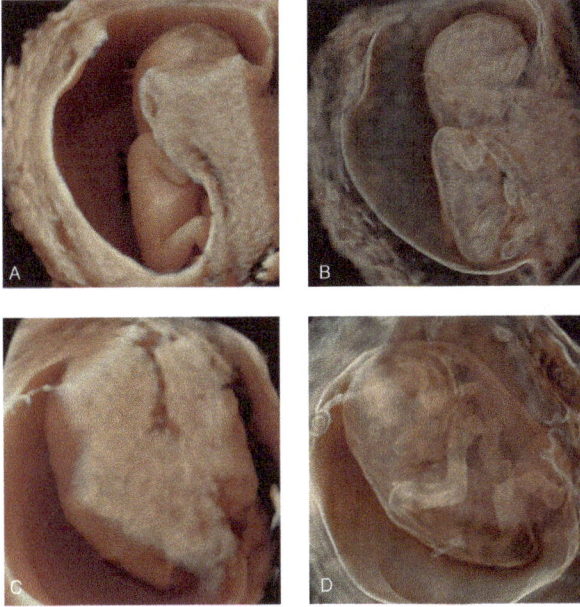

Fig. 11.7: Similar examples of using silhouette mode to make tissue transparent. In these two cases, a placenta covers the fetus in (A) and (C) in surface mode; after activating silhouette mode the shape of the fetus becomes visible in (B) and (D).

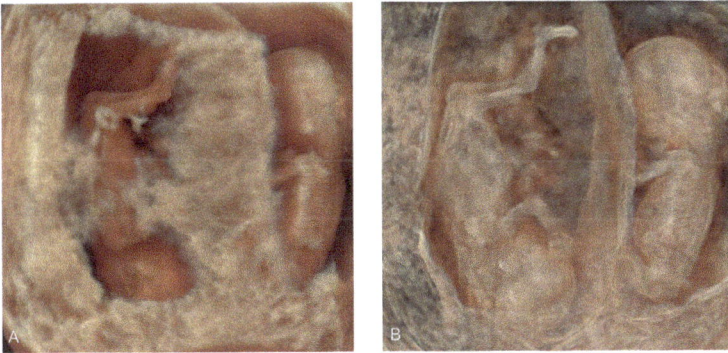

Fig. 11.8: Diamniotic twins shown in image A with the surface mode. Removing all structures in front of the fetuses with Magicut is tedious, while activating the silhouette mode directly provides a good overview of both fetuses.

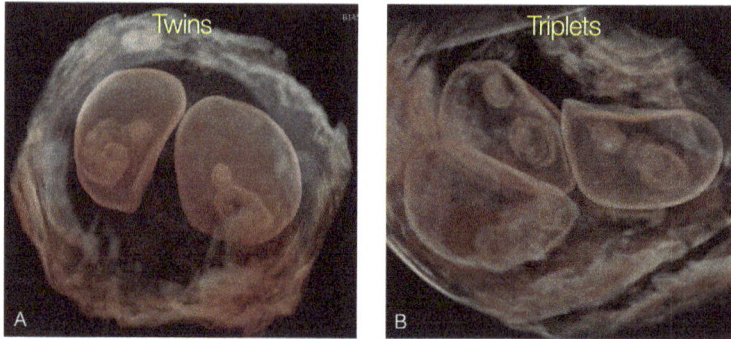

Fig. 11.9: Using the silhouette mode is very helpful for multiple pregnancies in the embryonic period. At one glance, the amniotic sacs and their contents can be visualized: in (A) dichorionic twins and in (B) trichorionic triplets.

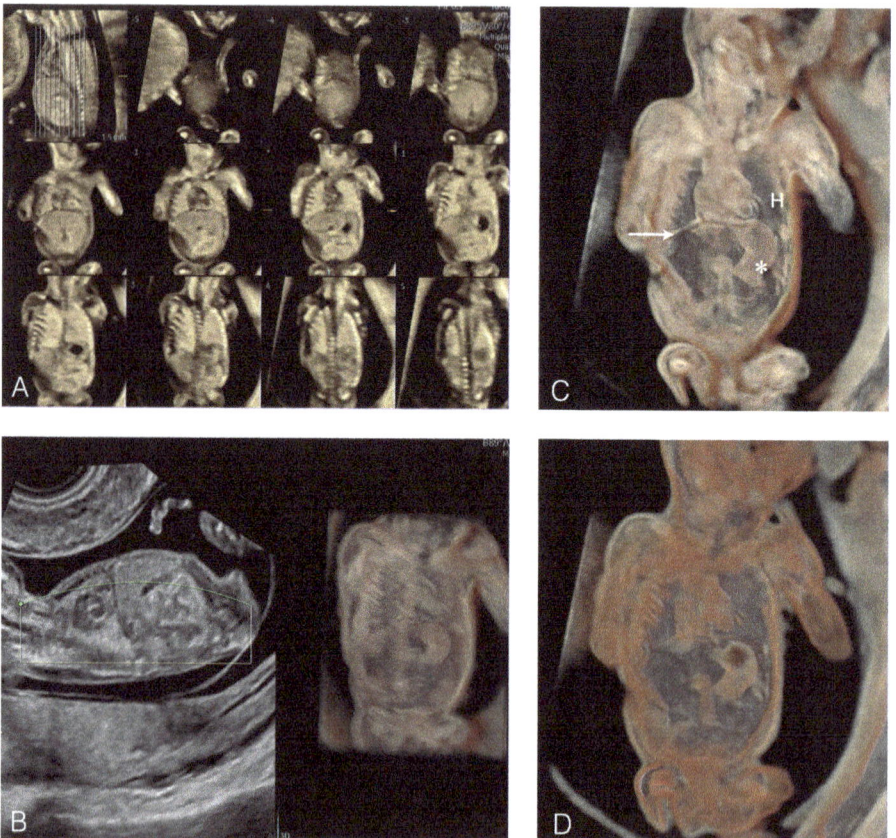

Fig. 11.10: Body of a fetus at 12 weeks' gestation shown in tomography mode (A) and then in 3D rendering (B, C and D). By activating the silhouette mode, the internal structures such as the diaphragm (arrow), the heart (H), the stomach (*) and more become transparent.

Normal   Holoprosencephaly

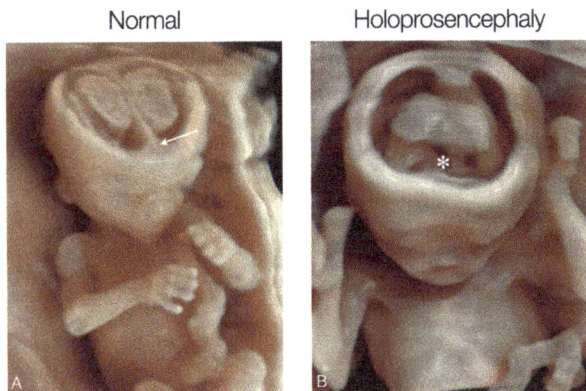

Fig. 11.11: 3D view of two fetal heads and faces at 12 weeks' gestation with the skull opened with Magicut and displayed in silhouette mode. Panel A shows a healthy fetus with a normal face and two hemispheres separated by the falx (arrow). Panel B shows a fetus with holoprosencephaly with fused ventricles (*) and a midface anomaly.

The skeletal system: Chapter 8 discussed the use of the silhouette mode to visualize the skeletal system. By making the skin transparent with a gray silhouette and increasing the silhouette threshold, it is possible to highlight a transparent skeleton, as shown in Figures 11.12 and 11.13. See also Chapter 8 for more details on the silhouette mode of bones.

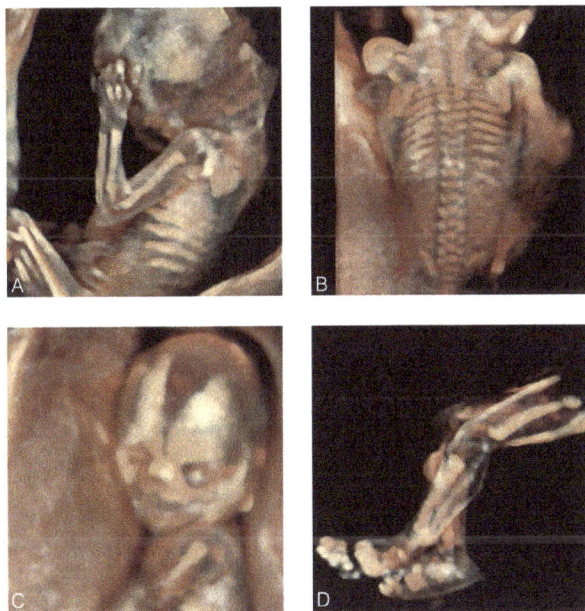

Fig. 11.12: Silhouette mode with high level of silhouette threshold between 120 and 200 increases the visibility of the skeletal system as shown in these cases. This tool is ideally used between 15 and 22 weeks before the skin becomes echogenic. Fetus in (A) is 15, fetus in (B) 17, fetus in (C) 18, and fetus in (D) 22 weeks' gestation.

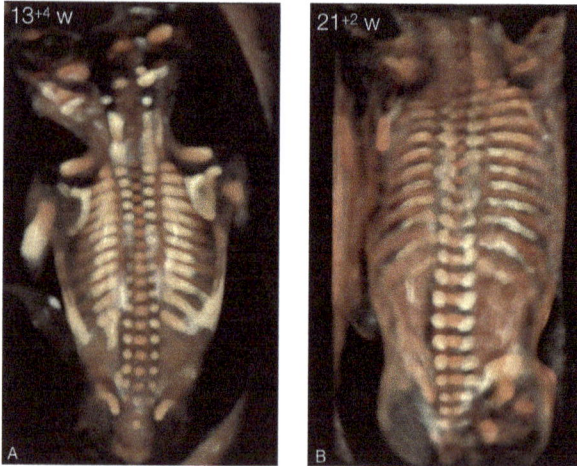

Fig. 11.13: Spine and ribs of a fetus at 13 and 21 weeks' gestation with silhouette mode and bone view with high silhouette threshold.

Outer body contours: Body contours are softened with the low level of silhouette mode. In the first, second or third trimester, the silhouette provides a soft "veil" on the surface (Figs. 11.1, 11.3, 11.14). For this purpose, silhouette mode can be useful in abnormal conditions where the body surface of the fetus is affected, such as a thickened nuchal translucency (Fig. 11.15), spina bifida (Fig. 11.16) and as shown in other chapters in omphalocele, gastroschisis, cleft lip and palate, and others.

Internal body structures: Silhouette mode can also be applied to the lungs and abdomen to highlight the surface of structures such as the liver, lungs, or intestines at low level silhouette (Fig. 11.17A) or to highlight fluid-filled organs such as the heart, stomach, gallbladder, intrahepatic vessels, dilated renal pelvis, and others by increasing transparency, as shown in Figures 11.17 to 11.21. The view may be frontal, lateral, or axial, as shown in these figures. In cases where a thin section is selected for the silhouette rendering mode, positioning the light from behind, as shown in Figures 11.19B and 11.21C, can add a special effect to the image. In particular, the use of the silhouette mode can be of great help in the case of enlarged anechoic spaces in the body, such as a dilated stomach (Figs. 11.20, 11.21), a multicystic kidney, hydronephrosis, and other fluid collections.

Fetal heart: Silhouette mode can also be used on a STIC heart volume in grayscale. This allows good visualization of the contours of the myocardium, valves, and papillary muscles (Fig. 11.22). Anomalies of the ventricles and great vessels can be highlighted. Silhouette can also be combined with color Doppler flow (see Chapter 12 and Chapter 19), with good smoothing of the grayscale information in the image. The more recently introduced silhouette mode of color Doppler is discussed in short later in this chapter.

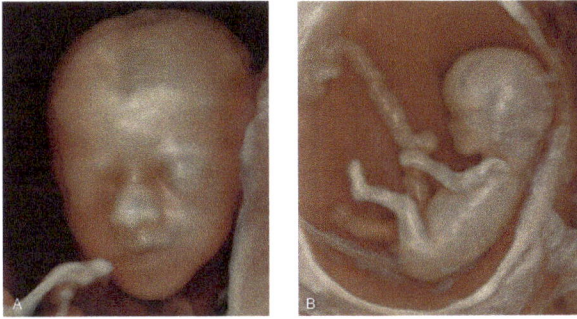

Fig. 11.14: Fetal face at 25 weeks' gestation and overview of a fetus at 12 weeks' gestation, shown in 3D surface mode and with the addition of a slight silhouette mode level, resulting in waxy skin. Increasing the silhouette level makes the skin transparent.

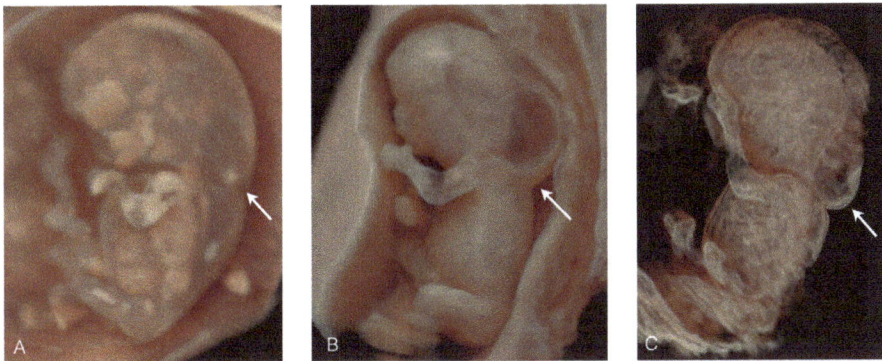

Fig. 11.15: Three first trimester fetuses with thickened nuchal translucency (arrow) of different shapes, shown in 3D surface mode along with silhouette mode. Using the silhouette mode allows a clear view of the nuchal translucency when more transparency is selected.

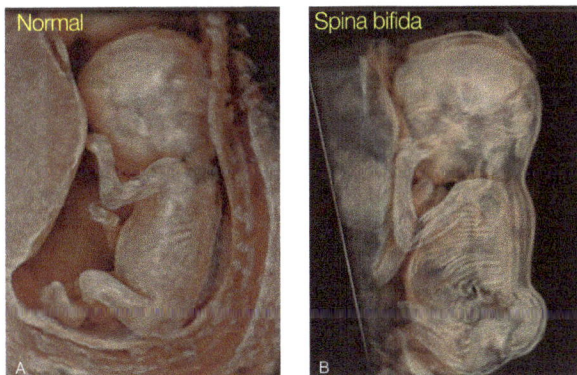

Fig. 11.16: Side view of two first trimester fetuses with normal back in (A) and with a large spina bifida in (B), shown in silhouette mode.

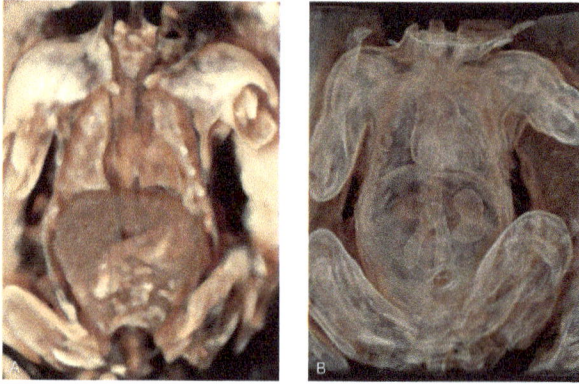

Fig. 11.17: Frontal view of the body of a fetus at 22 weeks' gestation in 3D in two different silhouette mode planes. In (A), the outline of the liver, intestine, diaphragm, heart, and lungs can be seen. If one increases the transparency of the silhouette (B), the organs become more transparent and the stomach, gallbladder and umbilical cord are visible.

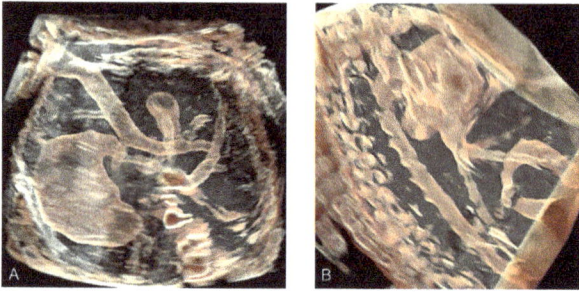

Fig. 11.18: Views of the abdominal cavity from cranial view (A) and lateral view (B) in silhouette mode. These views make the echolucent structures visible, such as stomach and vessels.

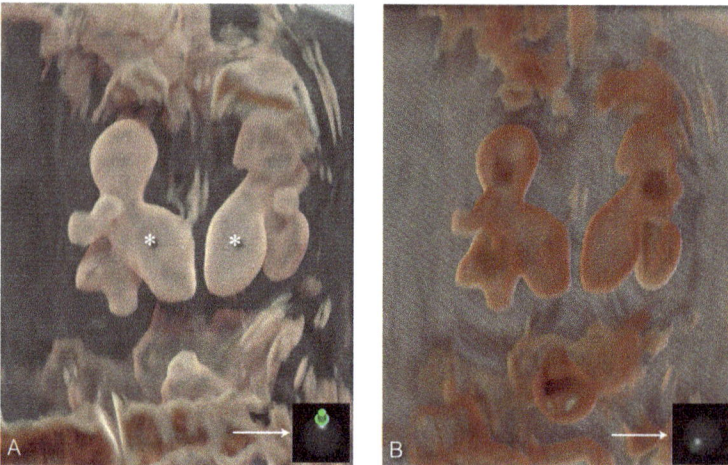

Fig. 11.19: A fetus with vesical-ureteral reflux and hydronephrosis in which the dilated renal pelvis is clearly visible in silhouette mode. The light source (arrow) is placed in (A) at the front and in (B) at the back.

Normal   Double Bubble

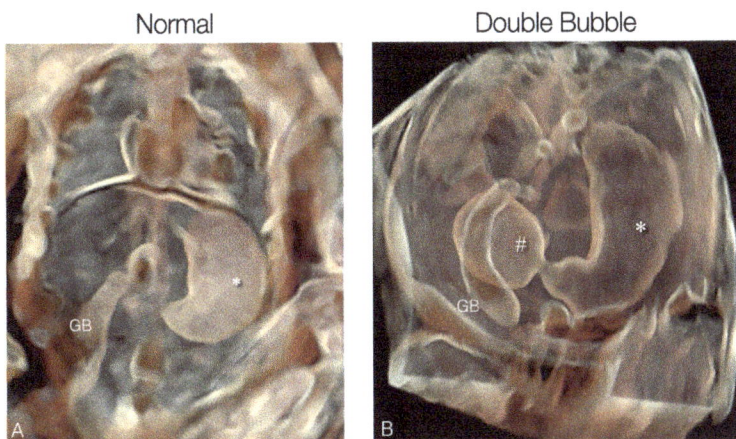

Fig. 11.20: The silhouette mode shows a projection of the fetal abdomen in two fetuses: a normal fetus in (A) and a fetus with double bubble sign in (B). In (A), the stomach bubble (*) can be seen, while in (B) the stomach (*) and the dilated duodenum (#) are clearly visible; gallbladder (GB).

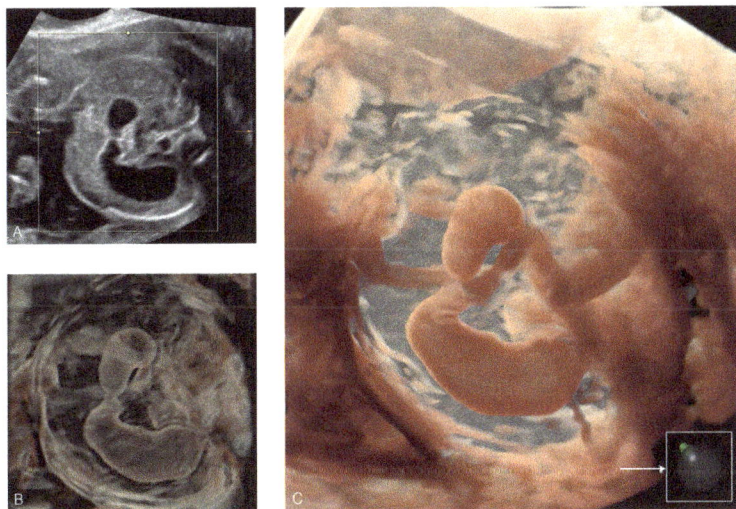

Fig. 11.21: Fetus with double bubble sign in duodenal atresia shown in 2D (A) and in silhouette mode as transparency (B, C). In (B), the light source is placed from the front, in (C) from the back (arrow).

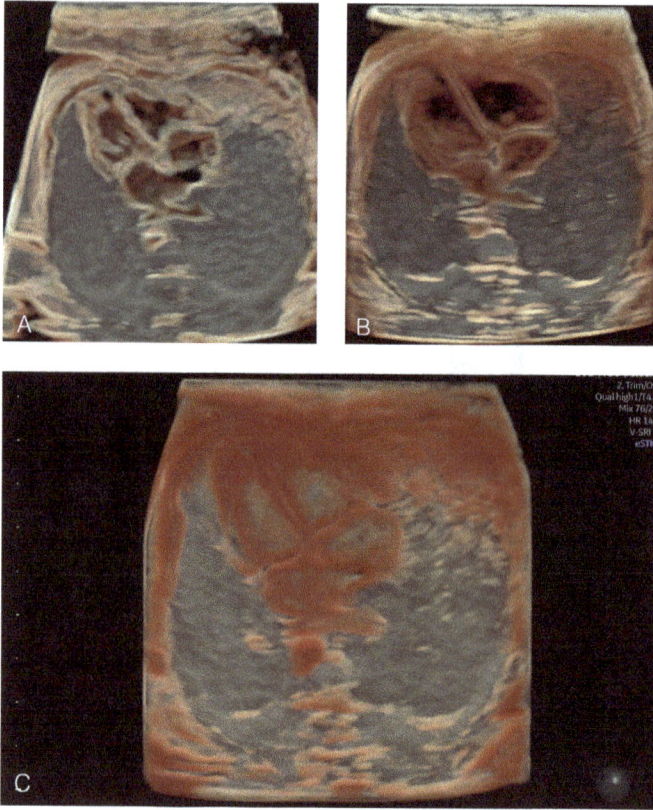

Fig. 11.22: Four-chamber view of the heart with silhouette and with different insonation, where the light source is from the front in (A), from above in (B) and from behind in (C).

Intracerebral ventricular system: Silhouette mode is an ideal tool for visualizing hypoechoic structures and can be used to demonstrate the intracerebral ventricular system in 3D mode, especially in early gestation (Fig. 11.23). The silhouette mode is ideal for the spatial visualization of the embryonic ventricular system at a time when ossification of the cranial bones has not yet occurred; Figures 11.24 and 11.25 illustrate such conditions. Later in gestation, the ventricular system can be best visualized through the fontanelles and conditions such as ventriculomegaly, holoprosencephaly, dilated posterior fossa can be visualized.

Thick slice silhouette: Dr. Ritsuko Pooh (Japan) introduced the concept of thick slice image in combination with silhouette a few years ago. For this purpose, a slice is selected and visualized with the silhouette, changing the position of the light source (Fig. 11.26). We think this can be applied very well to the transvaginally examined brain in sagittal and coronal views (Fig. 11.27), to the early fetus, and to other regions and organs, as shown in the overview in Figure 11.28.

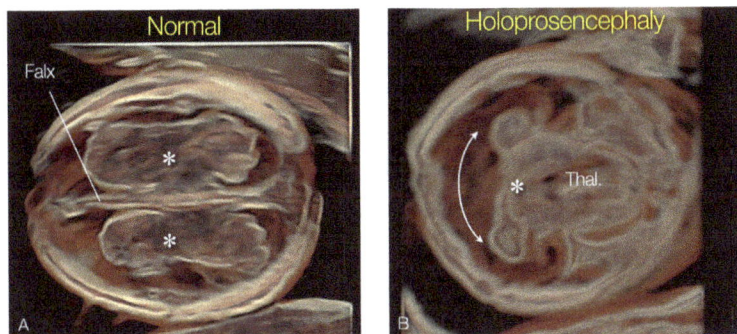

Fig. 11.23: Transventricular 3D view in silhouette mode at 13 weeks' gestation. It shows in (A) a fetus with normal anatomy in which the falx cerebri (arrow) separates both cerebral cavities with the two choroid plexuses (*), and in (B) a fetus with holoprosencephaly with fused choroid plexuses (*), lateral ventricles (double arrow) and fused thalami (Thal.).

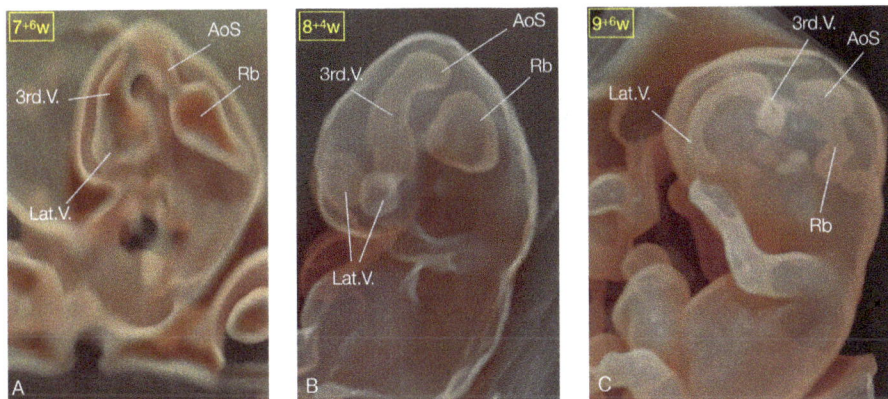

Fig. 11.24: Development of the cerebral ventricular system in three embryos at the seventh (A), eighth (B), and ninth (C) weeks of gestation, shown in silhouette mode. In this transparent view, the shape of the lateral ventricles (Lat.V.), third ventricle (3rd.V.), aqueduct of Sylvius (AoS), and rhombencephalon (Rb) can be clearly seen as they develop.

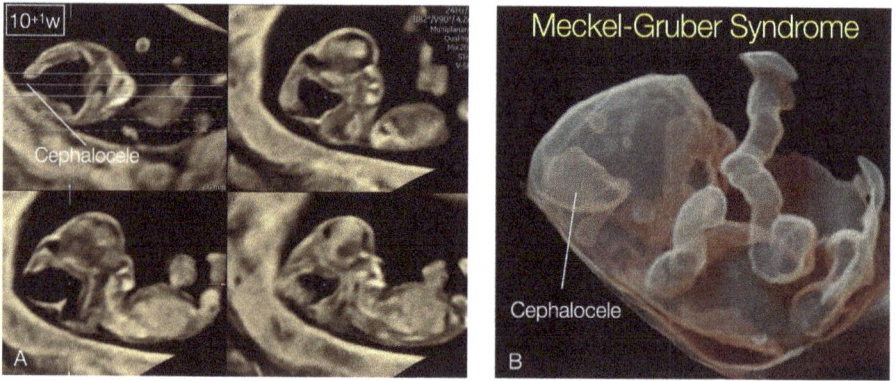

Fig. 11.25: Meckel-Gruber syndrome embryo at 10 weeks' gestation with a cephalocele shown in tomography mode (A) and rendered in silhouette mode, showing the dilated posterior fossa. Compare with the rhombencephalon of the embryo in Figure 11.24.

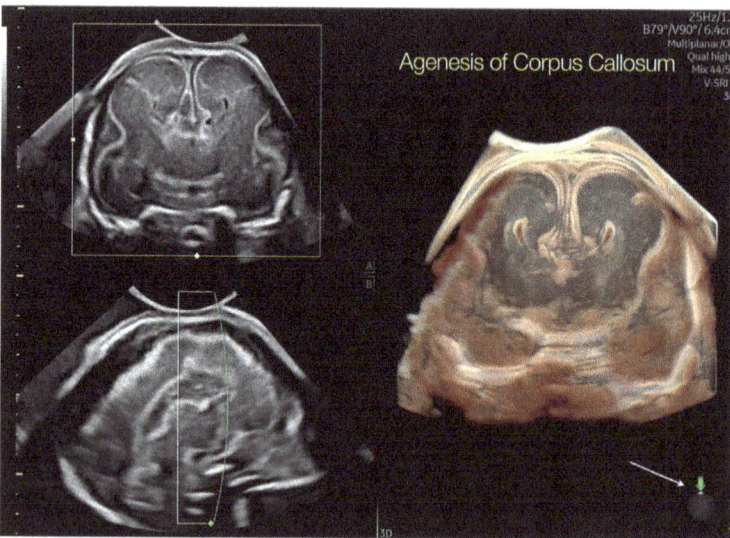

Fig. 11.26: The thick slice silhouette shown here is used to select a 3D layer of a structure (lower left panel); in this example a frontal brain slice in a fetus with agenesis of the corpus callosum. The transparent silhouette is applied, and the light source is placed on top at 12 o'clock (arrow) or even from behind.

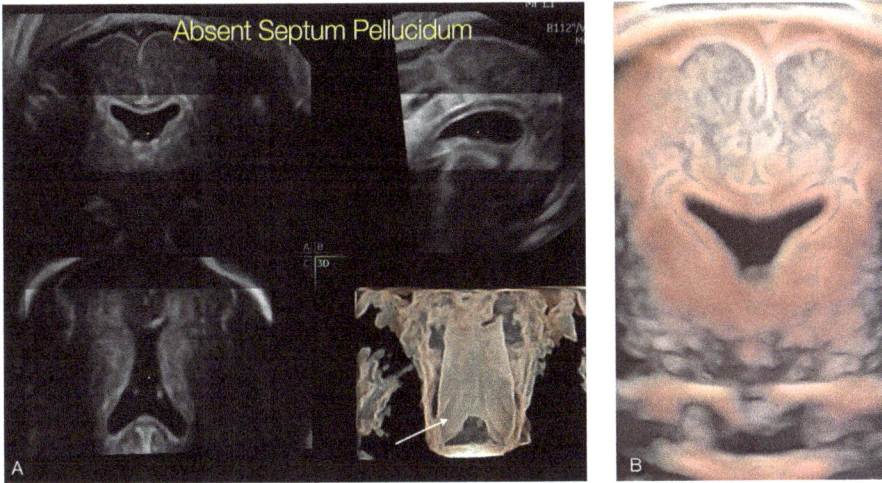

Fig. 11.27: Fetus with absent septum pellucidum shown in silhouette mode. The fusion of the two anterior horns can be seen in (A) in orthogonal mode and in 3D rendering with silhouette (arrow). The thick slice silhouette described in figure 11.26 is shown in (B).

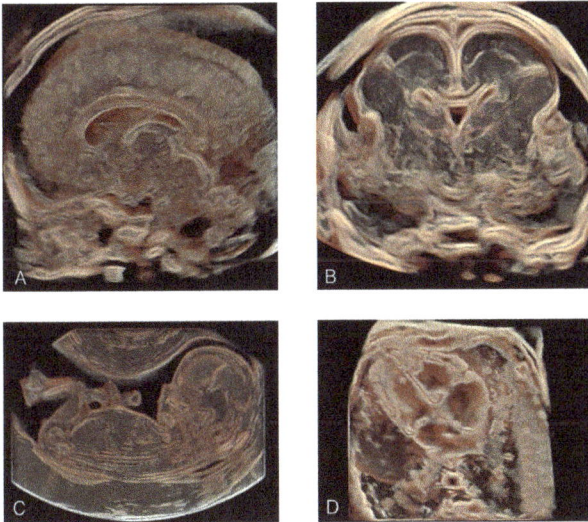

Fig. 11.28: With the thick slice silhouette it is possible to visualize different conditions. Shown here are a brain in sagittal view (A), a brain in coronal view (D), a sagittal view of a first trimester fetus (C), and the four chambers of the heart (D).

Color Doppler silhouette: With the release of a recent software, silhouette mode can now also be applied to color Doppler, making blood flow progressively more transparent and allowing the vessel edges to be easily seen. The color Doppler silhouette can be used as a stand-alone feature or in combination with the grayscale silhouette mode. Figure 11.29 shows examples of using the silhouette mode with color Doppler.

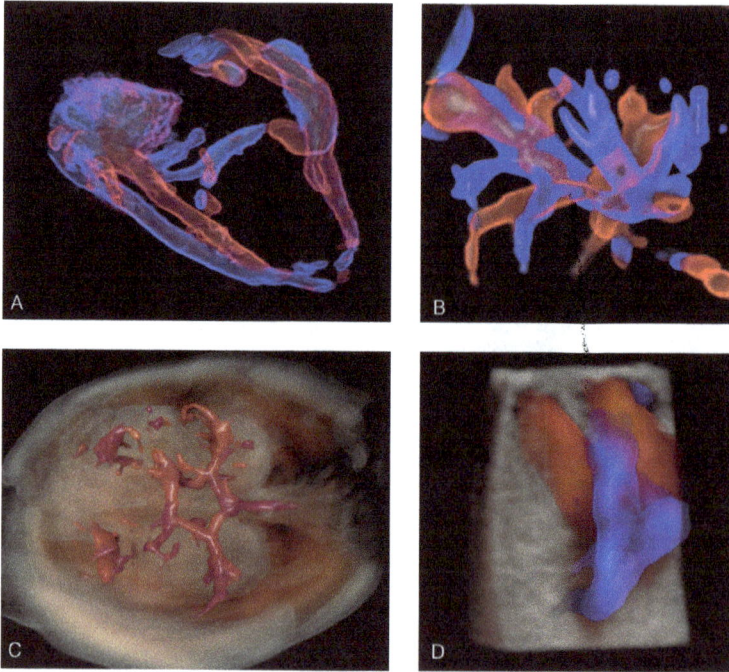

Fig. 11.29: Silhouette mode can also be used in combination with color Doppler: in (A) and (B) with color alone and in (C) and (D) together with grayscale background information as glass-body mode. In (A), one sees a right-sided view of the heart and abdominal vessels, in (B) a cranial view of the intrahepatic vessels, in (C) the Circle of Willis in monochrome, and in (D) a heart with the ventricles and crossing of the great vessels. Practically every color Doppler volume can be displayed in silhouette mode if required.

11.4 Conclusions

The recently updated silhouette mode displays images with an almost artistic effect, but with some experience the clinical benefits quickly become apparent. Using the silhouette in early gestation provides a quick overview of the position and shape of the embryo and fetus. Surface regions can be easily visualized with this tool, but its real power lies primarily in visualizing anechoic or hyperechoic structures within the render box. Unlike the inversion mode, the surrounding structures are visible when using the silhouette mode. One of the promising applications is the possibility to visualize the ventricular system of the embryo in early pregnancy or the thoracic and abdominal organs. After the learning curve is overcome, good results can be easily achieved.

12 The Glass-Body Mode

12.1 Principle

Color Doppler sonography with its various forms, such as color Doppler, high-definition (HD) bidirectional flow, power Doppler, or slow-flow HD can be used to study the cardiovascular system of the fetus with the umbilical vessels and placenta. In this chapter, the term *color Doppler* is used to refer to all four Doppler features. Color Doppler helps not only to detect cardiac abnormalities but also to visualize normal and abnormal vasculature in the various body organs. The arteries and veins of the human body generally have a spatial course, and 3D color Doppler can visualize this course and the branching of vessels better than the 2D image with color Doppler. The best 3D techniques include combining 3D or STIC with one of the color Doppler techniques. 3D imaging of vessels is well displayed with glass-body mode or with lower effort in a thin slice in multiplanar mode with the addition of the VCI slice, as explained in Chapter 4. In this chapter, the clinical use of glass-body mode will be discussed.

12.2 Practical approach

Glass-body mode: To achieve a good result, the operator should first optimize the color presets in order to improve the visualization of blood flow in the heart or vessels of interest. For volume acquisition in static 3D, both frame rate and persistence should be kept at a high level. The more images per second displayed in 2D, the more images with color information can then be acquired in a 3D volume. If the persistence is low and high pulsations are present, some images will be captured that do not contain color information. The 3D reconstruction of the vessel then shows interruptions in its course. An exception to this is STIC volumes, for which pulsations are required.

Prior to volume acquisition, it is advisable to perform a manual sweep with the transducer to verify that all vessels are clearly visible and potentially present in the volume to be acquired. The volume is then acquired with a middle volume quality using either static 3D or STIC. After seeing the result, the examiner can decide in a second attempt whether to use a higher or lower resolution during acquisition.

After acquiring the volume, the examiner can select the rendering mode which displays either grayscale only, color Doppler only, or a combination of both as glass-body mode (Fig. 12.1). To achieve a better result, the degree of transparency in glass-body mode should be adjusted as shown in Figure 12.2.

https://doi.org/10.1515/9783111249513-012

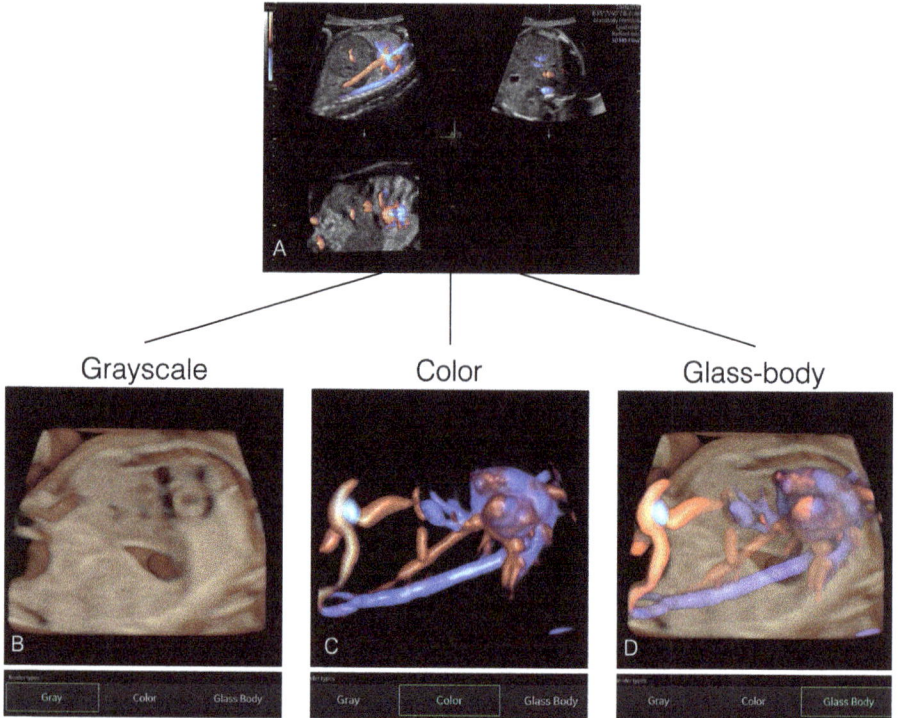

Fig. 12.1: 3D volume acquisition of thoracoabdominal vessels using static 3D in combination with color Doppler, shown in (A) in orthogonal mode. When activating the 3D rendering mode, the user can choose between different renderings in the rendering submenu: grayscale only (B), color Doppler information only (C), or a mixture of both as glass-body mode (D).

Magicut in glass-body mode: Magicut can also be used to selectively remove grayscale structures in front of or around the region of interest to highlight color Doppler information (Figs. 12.3–12.5). It is important to emphasize that Magicut offers additional features in glass-body mode, including the ability to delete either the grayscale or color Doppler information separately, or both together (Fig. 12.3).

The best way to learn these steps is to record an umbilical cord with the placenta in 3D glass-body mode and try out the different tools. Figures 12.3 through 12.8 show examples of umbilical cords where the Magicut was used to edit and selectively delete information. Artifacts caused by small signals from the vessels can also be selectively removed.

Monochrome color: The color Doppler used in glass-body mode can be converted in post-processing to a single color, called monochrome, which can be selected in the Render submenu. In this setting, the previous red color is slightly brighter than the previous blue color (Fig. 12.9C).

Mix Grayscale - Color Doppler

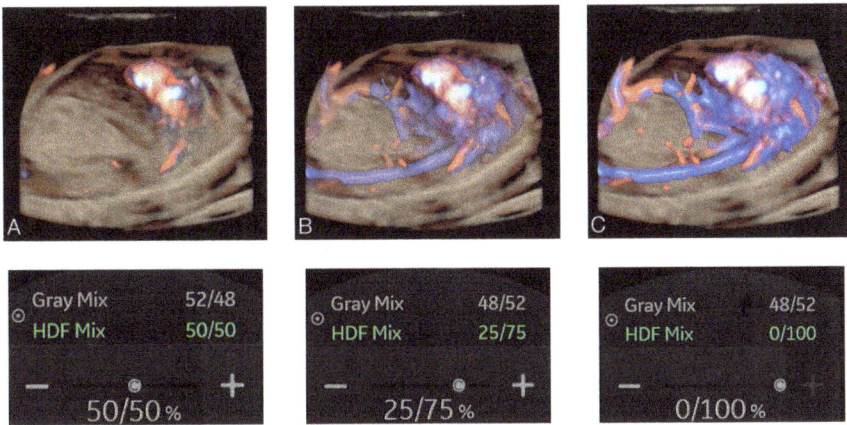

Fig. 12.2: 3D glass-body mode with color Doppler or High Definition Flow (HDF) with different transparency levels. In image optimization, the user can choose the blending level between grayscale and HDF separately (bottom panel), thus changing the appearance of the image. In (A) the mix is 50/50, in (B) 25/75, and in (C) 0/100, showing how the vasculature becomes progressively clearer from images A through C.

Magicut

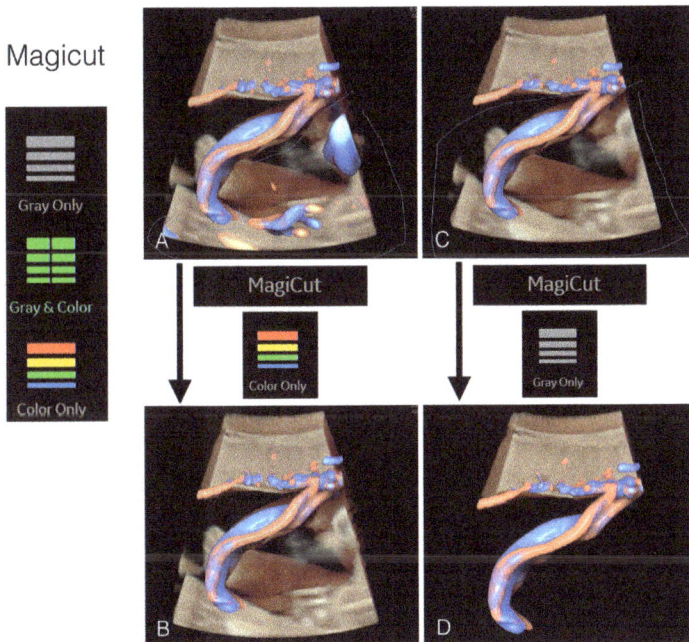

Fig. 12.3: 3D glass-body mode with the use of Magicut. When the Magicut function is activated in glass-body mode, different functions can be selected (left panel): grayscale only, color Doppler only, or both grayscale and color. (A) and (B) show the color Magicut before and after. Further use of the Magicut in (C) and (D) with only grayscale shows the removal of all structures except the placenta with the umbilical cord attachment.

Before   After Magicut

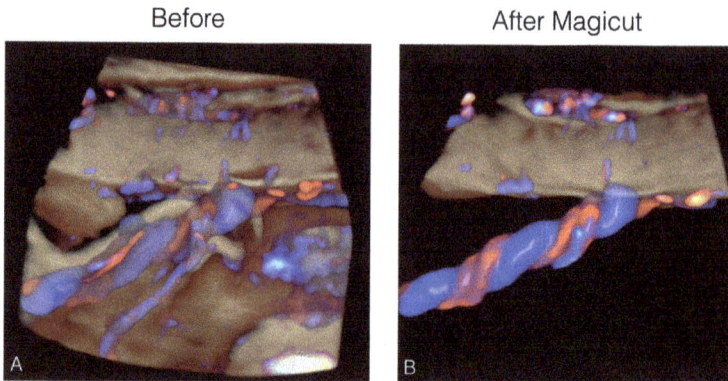

Fig. 12.4: Example of a placenta with umbilical cord insertion in 3D glass-body mode with surrounding information (A) and after cleanup with Magicut (B), as explained in Figure 12.3.

Silhouette mode for color Doppler: In a recent software release, the silhouette mode was also introduced for color Doppler independently of the activation of the grayscale silhouette mode. This can be used for all color Doppler types (Fig. 12.10). When using the color Doppler silhouette, the blood flow becomes transparent and the boundaries of the blood flow are displayed. This color silhouette of the blood flow makes it possible to see the shape of the blood flow even behind the vessels, as shown in the examples in Figure 12.10. To improve the image quality of the color Doppler silhouette, it is recommended to remove the grayscale information and lower the color Doppler threshold to increase the color information.

12.3 Typical applications of the glass-body mode

Umbilical vessels and placental vessels: Visualization of umbilical and placental vessels is generally easy to achieve (Figs. 12.3–12.10) because there are no interfering fetal movements. They are the ideal vessels to examine when learning the technique. From a clinical perspective, the origin and course of the umbilical cord can be assessed to demonstrate typical conditions, such as velamentous insertion (Fig. 12.7), vasa previa (Fig. 12.11), umbilical cord knot (Fig. 12.8), nuchal cord (Fig. 12.12), and others.

Liver and intraabdominal vessels: The intrahepatic veins, inferior vena cava, and descending aorta can be well visualized in both sagittal (Fig. 12.13) and axial cross-section views of the abdomen. From a clinical point of view, this approach can be used in cases of suspected abnormal course of the ductus venosus (Figs. 12.15, 12.16A) and in cases of interrupted inferior vena cava with azygos continuation (Fig. 12.16 B) as well as other rare, atypical vascular courses. In anomalies involving the ductus venosus, the examiner should focus on visualizing the portal venous system, which can be well visualized with 3D color Doppler in a cranial-caudal acquisition (Fig. 12.16).

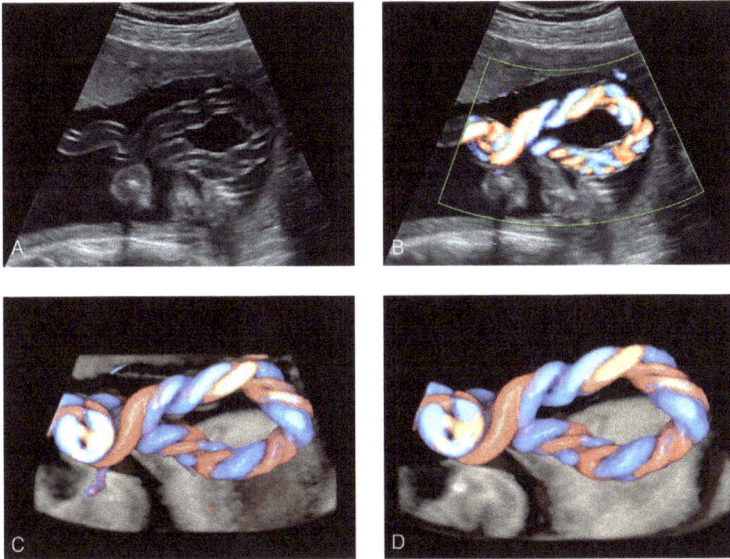

Fig. 12.5: In (A) an umbilical cord loop can be seen on the gray scale; in (B) blood flow in the umbilical cord is visualized with HDF; in (C) a static 3D volume is taken; and in (D) the result is shown after using Magicut.

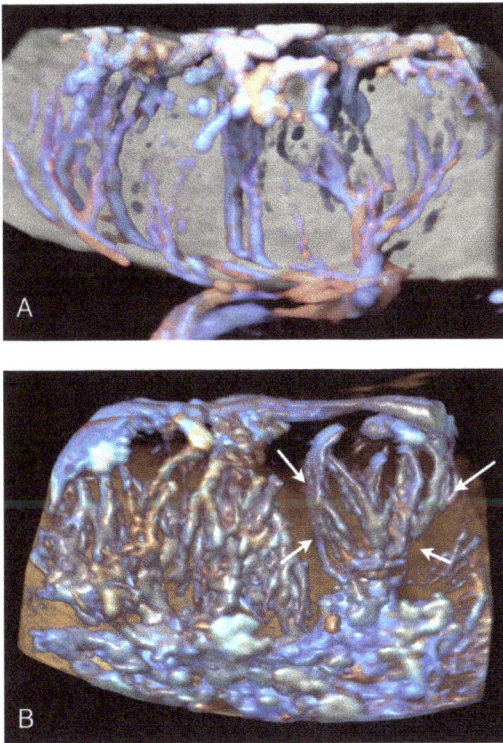

Fig. 12.6: 3D glass-body mode of intraplacental vessels in (A) with high-definition color Doppler and with slow flow in (B), allowing visualization of the vasculature within a cotyledon (arrows).

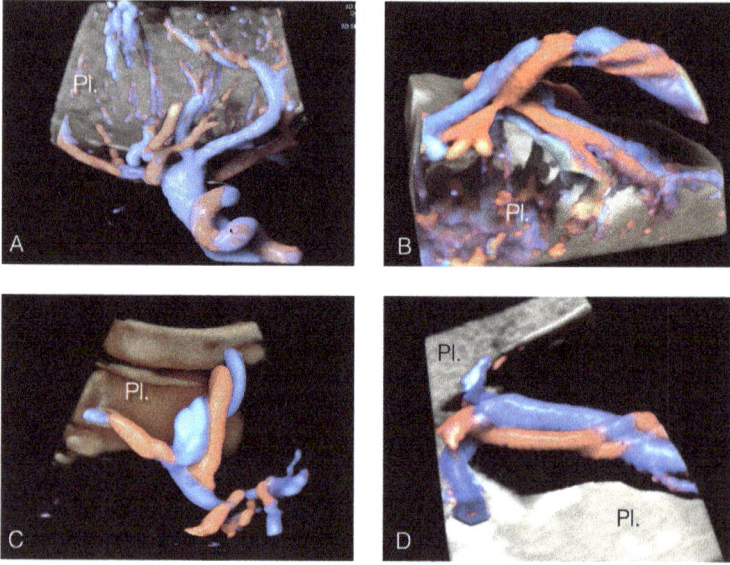

Fig. 12.7: 3D glass-body mode of placental cord insertion: in (A) insertion occurs at the anterior placenta (Pl.); in (B) at a posterior placenta; in (C) as a velamentous insertion; and in (D) as a placenta bipartita.

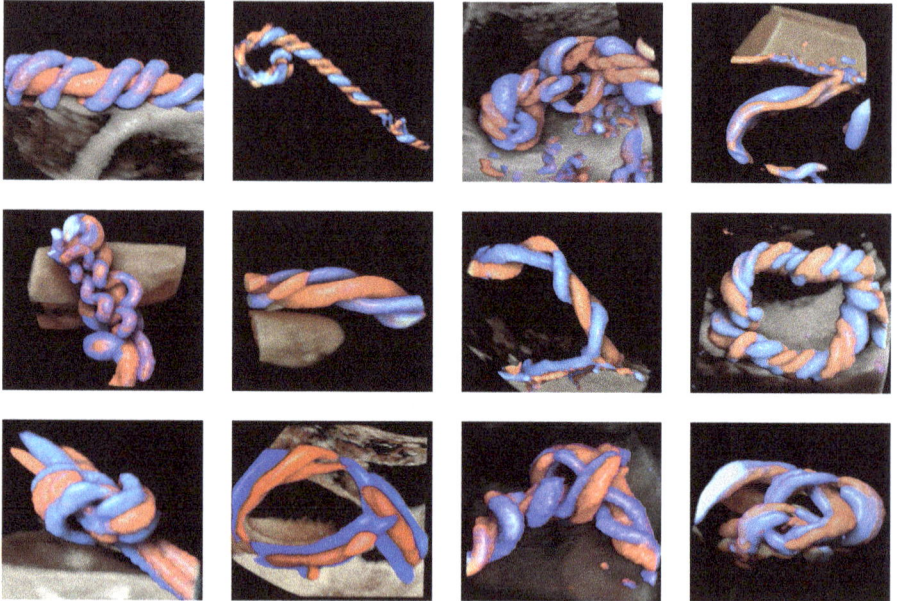

Fig. 12.8: 3D Glass-body mode in different umbilical cord variants with loops and knots.

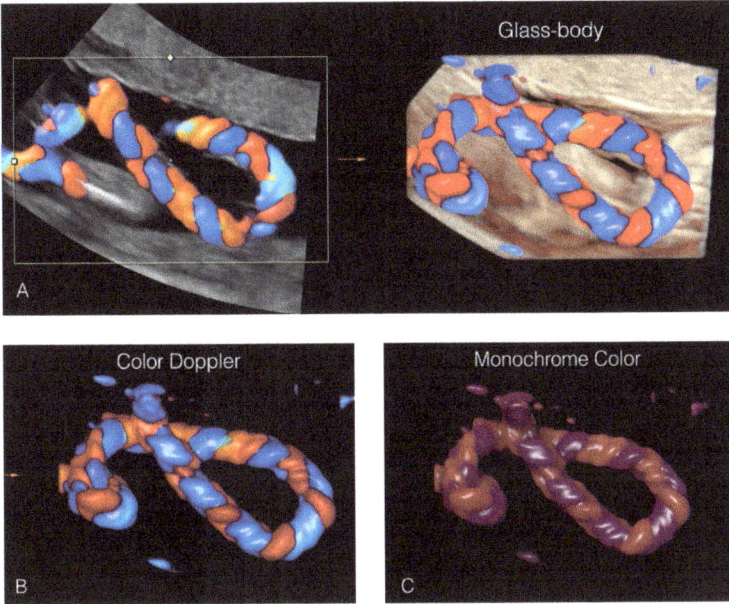

Fig. 12.9: Umbilical cord loop with color Doppler and glass-body mode (A), with color Doppler only (B), and monochrome only (C).

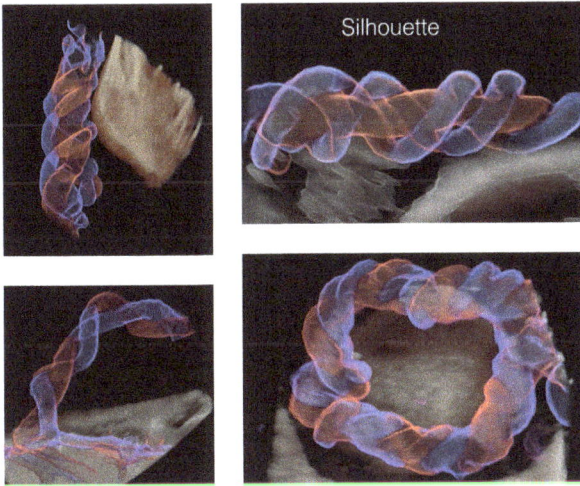

Fig. 12.10: Different umbilical cords in 3D glass-body mode in combination with silhouette mode making the vessels transparent.

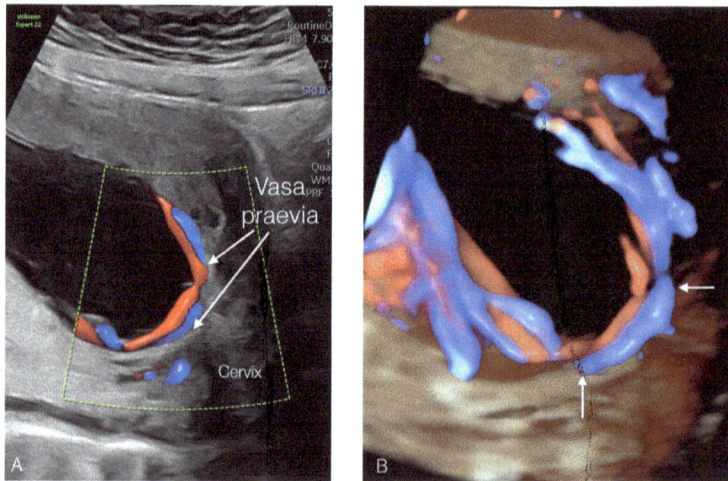

Fig. 12.11: Color Doppler in the lower uterine segment (A) shows free vessels along the cervix (arrows), as vasa previa. In (B), the spatial course of the vessels along the cervix can be seen in 3D glass-body mode (arrows).

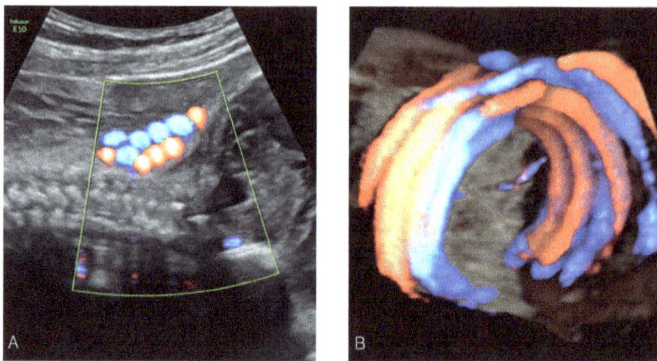

Fig. 12.12: Fetus with a single umbilical artery and fivefold umbilical cord around the neck in HDF (A) and in 3D glass-body mode (B).

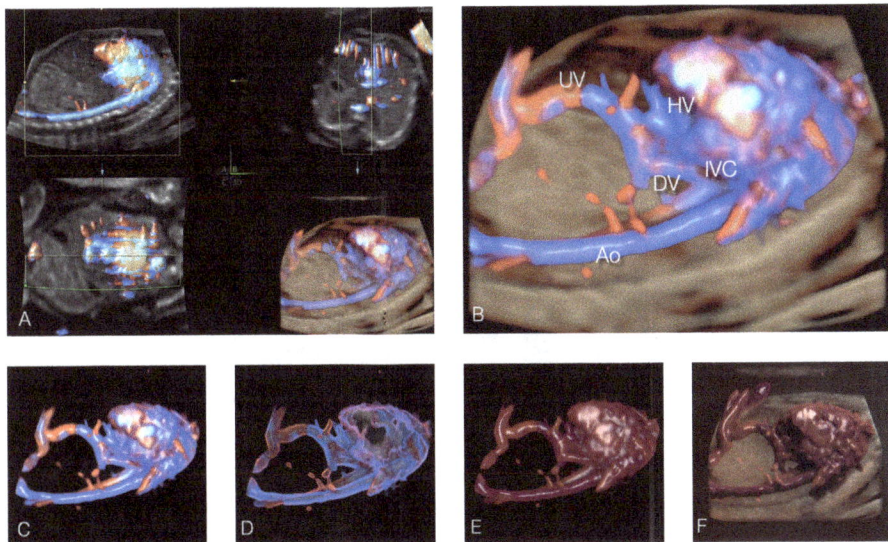

Fig. 12.13: Longitudinal section through the abdominal vessels showing the drainage of the ductus venosus (DV), inferior vena cava (IVC), and hepatic vein (HV) to the heart. The different displays are shown in (A) with less transparent mixture; in (B) in typical glass-body mode; in (C) with color Doppler only; in (D) with color Doppler and silhouette only; in (E) in monochrome mode; and in (F) in monochrome with grayscale silhouette. Aorta (Ao), umbilical vein (UV).

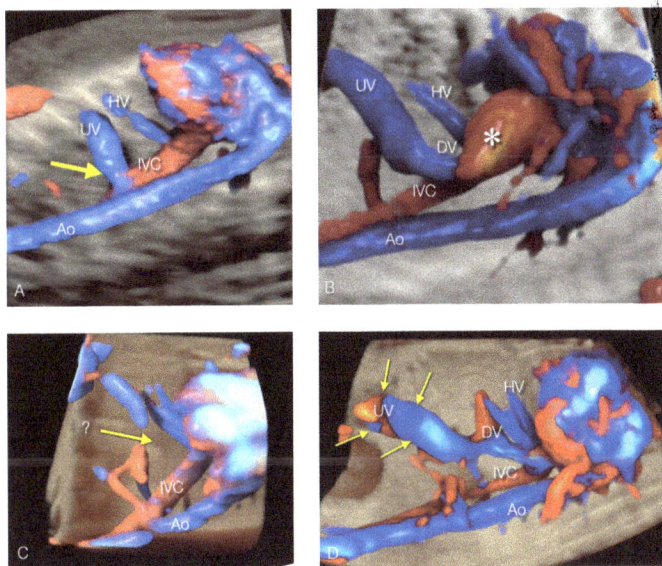

Fig. 12.14: 3D glass-body mode in four fetuses with abnormalities of the course of the umbilical vein (UV) and ductus venosus (DV). In (A), there is an anomalous connection of the UV directly into the inferior vena cava (IVC). In (B), there is also a direct connection of the DV into the IVC, resulting in its massive dilatation (*). In (C), the ductus venosus is absent (arrow, ?). In (D), the fetus has ectasia of the umbilical vein (arrows). Aorta (Ao), hepatic vein (HV).

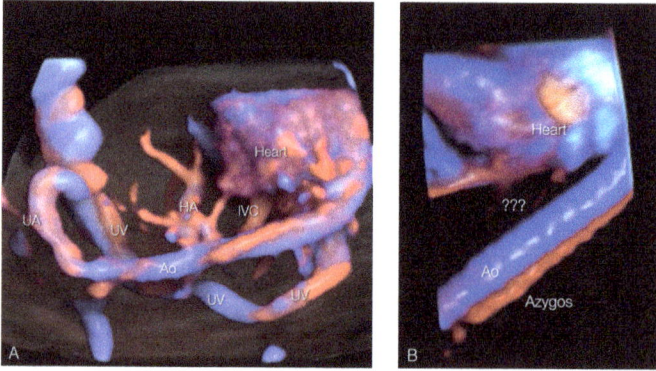

Fig. 12.15: (A) shows a lateral view of the abdomen and chest with color Doppler glass-body mode in a fetus with an abnormal connection between the umbilical vein (UV) and right atrium. (B) shows a view from the left side of a fetus with interrupted inferior vena cava (???) and azygos continuity showing aorta (Ao) and azygos side by side with opposite direction of blood flow. Umbilical artery (UA), hepatic artery (HA).

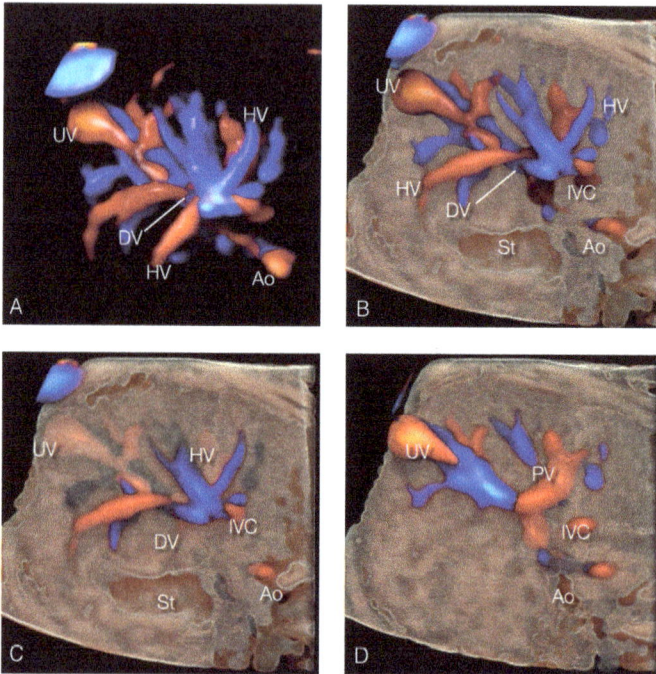

Fig. 12.16: 3D glass-body mode of the abdomen in a transverse view of the intrahepatic vasculature. (A) and (B) show the entire vasculature with color Doppler only in (A) and in glass-body mode in (B). Changing the transparency and scrolling through the volume, one can see in (C) the hepatic veins (HV) merging toward the inferior vena cava (IVC) at the level of the upper abdomen with the stomach (St) visible, while in (D) a lower plane with the umbilical vein (UV) is opening into the portal sinus (PV). Aorta (Ao), ductus venosus (DV), umbilical vein (UV).

Heart and great vessels: The greatest experience with glass-body mode is with the use of STIC in fetal echocardiography (Fig. 12.17) (see also Chapter 19). Anomalies involving the four-chamber anatomy can be visualized similarly to the 2D image with color Doppler, whereas anomalies involving the great vessels clearly demonstrate the superiority of 3D (Figs. 12.17, 12.18). Size difference, blood flow direction, spatial arrangement, or course of vessels are some of the information that can be visualized with the 3D glass-body mode. Typical anomalies enabling a good 3D image are transposition of the great arteries (Fig. 12.18B), right or double aortic arch, hypoplastic left heart syndrome, aortic coarctation; these can be well differentiated from a normal finding. The best view is generally obtained from a cranial-to-caudal acquisition from the mediastinum perspective or from the left upper side (Figs. 12.17, 12.18). Further examples are presented in Chapter 19.

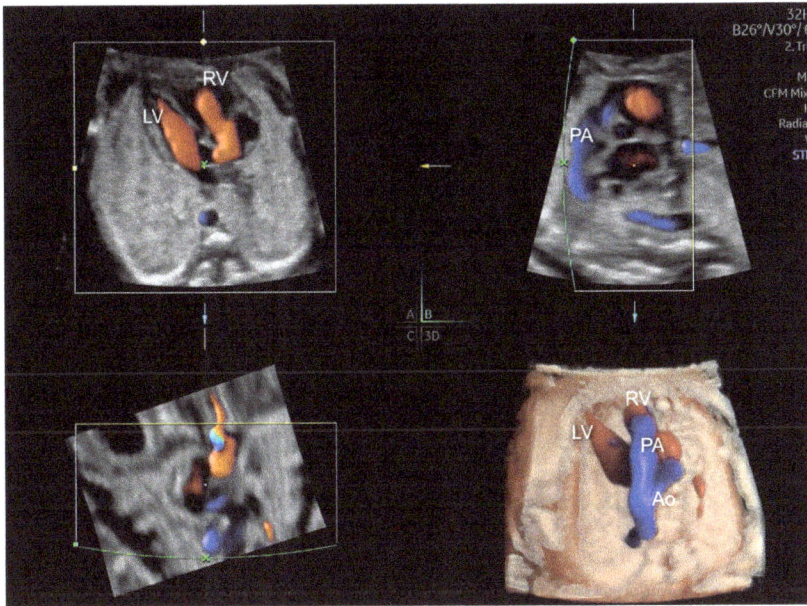

Fig. 12.17: STIC with color Doppler glass-body. The ventricles can be seen in the background, while the crossing of the great vessels appears in the foreground. Aorta (Ao), left ventricle (LV), pulmonary artery (PA), right ventricle (RV).

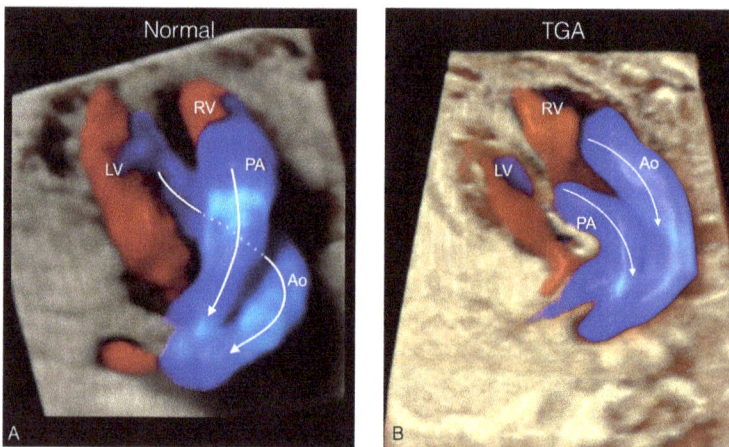

Fig. 12.18: STIC volume of a heart in glass-body mode with the view from cranial in a normal fetus (A) and in a fetus with d-transposition of the great arteries (TGA) (B). Note the normal crossing of the aorta (Ao) and pulmonary artery (PA) in (A) and its abnormal parallel course in (B). Left ventricle (LV), right ventricle (RV).

Intracerebral vessels: Intracerebral arteries and veins can be visualized with glass-body mode, ideally from a sagittal insonation in which the pericallosal artery along with the internal cerebral veins, the straight sinus, and the superior sagittal sinus can be demonstrated (Fig. 12.19). Another approach to the intracerebral arteries may be the axial view of the circle of Willis at the base of the skull (Fig. 12.20) or the transvaginal coronal view across the fontanelle (Fig. 12.21). Clinical conditions, such as the abnormal course of the anterior cerebral artery in complete or partial agenesis of the corpus callosum (see Chapter 16), abnormal vessels in aneurysmal malformation of the vein of Galen (Fig. 12.22), and other disorders can be well documented with this technique. Intracranial venous anatomy in 3D is a new area of research that examines the relationship between venous development and cortical maturation or focuses on the course of the veins in various brain anomalies. However, in these cases the best images are shown with the transvaginal approach (Fig. 12.21).

First trimester scan: The increasing importance of first trimester screening between 11 and 14 weeks of gestation was accompanied with the use of 3D in early pregnancy (see Chapter 20). Color Doppler is commonly used in the first trimester to examine the fetal heart and occasionally the umbilical cord, body, and cerebral vessels. These areas can also be examined with 3D glass-body mode. The approach is very similar to the regions described earlier in this chapter. Figures 12.23 and 12.24 show a glass-body mode of the fetal heart and Figure 12.25 of the fetal thorax and abdomen.

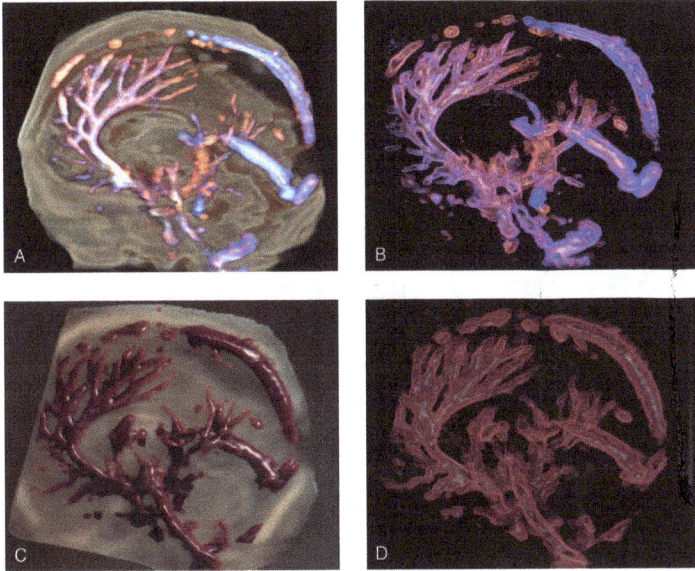

Fig. 12.19: Midsagittal view of intracranial arteries and veins in 3D glass-body display showing bidirectional flow in (A) and (B) and monochrome color in (C) and (D). In (A) and (C), the grayscale information is shown in silhouette mode, while in (B) and (D), only the color information is shown with the additional use of color silhouette mode.

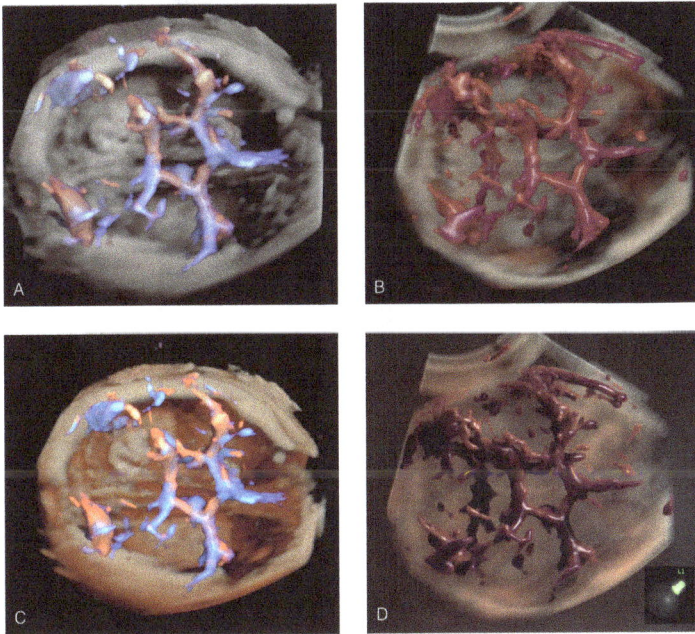

Fig. 12.20: Axial view of the circle of Willis in 3D glass-body mode with bidirectional color (A and C) and monochrome color (B and D) and different renderings additionally using silhouette mode for grayscale with transparency and light effects.

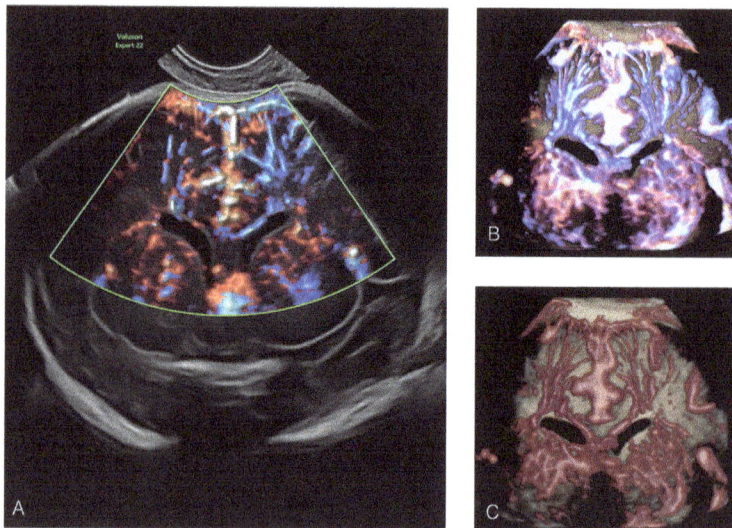

Fig. 12.21: Transvaginal examination of the vasculature of the brain parenchyma with slow-flow HD color Doppler allowing visualization of tiny medullary veins. In (B) and (C) after volume acquisition with glass-body mode in bidirectional and monochrome color, respectively.

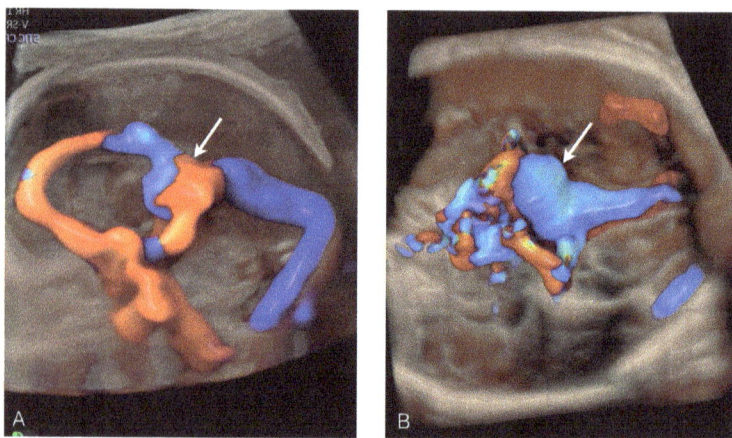

Fig. 12.22: Two fetuses with aneurysmal malformation of the vein of Galen (arrow) at 22 weeks (A) and 33 weeks of gestation (B), shown in glass-body mode. The view in (A) is from the side and in (B) from cranial.

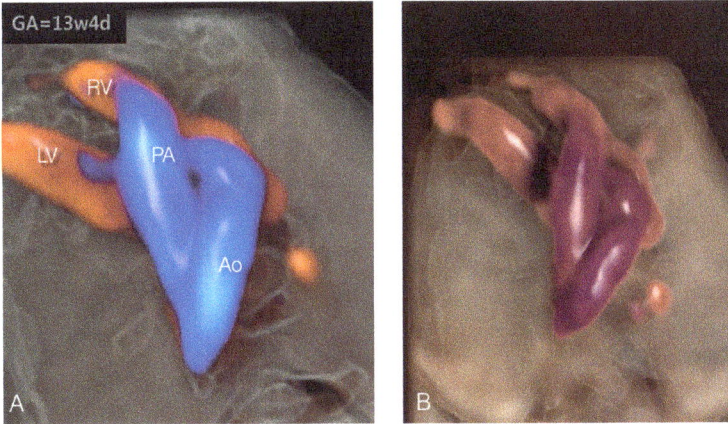

Fig. 12.23: STIC volumes of a normal heart at 13 weeks' gestation in glass-body mode with the filling of the right ventricle (RV) and left ventricle (LV) in the background and crossing of the pulmonary artery (PA) and aorta (Ao). (A) shows bidirectional flow and (B) monochrome flow. The images are similar to second trimester information (see Fig. 12.18) but are often more difficult to obtain due to the moving fetus in early pregnancy.

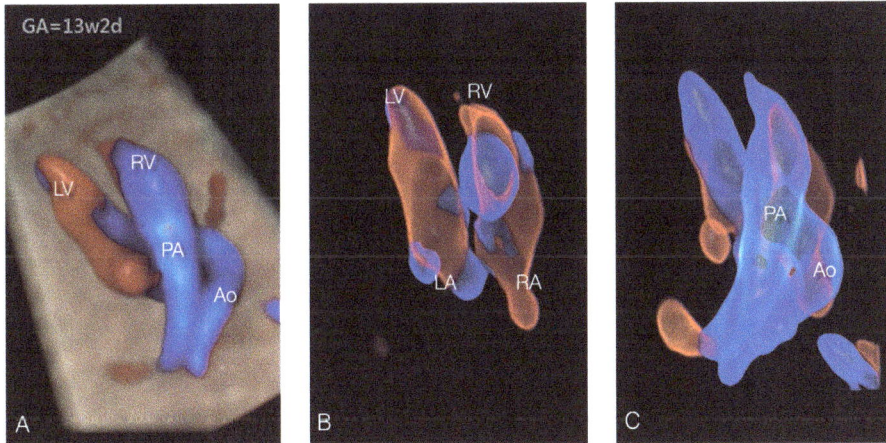

Fig. 12.24: STIC volume with color Doppler of a heart at 13 weeks, displayed in glass-body mode and showing both ventricles and the crossing of the great arteries in (A). In (B) and (C), the grayscale information was removed and the color Doppler silhouette mode was activated, showing four-chamber perfusion in diastole in (B) and crossing of the great vessels in systole in (C). Aorta (Ao), left atrium (LA), left ventricle (LV), pulmonary artery (PA), right atrium (RA), right ventricle (RV).

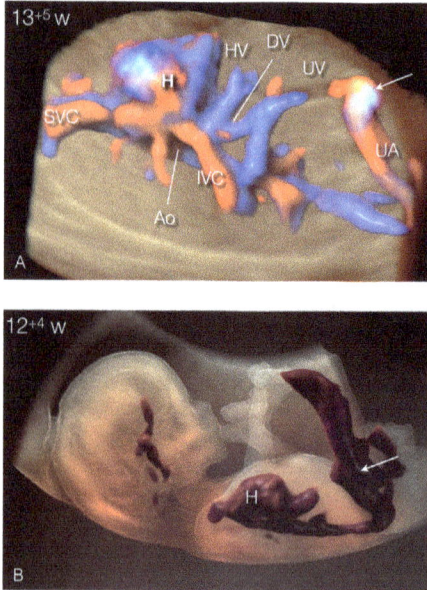

Fig. 12.25: Glass-body mode in the first trimester. (A) is a view from the right side of the body, similar to the second trimester, showing the abdominal and thoracic vasculature including the inferior vena cava (IVC) and superior vena cava (SVC), umbilical vein (UV) with ductus venosus (DV) and other vessels. In (B), an overview of the entire fetus at 12 weeks of gestation is displayed in silhouette mode and shows the vasculature in monochrome silhouette mode. The arrow points to the umbilical cord attachment on the abdominal wall. Aorta (Ao), heart (H), hepatic vein (HV), umbilical artery (UA).

12.4 Conclusions

Glass-body mode is generally used to visualize blood flow in the heart and vessels by combining color Doppler and 3D. Vessels can be viewed alone or together with neighboring structures displayed in grayscale. Not only the heart, but also other regions with well-developed vasculature such as the liver, brain, lungs, or placenta are regions of interest for the use of glass-body mode. Fetal cardiac examination provides spatial visualization of the heart with the crossing of the great vessels and can be useful for detailed fetal echocardiography.

13 Calculation of 3D Volumes

13.1 Principle

Fetal measurements are an integral part of prenatal ultrasound. During a routine examination, diameters, circumferences, or areas are measured and compared to reference ranges. Volume calculations are never performed during a screening examination; when necessary, the examiner simply makes an assessment based on an ideal shape of the region of interest, calculating distances and areas. Acquisition of a 3D volume is a good prerequisite for any reliable volume measurement. In the current available 3D software, there are a few techniques for volume calculation which, depending on the region of interest, can be quick and easy or time-consuming. In this chapter, two important tools for volume calculation are presented.

13.2 Practical approach

3D volume measurements can be performed in a variety of ways. The best known and most widely used method is the software VOCAL (see below). In recent years, additional tools have been introduced that allow automatic and rapid measurement of echolucent regions. It is likely that volume measurements in prenatal diagnosis will increase in the future so that there will be a need for simplified tools for that purpose. The few techniques available for performing volume measurements are quite time consuming in the implementation; this certainly explains in large part why most volume calculations are reported in research studies but not used in clinical practice. Two methods are presented below, namely the software VOCAL and Sono-AVC.

13.2.1 Virtual Organ Computer-aided Analysis (VOCAL) Software

VOCAL software is the commonly used technique to calculate a volume. Once a static 3D volume acquisition is stored, the structure to be measured is displayed in the orthogonal mode and magnified to be placed in the center of the image. After VOCAL is activated, a vertical line with two triangles at its two poles appears. The user manually moves each triangle and places it on the poles of the region to be measured (Fig. 13.1). In the next step, the contour drawing is selected: either manually (Fig. 13.2), semi-automatically, or automatically. Automatic contour drawing is reliable when a single echolucent structure with well-defined boundaries is selected, such as the stomach, bladder, or cyst. This is rarely the case. In most cases, such as the assessment of kidneys, lungs, placenta, and other structures, automatic detection of contours is difficult, so that selecting the manual or semi-automatic function is recommended. The user can then draw or modify the outline according to the ultrasound information on the screen (Fig.

https://doi.org/10.1515/9783111249513-013

13.2). Once drawing the outline is finished, this step is confirmed manually, and the image automatically changes to the next image by rotating it a few degrees around the longitudinal axis. The same steps are confirmed in each plane and manually corrected (Figs. 13.3, 13.4) until a complete rotation of 180° is achieved. The more rotation steps are selected, the more accurate the volume calculation becomes. Figures 13.1 through 13.5 show the step by step procedure for lung volume measurement with VOCAL. The visualization of the calculated volume is displayed on the screen at the end with either a solid or a mesh-like envelope (Fig. 13.5).

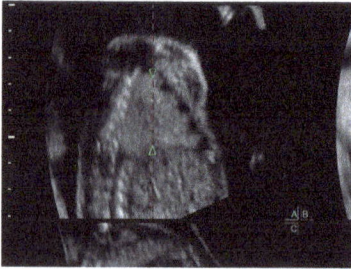

Fig. 13.1: 3D volume calculation with VOCAL step by step: after the region of interest has been displayed in orthogonal mode, the VOCAL tool is selected. A vertical line with two triangles appears. These are manually placed at the two poles of the selected region, in this case the lung.

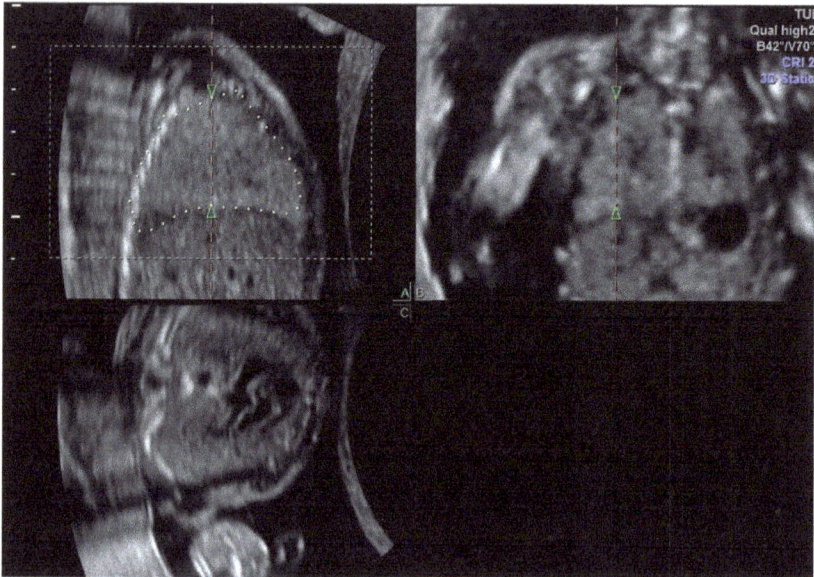

Fig. 13.2: The next step of the VOCAL volume calculation (see Fig. 13.1) involves zooming in on the region of interest and placing the triangles at the poles; the type of outline drawing is then selected, either manually or semi-automatically. Once the outline is well drawn, the measurement is confirmed and the volume is automatically rotated to the next image.

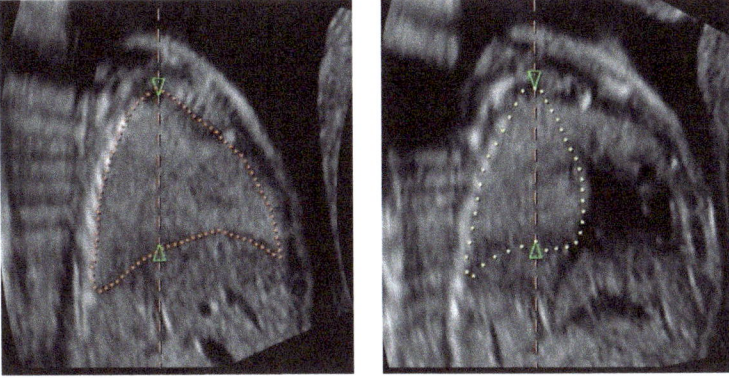

Fig. 13.3: In the next step of the VOCAL volume calculation (see Figs. 13.1 and 13.2) the user now proceeds image by image similarly to Figure 13.2, draws the outline and confirms the result until all steps are done. The number of rotations is selected by the operator before the volume calculation.

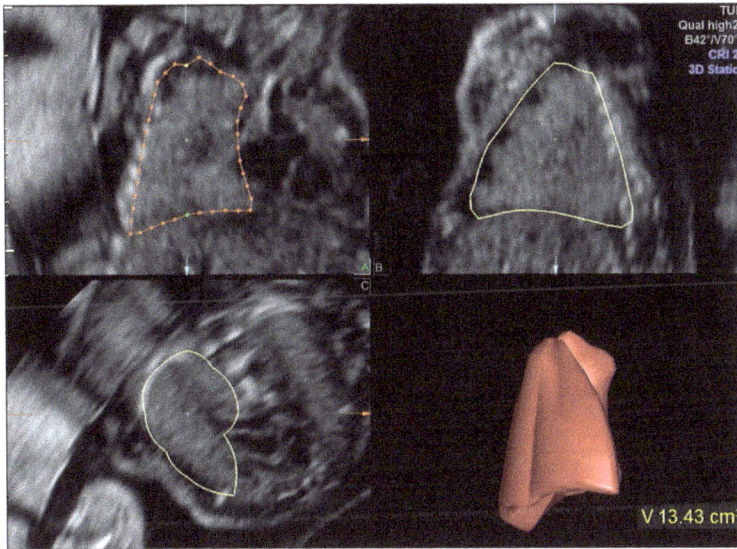

Fig. 13.4: In the next step of the VOCAL volume calculation (see Figs. 13.1 to 13.3), after finishing the previous steps of drawing the lines and rotating the volume, the result of the calculation is displayed on the screen in the bottom right panel, here the lung. Some corrections can be made on the screen by checking one or another plane to adjust the contour drawings.

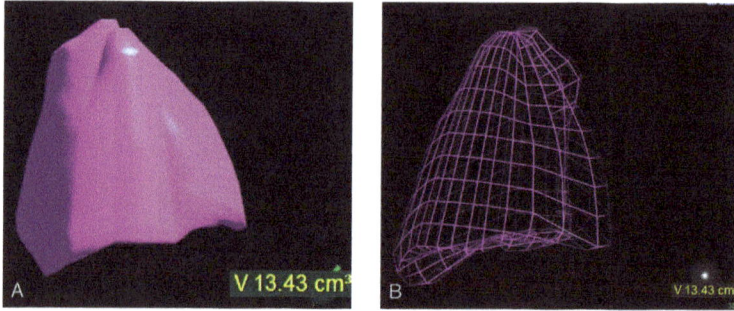

Fig. 13.5: 3D VOCAL result for the previously calculated lung. The result can be displayed in different colors as a solid surface (left) or as a mesh (right).

13.2.2 Sonographic Automatic Volume Calculation (Sono-AVC)

Another volume calculation software is more commonly used in gynecologic ultrasound for automatic measurement of cysts and follicles. The software automatically recognizes single or multiple echolucent areas as cysts and calculates the corresponding volumes accordingly (Figs. 13.6–13.10). The user selects the area containing the organs to be examined by inserting them into the render box. The structures to be measured can be selectively added or removed by a simple mouse click and a button on the trackball. It should be noted that the software automatically detects echolucent areas and

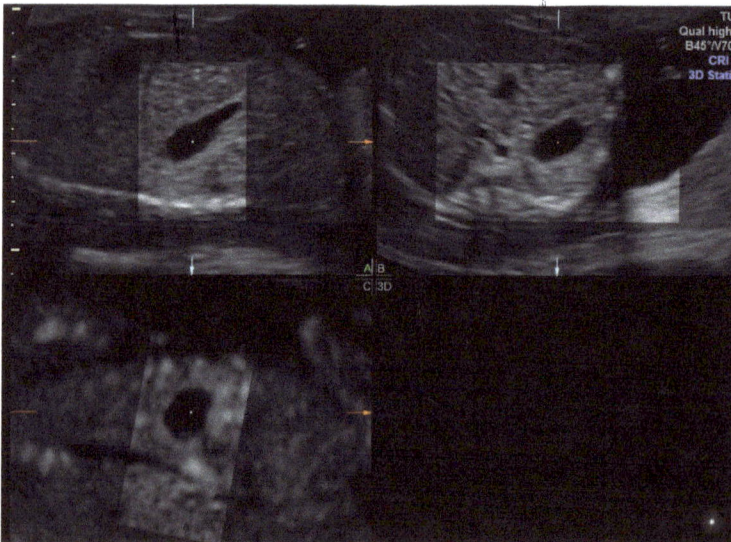

Fig. 13.6: 3D volume calculation with Sonographic Automatic Volume Calculation (Sono-AVC). After selecting the region of interest where the fluid is to be measured (here the stomach), the region can be selectively clicked with the mouse, activating Sono-AVC (see Fig. 13.7).

therefore shadows may cause artifacts. On the other hand, this technique is the fastest technique for volume calculation of fluid filled structures, especially when multiple cysts need to be measured (Fig. 13.10). Therefore, measurement of a filled stomach (Figs. 13.7, 13.8), fluid volume in the dilated renal pelvis (Fig. 13.9), or cyst volume in multicystic kidneys (Fig. 13.10) can be easily calculated.

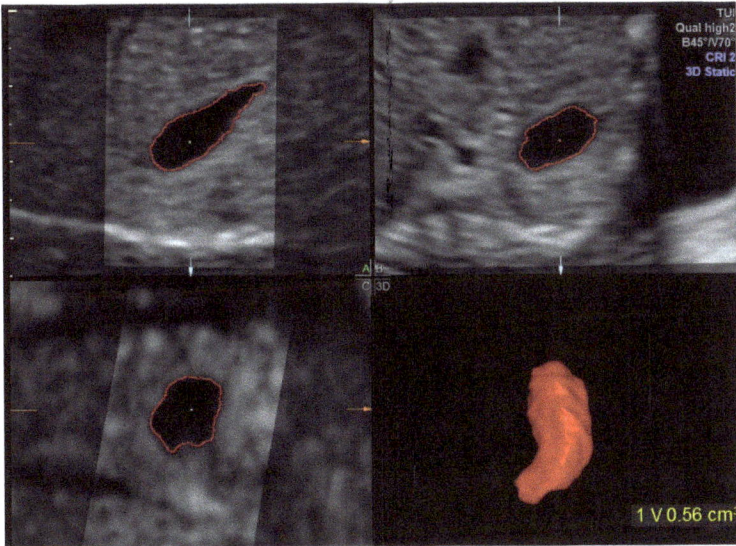

Fig. 13.7: 3D volume calculation with Sono-AVC. After a mouse click, the liquid is identified and the volume is displayed. The 3D shape of the stomach is displayed and the volume is calculated.

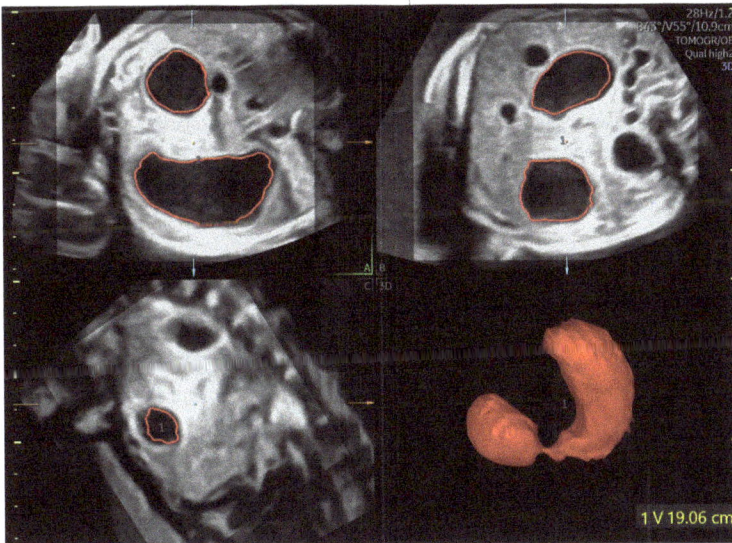

Fig. 13.8: 3D volume calculation with Sono-AVC, here in a fetus with double bubble sign in duodenal atresia.

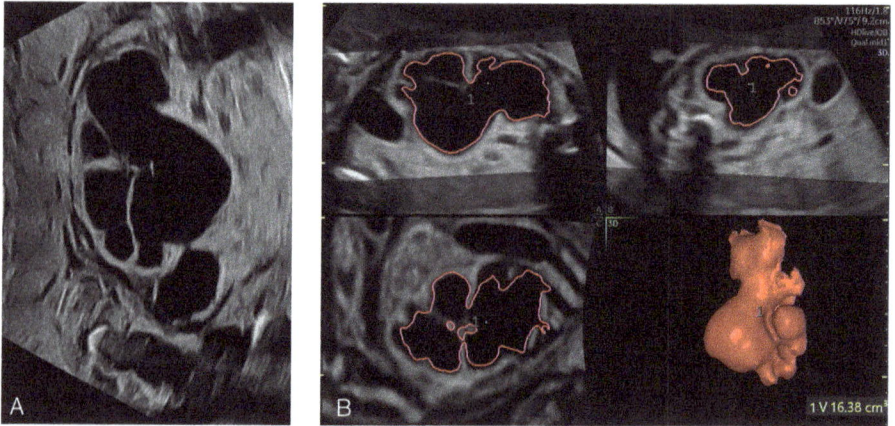

Fig. 13.9: 3D volume calculation with Sono-AVC in a fetus with hydronephrosis in pelvic ureteral junction obstruction.

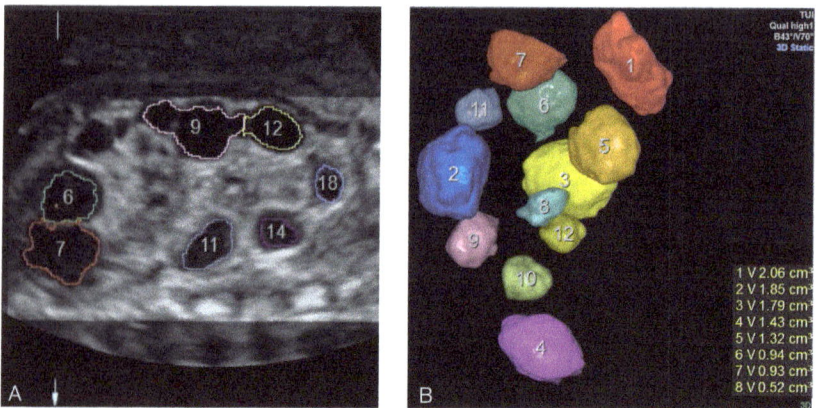

Fig. 13.10: 3D volume calculation with Sono-AVC in a fetus with multicystic renal dysplasia. The volumes of the different cysts can be calculated and displayed separately. The measurements are shown in different colors for the different cysts and the numbers refer to the measured region.

13.3 Typical applications of volume calculations

Volume calculations and corresponding reference ranges for early gestation were published and include volume of placenta, amniotic sac, and embryo. The lung is another organ commonly measured in normal fetuses and in fetuses at high risk for pulmonary hypoplasia. Volume measurements have been performed for various fetal structures, such as the liver, brain, placenta, kidneys, lateral ventricles, cardiac cavities, and others. One of the main applications of volume measurements is to estimate fetal weight by calculating the volume of an extremity or in combination with other volume measurements. However, routine use of volume calculation is still uncommon and is performed in obstetrics mainly in research studies.

13.4 Conclusions

In selected cases 3D volume measurements are becoming important in prenatal ultrasound, but performing such calculations is still time consuming. VOCAL and Sono-AVC are the most often used instruments and require a certain level of experience before they can be used effectively and easily, limiting their application in routine ultrasound examinations.

14 The Electronic Matrix Transducer

14.1 Principle

One of the special features of an electronic matrix probe is that the transducer has multiple rows of crystals instead of one as found in conventional mechanical transducers. With these multiple rows of crystals (64 rows in some cases), the transducer has a footprint of more than 8,000 elements, hence the term *matrix array transducers*. In conventional mechanical 3D probe, a single row of crystals is used to generate the 2D image. Once the 3D acquisition is selected, a mechanical motor sweeps the ultrasound beam, creating multiple 2D planes that are assembled into a 3D volume. By using fast computer processors, matrix probes can electronically steer the ultrasound beam through a selected volume box and acquire volumes two to four times faster than a mechanical 3D transducer. For this reason, an electronic volume transducer offers several advantages over a conventional mechanical volume transducer. These include the following:

– The high number of electronically controllable crystal elements is reflected in an improved image in both B-mode and color Doppler.
– Acquisition of 3D/4D volumes is significantly faster with the electronic transducer. For example, STIC volume acquisition with an electronic transducer takes only 2–3 seconds compared to 7.5–15 seconds with a mechanical 3D transducer. This is the reason why even an examination in real-time 4D or with VCI-A runs much smoother and with a higher frame rate than with a mechanical 3D transducer.
– With the electronic 3D/4D transducer, it is possible to perform the examination with a slice thickness. This is now also possible during the 2D examination. The software highlights certain image contents (bones, soft tissues) that are defined by the examiner and hides other areas. The slice thickness can be defined with a selection from 2 to 20 mm.
– Another important application that is only possible with a matrix transducer is the simultaneous display of two orthogonal planes as a so-called biplane display. This allows the operator to examine in real-time one plane for a structure of interest and simultaneously the corresponding perpendicular sectional image in dual mode. In contrast to the sectional images in the context of a 3D volume image, these are two original and not digitally reconstructed ultrasound images. Depending on the question of interest, the examiner places the camera line in the first image, generates the corresponding orthogonal image in real-time, and can change the position of the line.

https://doi.org/10.1515/9783111249513-014

14.2 Biplane display

14.2.1 Practical approach

The examination is first performed in 2D with the matrix transducer and the area to be examined is selected. In addition to optimizing the image, it is helpful to keep the aperture angle of the image as narrow as possible before switching to the biplane function. The image is divided into two images, A and B (dual image) (Fig. 14.1). The left image (plane A) shows the native image. In addition, a vertical line ("camera line") is placed by the examiner on the structure to be examined. The right image (plane B) corresponds to the orthogonal image along the line in image A (Fig. 14.1). During the examination in plane A, images are created simultaneously in plane B along the camera line at 90° angle to image A. The biplane examination can be performed in grayscale or in combination with color Doppler. The authors recommend that the user simply try working with this interesting imaging tool.

14.2.2 Typical applications of the biplane display

Once the user has practiced the biplane display in many examinations, he or she will realize that this new scanning modality is not limited to screening examinations but can also be used in cases of suspected fetal anomalies.

Examination of the head and face: Head and face are routinely examined in multiple planes in 2D and 3D multiplanar modes. The biplane mode therefore provides an ideal tool for visualizing many anatomical structures. For example, while the head is examined in a transverse plane, the biplane image can simultaneously visualize the cavum septi pellucidi, lateral ventricles, Sylvian fissure, or posterior fossa. Anomalies of the brain can be well visualized and verified with the biplane mode in both planes, such as agenesis of the corpus callosum, absent septum pellucidum, and others. Figures 14.11 to 14.3 illustrate the use of the biplane in brain assessment.

The biplane mode is particularly useful in the evaluation of the fetal face, where examination best starts from the profile with sagittal insonation. It is probably easier to obtain a profile while tilting the biplane line from the plane of the eyes to the nose and then to the maxilla and mandible (Figs. 14.4, 14.5). Facial anomalies such as cleft lip and palate (Fig. 14.6) and other malformations can be clearly visualized and identified with the biplane mode. A similar approach can already be taken in a first trimester screening examination (Fig. 14.7).

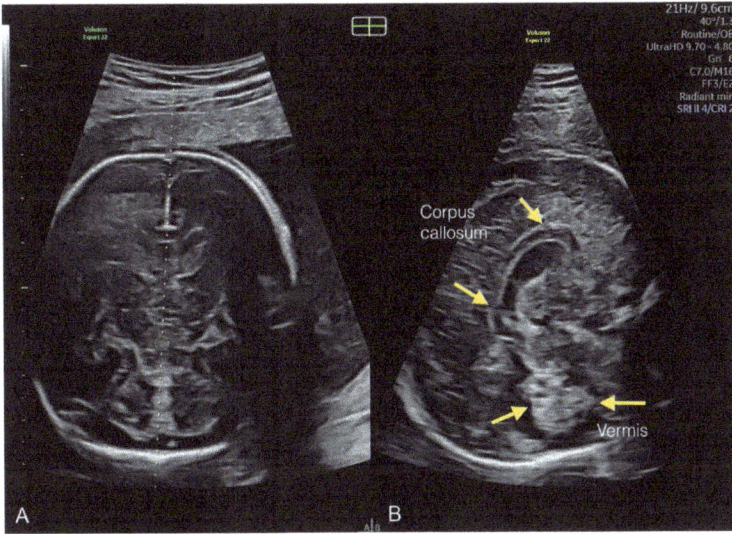

Fig. 14.1: Examination of the head with the biplane through the forehead in (A), showing the midsagittal view of the corpus callosum (arrows) in (B).

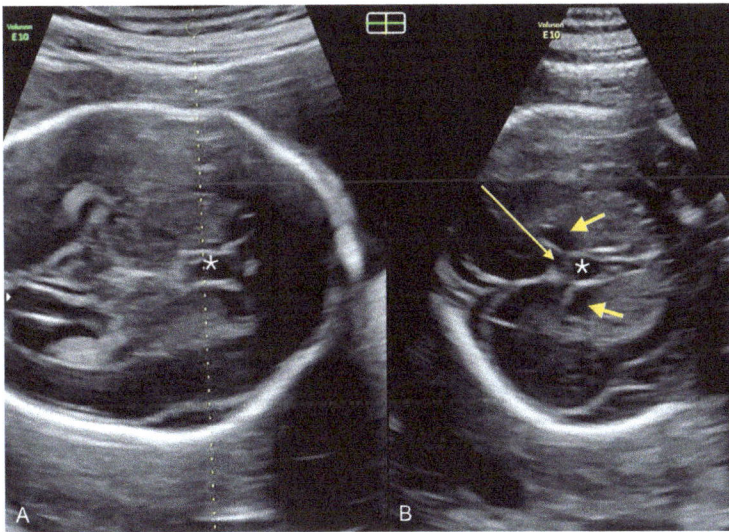

Fig. 14.2: Examination of the brain in biplane mode at the level of the cavum septi pellucidi (*) in both orthogonal planes. The plane on the left (A) is the standard axial plane of the head. The image on the right (B) shows the two anterior horns (short arrows) and the corpus callosum (long arrow).

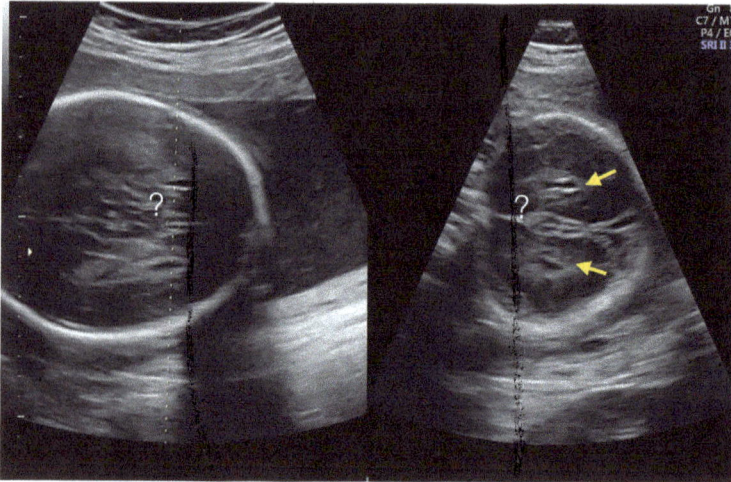

Fig. 14.3: Agenesis of the corpus callosum shown in biplane mode. The head is examined in the standard axial plane, as in Figure 14.2, but in this case the cavum septi pellucidi is absent in both planes (?). In the bi-plane image on the right, the anterior horns are displaced laterally.

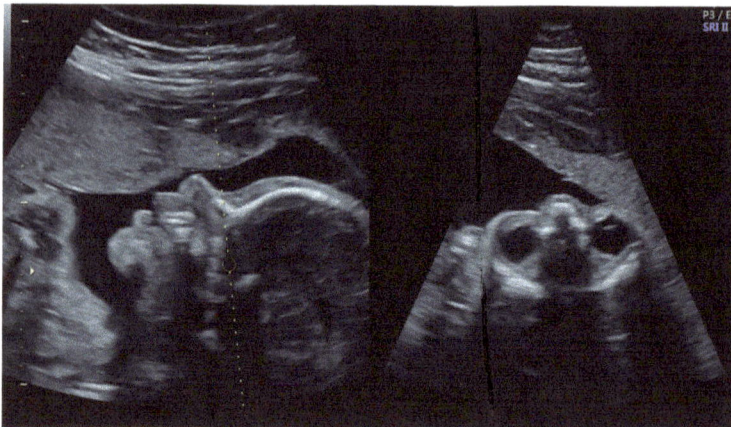

Fig. 14.4: Examination of the fetal face in biplane mode. The profile of the fetus is visualized and the bi-plane is placed at the level of the eyes. The eyes are not visible in plane A, but the orthogonal biplane image shows both the eyes and the orbits.

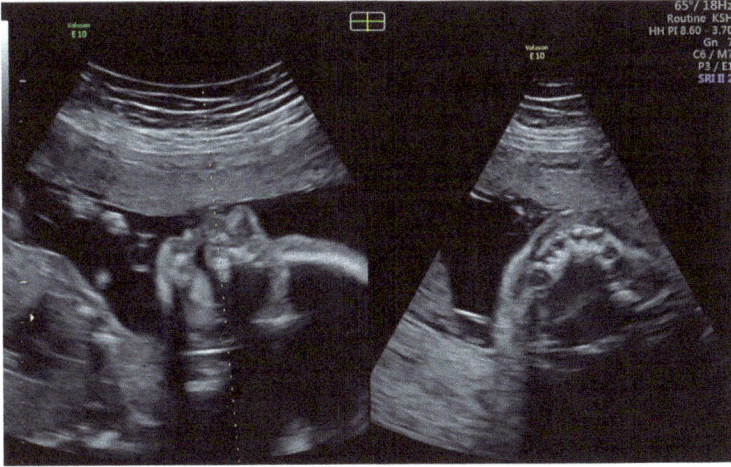

Fig. 14.5: Biplane mode of the face. The profile is as in Figure 14.4, but the biplane line is now at the level of the mouth so that the intact upper jaw is visible.

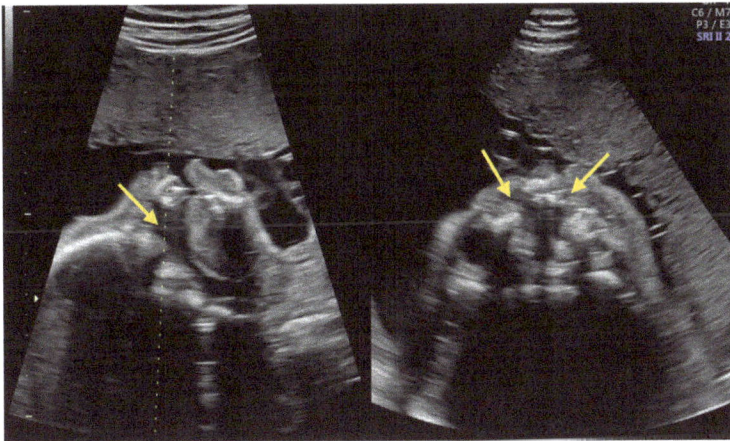

Fig. 14.6: Biplane visualization of the face in bilateral cleft lip and palate (arrows). The biplane examination is performed by visualizing the profile and placing the line along the maxilla.

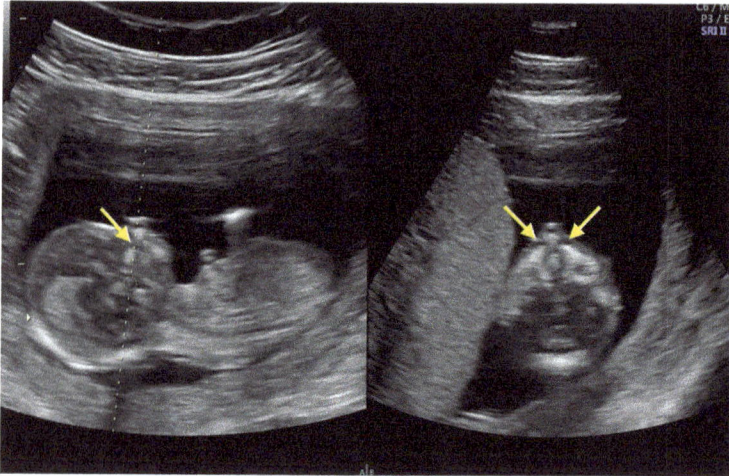

Fig. 14.7: Biplane mode in a bilateral cleft lip and palate (arrows) in a fetus at 13 weeks of gestation. The left image shows the "maxillary gap" where the line is placed, and the suspicion is confirmed in the resulting biplane image.

Examination of the heart: The biplane mode is an interesting tool for the examination of the heart, thorax, and mediastinum. At the level of the heart, the four-chamber view or the three-vessel and trachea view can be examined, while at the same time a sagittal section of the aortic arch or ductal arch (Fig. 14.8) can be visualized. The visualization of the interventricular septum in two planes is interesting, especially the direct view of the septal surface (Fig. 14.9). This novel view allows the integrity of the interventricular septum to be checked in grayscale or in combination with color Doppler (Fig. 14.10). Figures 14.8 to 14.10 show examples of fetal hearts under normal and abnormal conditions.

Examination of the chest, abdomen, skeletal system, and other areas: Biplane display can be used for other body organs as well. Visualization of the spine in two planes can be well achieved and can be helpful in assessing the level of a spinal defect or hemivertebra. The lungs and abdominal organs can also be examined in biplane mode, and this visualization makes it easier to get a better overview of normal and abnormal conditions. Figure 14.11 shows an example of a fetus with pleural effusion in biplane mode.

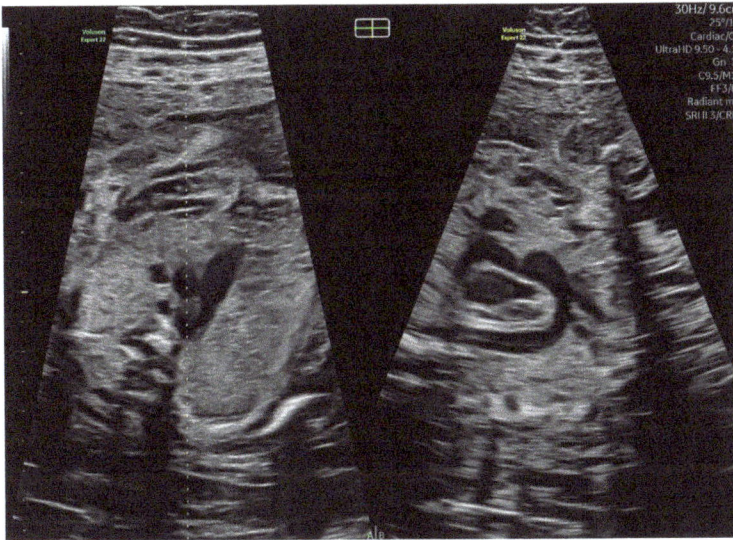

Fig. 14.8: Biplane mode in a normal heart. The examination is performed in the three-vessel trachea view plane (left). In the biplane view, the aortic arch is displayed simultaneously.

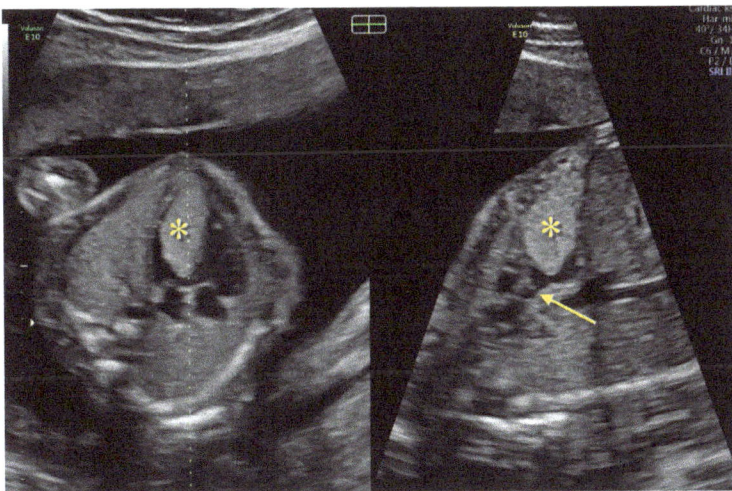

Fig. 14.9: Biplane view of the interventricular septum in a fetus with rhabdomyoma. A large rhabdomyoma (*) is in the region of the interventricular septum and left ventricle. In biplane mode, it is seen that the aortic valve is not obstructed by the tumor (arrow).

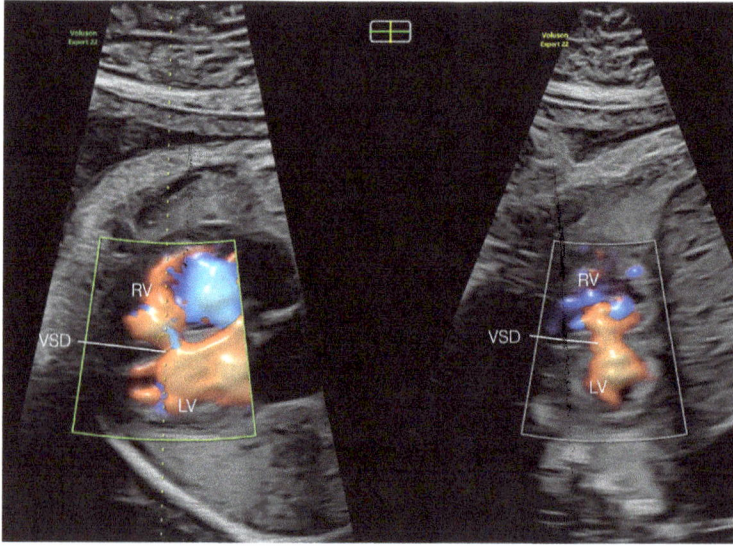

Fig. 14.10: Biplane imaging in color Doppler in a heart with a muscular ventricular septal defect (VSD). The defect is suspected in the left image and confirmed in the right image. Left ventricle (LV), right ventricle (RV).

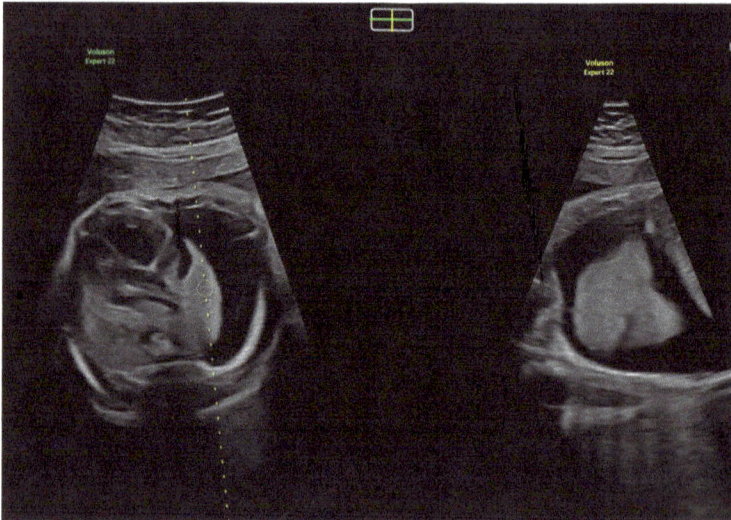

Fig. 14.11: Biplane visualization of a right-sided hydrothorax. In the left image, the pleural effusion can be seen; its extent can be seen better in the orthogonal sagittal plane.

14.3 Volume Contrast Imaging of the A-plane (VCI-A)

14.3.1 Practical approach

The principle of VCI was explained in Chapter 4 and is based on highlighting a thin layer (1–20 mm) from the static 3D volume data set to improve detail detection while reducing artifacts. In static 3D (see Chapter 4), all three orthogonal planes A, B and C are highlighted simultaneously. VCI can also be applied in a real-time 4D examination in which only the examination plane, namely plane A, is highlighted; it is therefore called VCI-A. VCI-A can be used with a mechanical transducer, but the full power of this tool in terms of frame rate and resolution can be better achieved with the electronic matrix transducer. The slice thickness as well as the rendering used to visualize the organ of interest can be selected live during the examination. Different rendering modes, such as tissue mode (X-Ray), maximum mode (skeleton), minimum mode, surface mode, and inversion mode can be selected, as explained in Chapter 4 for static VCI (see Fig. 4.3). From our clinical experience, we mainly use the VCI-A in tissue mode with a thin slice for soft tissue organ examination and in maximum mode with a thick slice for bones imaging, as explained below.

14.3.2 Typical applications of the VCI-A display

VCI-A tissue mode for soft tissue examination: When activating this function, the operator examines in the usual examination plane (plane A), but with 3D slice thickness activated. The tissue rendering mode (X-Ray) can focus on increasing soft tissue contrast by selecting a slice of a few millimeters (1–5 mm). This contrast enhancement significantly increases the plasticity of the images obtained (Figs. 14.12–14.14). This tool is appropriate for the examination of the fetal heart (Figs. 14.12, 14.13), brain (Fig. 14.15), abdomen (Fig. 14.16), and thorax. In the thorax, the contrast between myocardium, lumen and lungs can be well discriminated (Figs. 14.12–14.14). In the abdomen, the bowel, kidneys, liver, and diaphragm have different echogenicities and can also be well delineated with VCI-A for tissue (Figs. 14.14, 14.16). For these indications, we usually use a slice thickness between 2–5 mm, depending on the clinical case and gestational age. Figures 14.12 to 14.16 show images acquired with VCI-A for soft tissue.

VCI-A maximum mode for skeletal examination: The VCI-A examination technique explained above is particularly appropriate for imaging the bony skeleton. The operator selects a slice from 8 mm to 20 mm in the second or third trimester. At a 10 mm thickness for example, 5 mm are in front of the examination plane and 5 mm are behind; it is then processed in the 3D calculation. The layer content is then rendered in real-time in maximum mode (see Chapter 8). In clinical practice, the authors choose a slice thickness of 8 mm to 14 mm and use VCI-A when visualizing the extremities, the spine, as well as the cranial bones (Figs. 14.17–14.22). With this approach, the entire hand can be imaged, even when the fingers are flexed. Similarly, imaging of the cranial bones and sutures can be routinely performed. It is important to emphasize that this volume imaging also has great potential in the first trimester, as the entire fetus can be imaged using the skeletal mode.

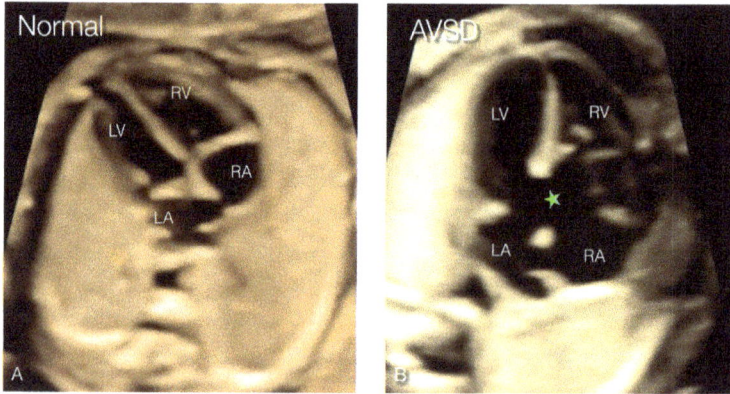

Fig. 14.12: Volume Contrast Imaging (VCI) in the A-plane, called VCI-A, shown here with soft tissue enhancement in two fetal hearts at a slice thickness of 4 mm and with X-Ray mode display. (A) shows a normal four-chamber view, whereas (B) shows a heart with an atrioventricular septal defect (AVSD), where the defect (star) is clearly visible. Left atrium (LA), left ventricle (LV), right atrium (RA), right ventricle (RV).

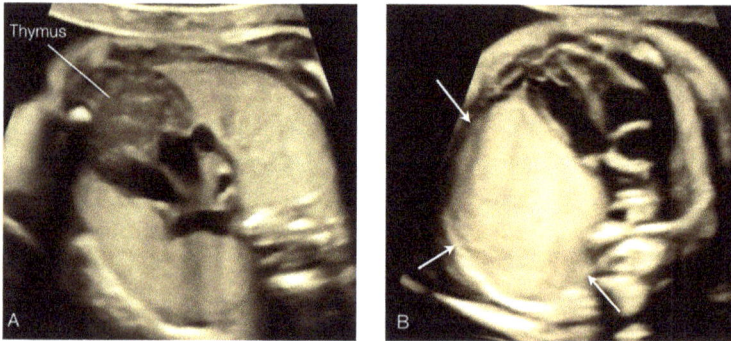

Fig. 14.13: VCI-A of two hearts showing soft tissue enhancement in (A) at the level of the three-vessel trachea view with the dark-appearing thymus clearly visible between the two bright lungs. In (B), the heart is displaced to the right by an enlarged hyperechogenic left lung (arrows).

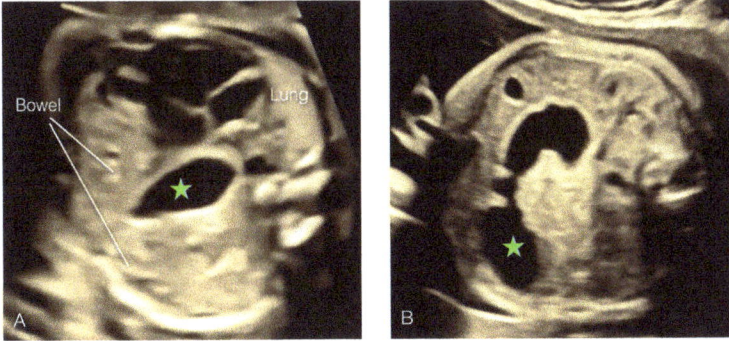

Fig. 14.14: VCI-A of two stomachs in fetal anomalies: in (A) congenital diaphragmatic hernia and in (B) double bubble sign in duodenal atresia. The increased contrast in (A) allows good differentiation of the tissue not only of the stomach (star) shape, but also between the intestine and the lung. (B) shows double bubble (star) with dilated stomach and duodenum.

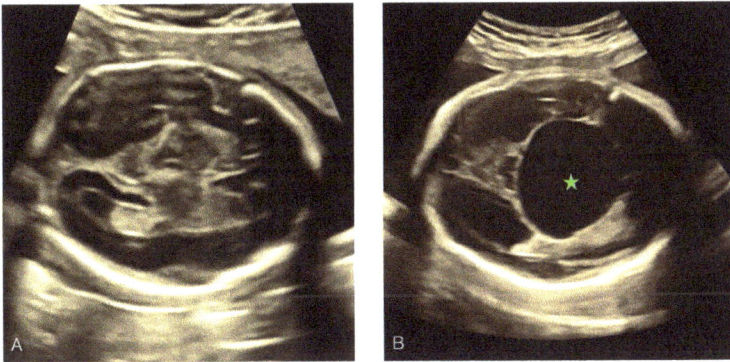

Fig. 14.15: VCI-A of the fetal head with brain in a normal fetus showing the symmetrical intracerebral structures in (A) and (B) showing a large interhemispheric cyst (star).

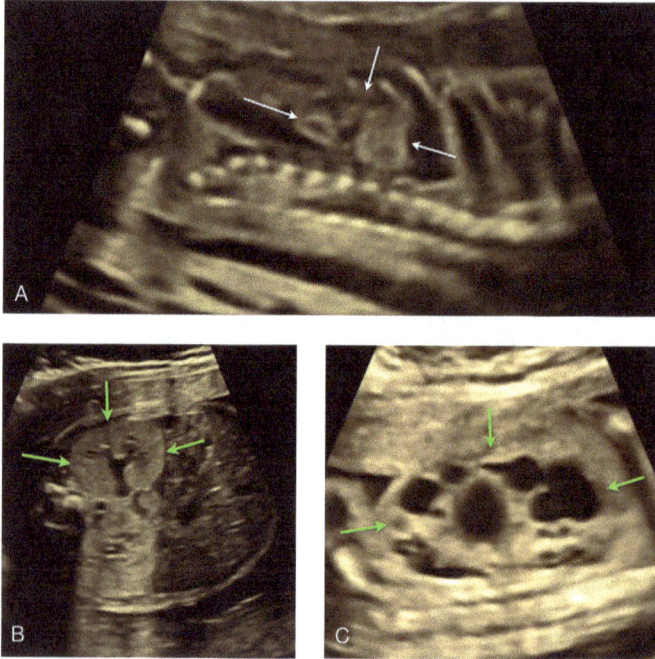

Fig. 14.16: VCI-A of a fetus with normal kidney (A) (white arrows) and two fetuses with abnormal kidney anatomy. The fetus in (B) had enlarged hyperechogenic kidneys (arrows) and the fetus in (C) had multicystic renal dysplasia with numerous cysts of different sizes.

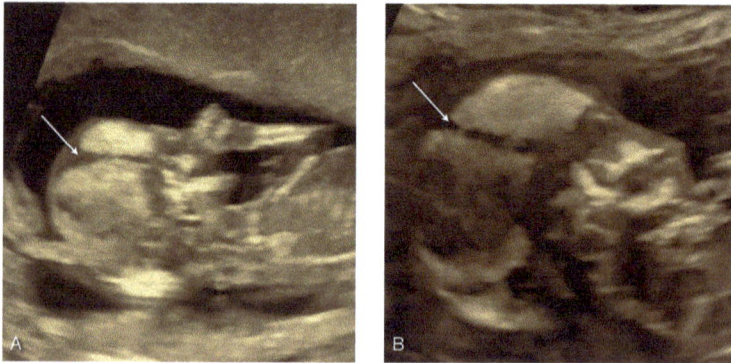

Fig. 14.17: VCI-A for bones shows a parasagittal view of the face with a lateral view of the skull in two fetuses at 14 and 22 weeks of gestation. Note the coronal suture (arrow) in both fetuses and some of the facial bones in these views. In (A) the slice thickness is 12 mm and in (B) 13 mm.

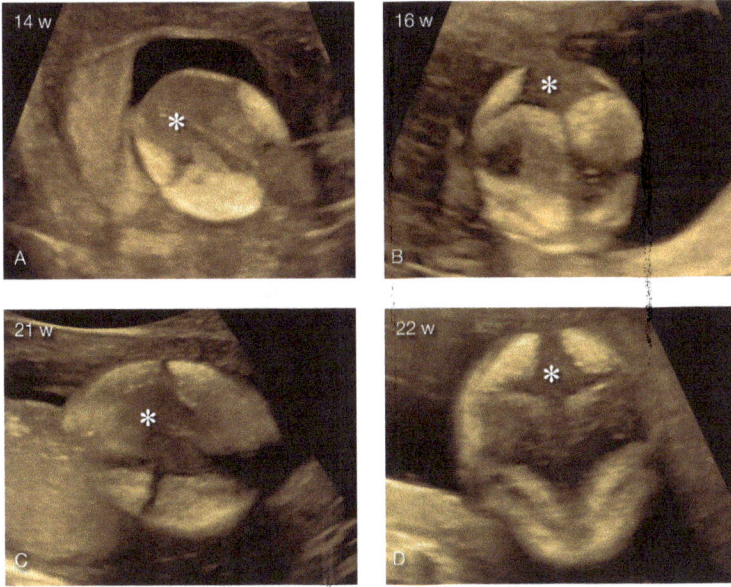

Fig. 14.18: VCI-A for bones shows a view of the top of the skull with the fontanelle (*) well demonstrated at different gestational ages. The layer thickness is 10 mm in all four cases.

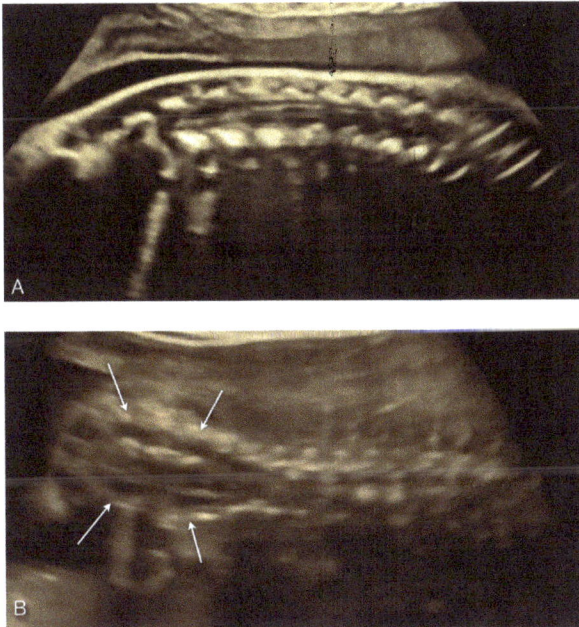

Fig. 14.19: VCI-A for bones shows a lumbar spine in a normal fetus (A) and in (B) a fetus with open spina bifida (arrows) with a frontal view of the lesion.

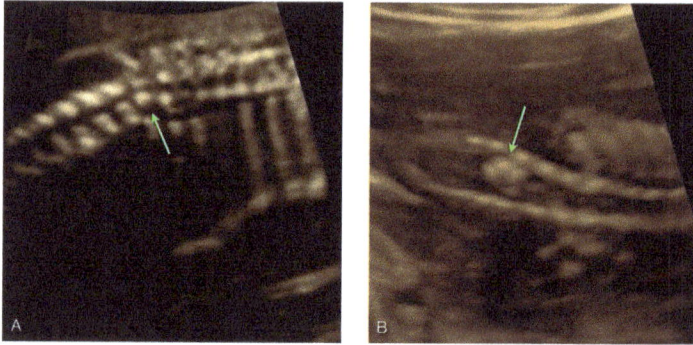

Fig. 14.20: VCI-A for bones showing a frontal view in a fetus (A) with hemivertebra (arrow) and in a fetus (B) with a bone spur in diastematomyelia (arrow).

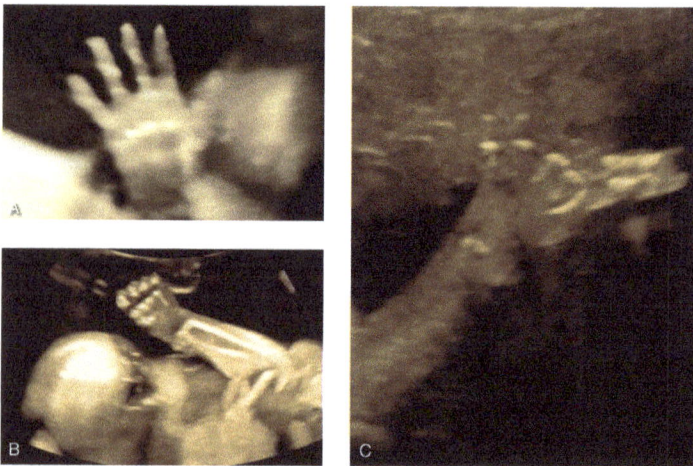

Fig. 14.21: VCI-A for bones showing the hands in two normal fetuses (A and B) and one abnormal case (C). In (A) the hand and in (B) the forearm with hand can be seen, while in fetus (C) a split hand can be recognized.

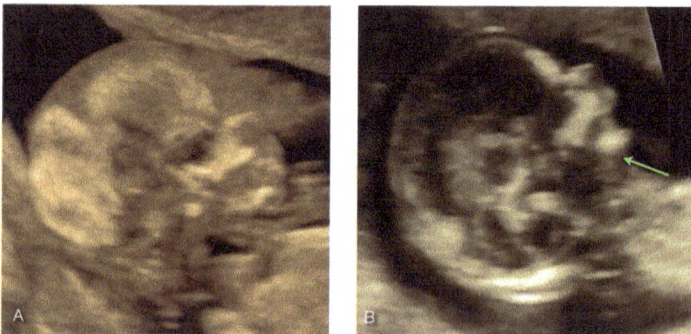

Fig. 14.22: VCI-A for bones showing the profile of two fetuses: in (A) with normal maxilla and mandible and in (B) with retrognathia (arrow).

14.4 The new tool VCI-2D

Recently, new software for the electronic matrix transducer was introduced, based on the experience of VCI-A rendering. Like the VCI-A approach, the matrix transducer uses a layer of a few millimeters instead of a single plane to perform the 2D examination. With this software, called VCI-2D, the image resolution is higher than that of a simple 2D or VCI-A image, and the operator can choose the slice thickness (1–20 mm) and image quality (tissue or bone). This is a promising new approach that uses 3D imaging algorithms for a 2D examination. Figures 14.23 and 14.24 show first examples of this new technique.

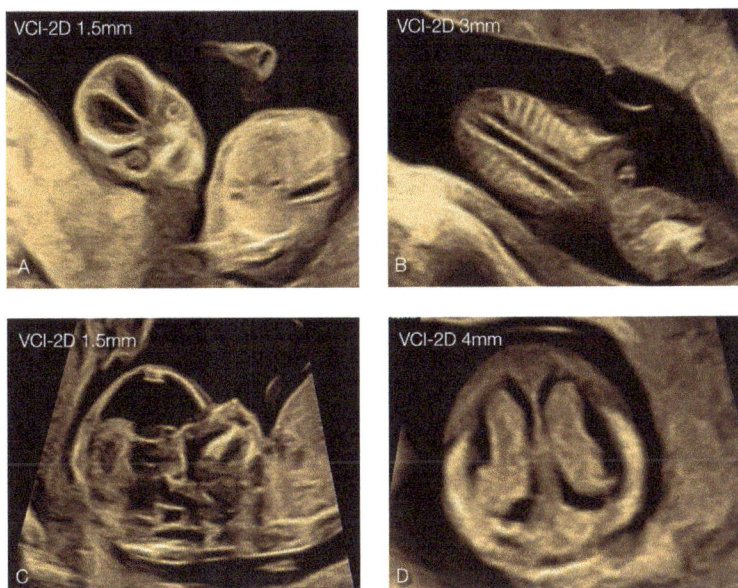

Fig. 14.23: A recent technological development of the electronic matrix probe is the ability to examine in 2D with a layer instead of a simple plane. This thickness approach is called VCI-2D, and the thickness can be selected. Images of these first trimester fetuses show increased contrast and detail. The selected slice thickness is displayed.

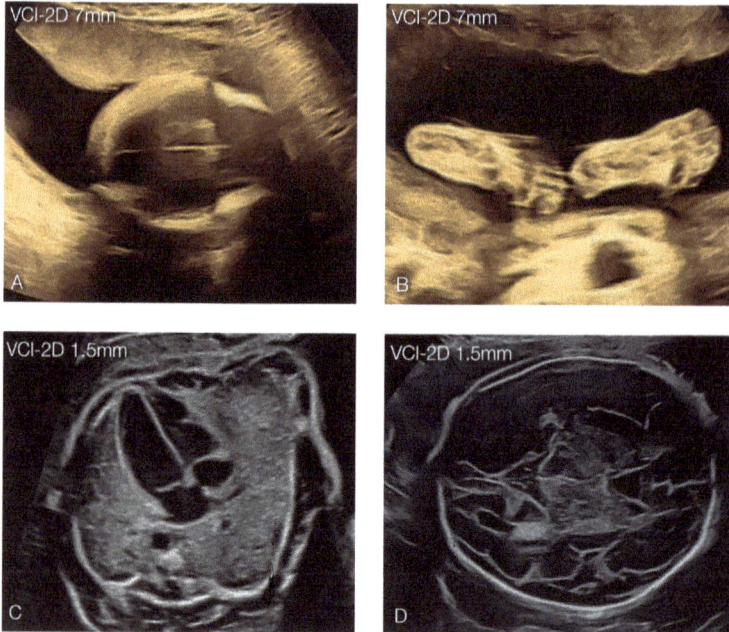

Fig. 14.24: As explained in Figure 14.23, these are additional examples of the use of VCI-2D. These examinations were performed at 22 weeks (A to C) and 28 weeks of gestation. Note how slice thickness increases resolution and contrast.

14.5 Conclusions

The basics of the electronic matrix transducer have already been explained in Chapter 1, and the application of real-time 4D has been discussed in Chapter 1 and Chapter 15. The most important aspect to emphasize is that with an electronic transducer and with the increasing computational capacity of today's processors, 4D image sequences can be acquired and displayed in near real-time. Therefore, we prefer the matrix to the mechanical probe for a 4D examination, especially since the images can be displayed at higher resolution throughout the pregnancy. See Chapter 15 for examples of fetal facial expressions and grimaces acquired with this transducer in the third trimester. Real-time 4D is also a good tool for live 4D examination of the fetal heart, but eSTIC acquisition is recommended because of its better postprocessing capabilities. The eSTIC acquisition is not only very fast, but also has a higher resolution. Unfortunately, the fine details discussed in this chapter on 4D live acquisition are difficult to capture in still images as showed in this book. Therefore, we recommend that the operator tries out the electronic transducer and discovers what this probe can do with the various tools presented in this chapter.

Part III: **Clinical Applications in Prenatal Diagnosis**

15 The Fetal Face in 3D

15.1 Examination of the face in 2D and 3D ultrasound

A comprehensive examination of the fetal face with 2D ultrasound usually includes the midsagittal view, which is the profile, and a series of parallel axial views showing both orbits, the nose, the upper and lower lip, the maxilla, the mandible, and ideally the hard palate. In addition, one or both ears may be visualized if possible. The profile is one of the most important views a pregnant woman expects to see, as it is one of the few ultrasound images that a layperson can easily recognize. Today, the best way to visualize a fetal face in 3D is with surface rendering (see Chapter 7). One of the main advantages of 3D surface rendering is the ability to represent the entire face in a single realistic view, thus personifying the fetus and intensifying the bond between the parents and the unborn child. It is also interesting to observe how the facial features change as the pregnancy progresses (Fig. 15.1). At the beginning of the third trimester, the images of the face remarkably resemble the newborn´s facial features (see below). The operator using 3D ultrasound will perform more than 80% of 3D/4D imaging of the fetal face compared to other organs during his or her practice. For this reason, we have

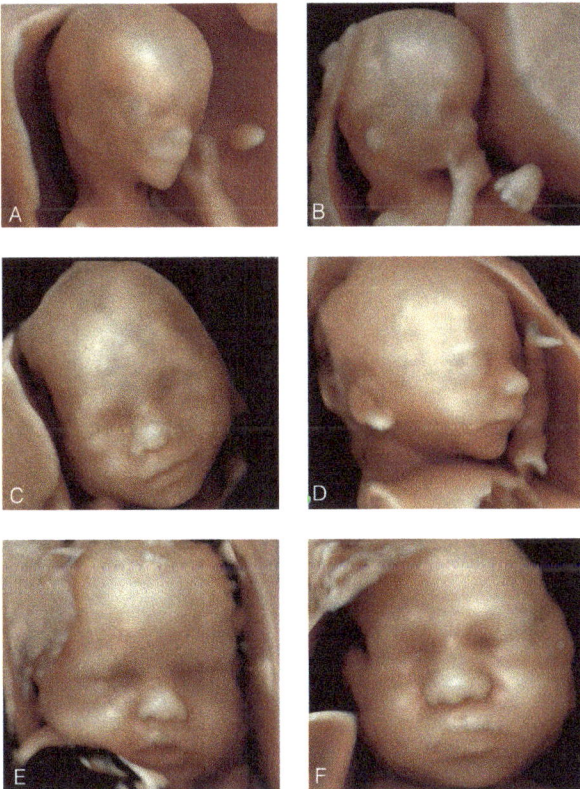

Fig. 15.1: Fetal faces in 3D surface mode. The appearance of the fetal face changes significantly during gestation, with subcutaneous tissue increasing in the third trimester. See the difference between 12 weeks (A and B), 22 weeks (C and D) and after 30 weeks of gestation (E and F).

https://doi.org/10.1515/9783111249513-015

dedicated a separate chapter to the fetal face. Examination of the fetal face can be performed using surface mode, multiplanar mode, and skeletal mode. In this chapter, we will discuss the first two, highlighting normal and abnormal findings, while the bony face and skull will be discussed separately in Chapter 17.

15.2 The normal face in 3D surface mode

Visualization of the fetal face with 3D/4D ultrasound is often synonymous with 3D ultrasound and is expected by most patients undergoing ultrasound screening in pregnancy. Four steps must be followed to achieve a good result. These are:
1. An optimal 2D image prior to 3D/4D acquisition
2. An insonation angle of the face considering the surrounding structures
3. Good presets before 3D/4D acquisition
4. Post-processing 3D display and volume manipulation

These steps are explained in this section. See also Chapter 7 on surface mode.

15.2.1 2D image before 3D acquisition

Before starting a 3D acquisition, make sure that the 2D image has a high resolution to allow good delineation of facial features. The image contrast can be increased so that the amniotic fluid is displayed clearly and without speckles (see Fig. 1.2 in Chapter 1).

15.2.2 The insonation angle

The examiner should make sure there is enough amniotic fluid in front of the face and that no objects such as hands or umbilical cord obscure the face during volume acquisition. Before volume acquisition, it may be helpful to perform a free hand sweep for the demonstration of the regions left and right of the reference plane. To achieve a perfect result, it is better to approach the face from the side and not from the direct midsagittal profile view (compare Figs. 15.2 and 15.3). It is helpful imagining a photographer taking a classic portrait shot. For a good 3D result, the examiner should approach the face from a slightly anterolateral position. For this purpose, we recommend keeping the chin, mouth, nose, and forehead on the same horizontal plane (Figs. 7.6, 15.3); otherwise, the mouth-chin region will not be visible in 3D if the mouth region is lower, as shown in Figure 15.2.

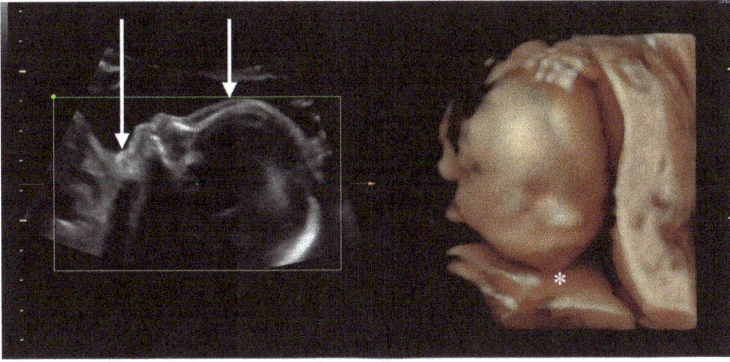

Fig. 15.2: In this example, the 2D profile image is acceptable, but the position could be improved for the 3D volume visualization. In this 3D acquisition, the mouth and chin area are low compared to the head (long versus short arrow). The result in 3D shows that the mouth-chin area (*) cannot be displayed optimally. See Figure 15.3.

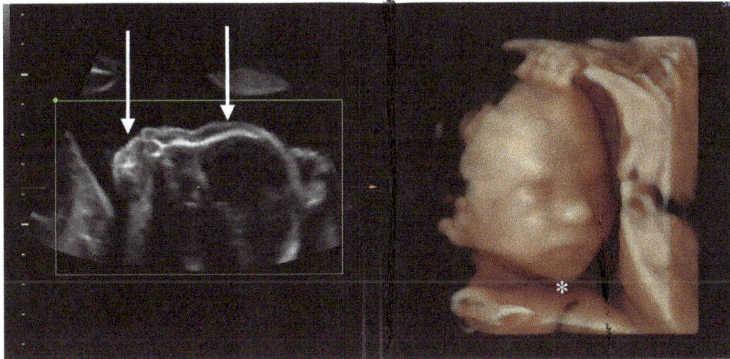

Fig. 15.3: In this 3D acquisition, care was taken to ensure that the fetal face is almost horizontal and that the mouth, chin, and forehead are almost at the same level in the 2D image (left). Compared to the image in Figure 15.2, this results in a good 3D rendering of the entire face, especially of the mouth and chin area (*).

15.2.3 3D presets before acquisition

Pre-programmed 3D rendering presets for the fetal face view are available in the ultrasound system. In general, three features need to be selected ahead, namely acquisition box size, volume depth, and volume resolution. We recommend a larger box and sufficient depth to capture as much information as possible (see Fig. 7.8). For volume resolution, we prefer a middle range (mid-1, mid-2) to allow a soft facial image. For a 3D visualization of hands or ears, we recommend increasing the resolution.

15.2.4 Post processing 3D rendering and volume manipulation

An important function for a successful 3D rendering of the face is to adjust the softness of the image in HDlive. For this purpose, we select V-SRI at level 1 for sharper contours to level 5 for soft contours (see Fig. 7.10). Another soft color is obtained by increasing the shadow level to, e. g., 130. The additional use of silhouette mode makes the image

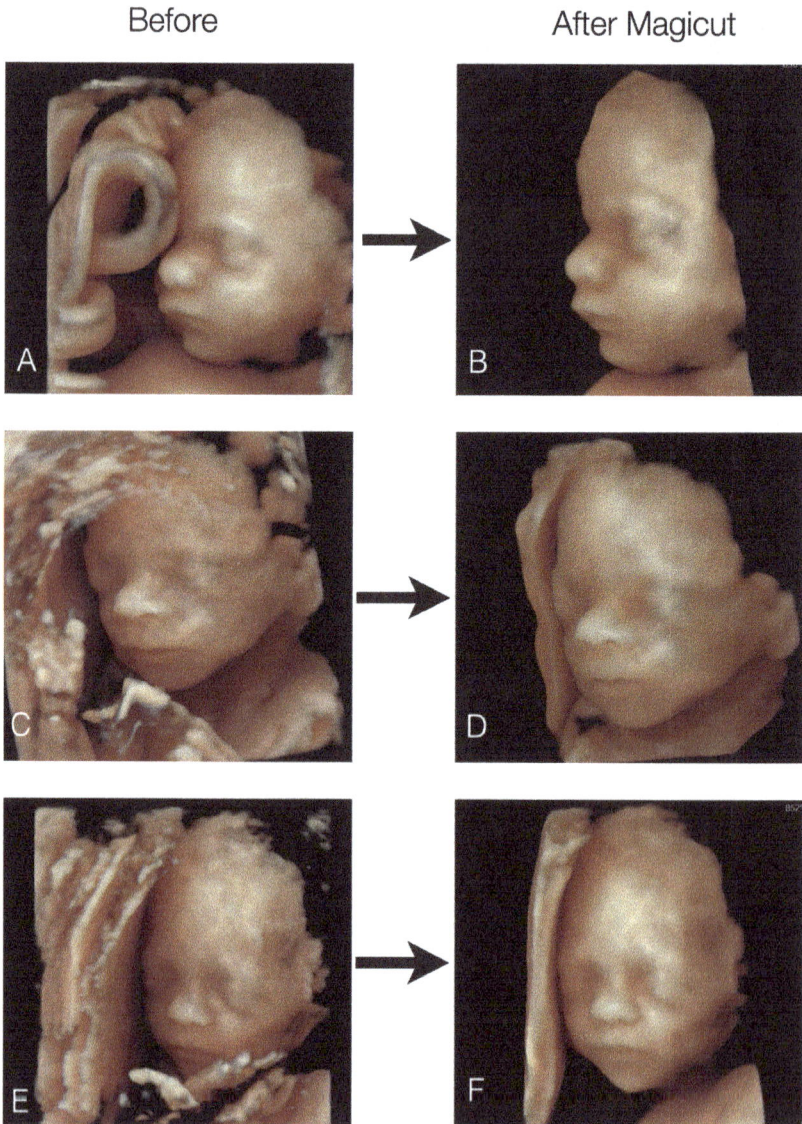

Before   After Magicut

Fig. 15.4: Most face images are manipulated with the Magicut tool to enhance the image. Here are three examples before Magicut (A, C and E) and after Magicut (B, D and F).

even softer, as described in detail in Chapter 11. Often the Magicut tool is needed to remove adjacent artifacts from the 3D image. For this purpose, the 3D volume is first fixed and "unneeded" structures are removed with Magicut (Fig. 15.4). In some cases, changing the gain and threshold can help reduce the presence of a disturbing umbilical cord. The position of the light source can be adjusted so that the face is illuminated from above and not from the front (see Fig. 3.16). Figures 15.4 through 15.7 show a collection of images created and processed using the steps explained in the previous section.

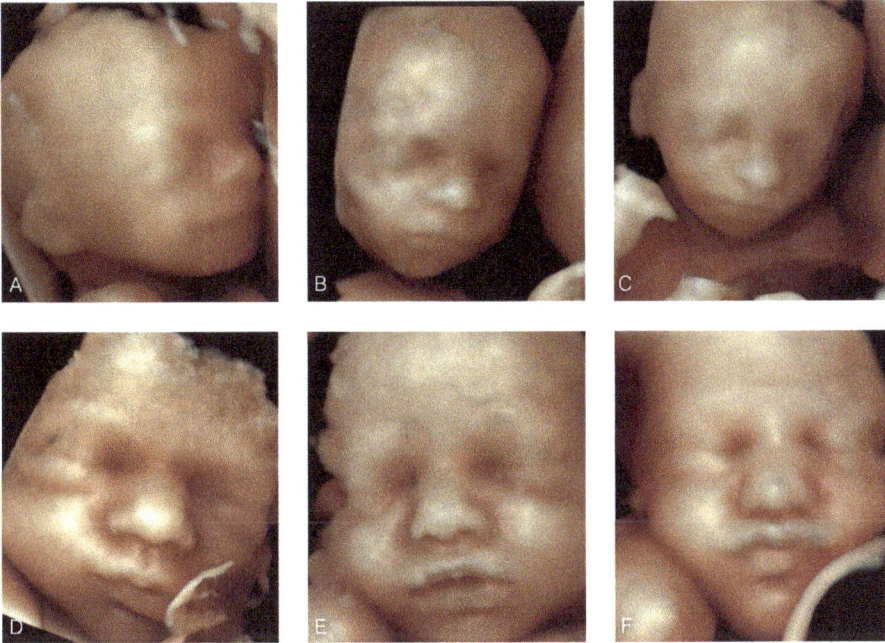

Fig. 15.5: In the resting phase, the fetuses appear as if they were sleeping; here at 22 weeks (A, B and C), at 30 weeks (D and E), and at 32 weeks (F).

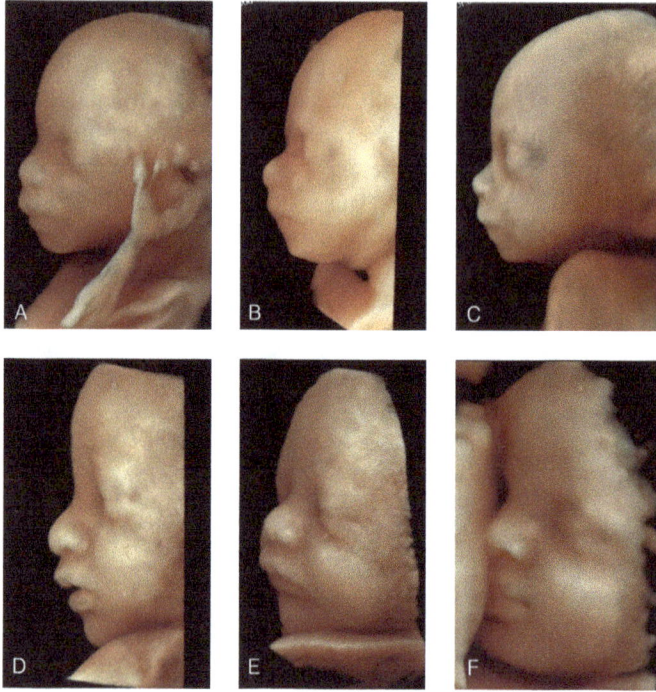

Fig. 15.6: Fetal profiles created by cutting the background with Magicut. In (A), (B) and (C) the fetuses are at 22 weeks of gestation and in (D), (E) and (F) at 30 weeks of gestation. Note the development of facial features after 28 weeks.

Face with Hand

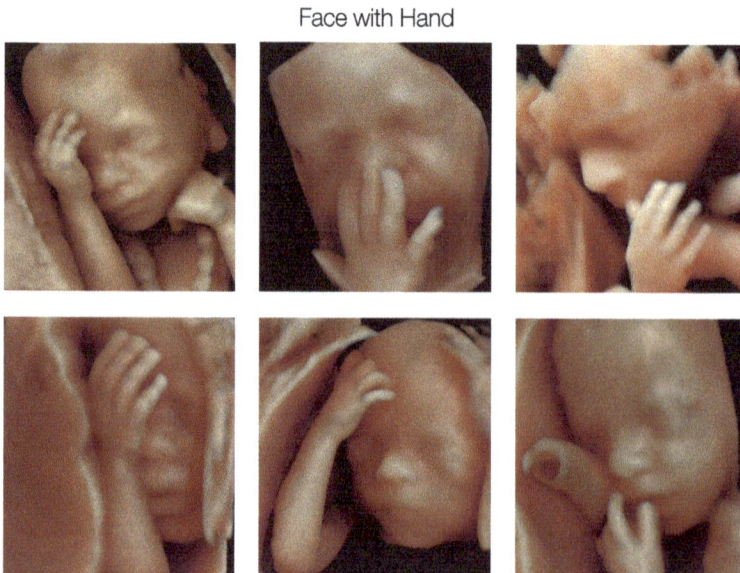

Fig. 15.7: A typical behavior of fetuses is holding the hand in front of the head and face, which can be well visualized in 3D.

15.3 The normal face in 4D surface mode

The examination of the face with real-time 4D is somewhat different from a static 3D examination. While the previous steps 1 and 2 are similar, in step 3 the size of the box is chosen close to the face and placed in the amniotic fluid to provide a direct view of the face. Intensive use of Magicut and other features is limited in a 4D examination due to the moving fetus. Therefore, for a real-time 4D examination, the examiner should prepare ahead the various features such as light source, image smoothing with V-SRI, and others as discussed in step 4. Instead of Magicut, the examiner can activate the SonoRender live tool (see Chapter 3), which allows real-time adjustment of the render line to the moving fetus. The great advantage of real-time 4D is, on the one hand, the simplicity of obtaining the result directly, but more importantly, that both the examiner and the parents can focus on the facial movements, such as the opening of the mouth or eyes, facial expressions (Fig. 15.8), or hand movements in front of the face. Figures 15.8 and 15.9 show examples of changes in fetal facial expression as observed in a sequence of serial images extracted from 4D volumes. The 4D examination is of particular interest in the third trimester, when facial features and grimaces become more prominent.

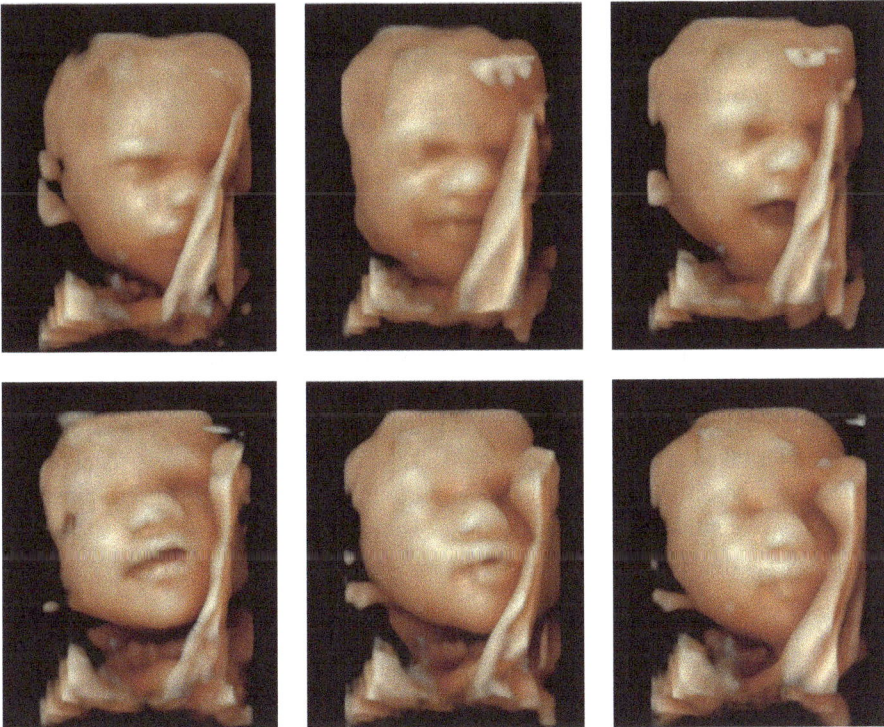

Fig. 15.8: A series of images from a cineloop of 4D volumes illustrating fetal facial expressions. The fetus is drinking, yawning, or simply grimacing.

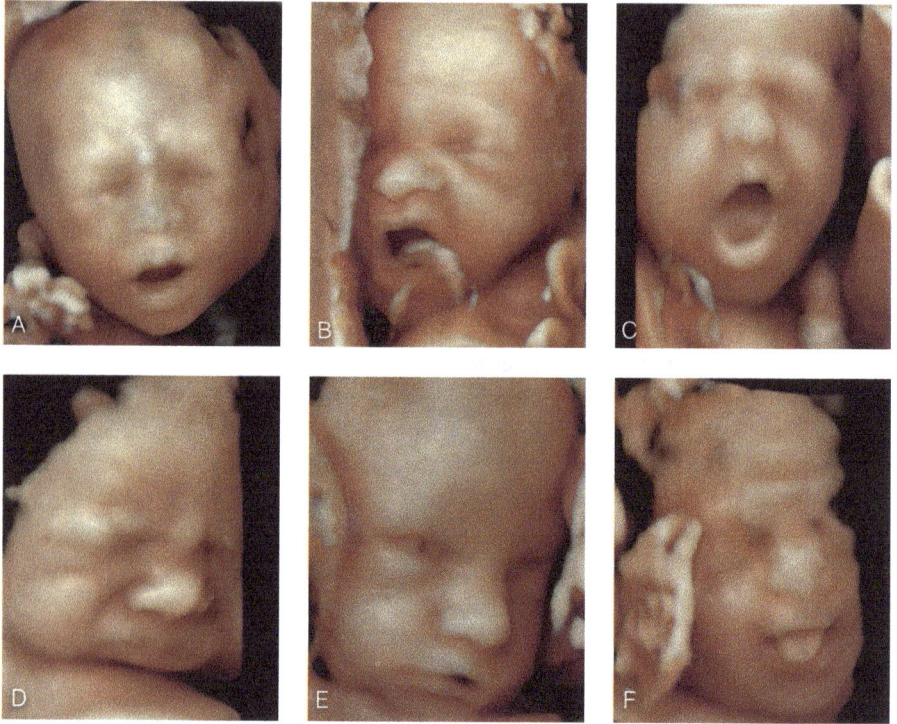

Fig. 15.9: During a 4D real-time examination, facial expressions such as drinking (A and B), yawning (C), crying (D), thinking with eyes open (E), or showing the tongue (F) can be frequently observed, especially in the third trimester.

15.4 The normal face at different gestational ages

3D face in the first trimester and early second trimester: In a fetus before 19 weeks of gestation, the subcutaneous fat is not yet sufficiently developed, and the size of the fetus is too small to capture certain facial features with good resolution. Therefore, to improve the image result, the examination is better performed transvaginally, and the acquisition is taken at a higher resolution (level high-1 or high-2). If a clear fetal face is needed for medical indication to exclude or confirm an anomaly, we recommend a transvaginal examination. Figure 15.10 shows examples of fetal faces between 11 and 14 weeks of gestation.

3D face in mid-pregnancy: The presets discussed in Chapter 7 focused on the most common scenario of a second trimester examination. A collection of images is shown in Figure 15.11 and in the upper row of Figures 15.5 and 15.6. During the midtrimester scan, facial movements are not very common, and the subcutaneous tissue is not sufficiently developed to provide an acceptable differentiation between fetal face features

3D Faces in First-Trimester

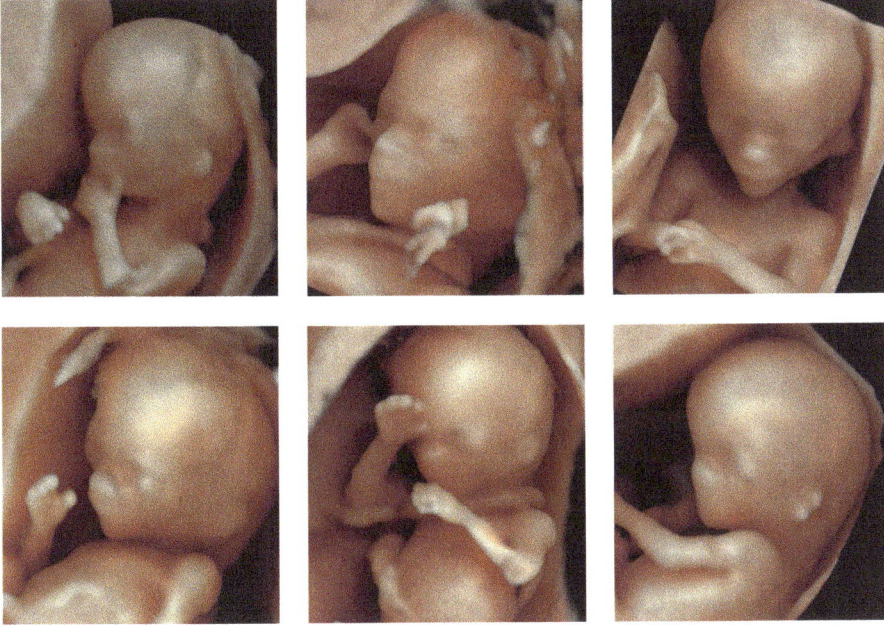

Fig. 15.10: Fetal facial images in 3D surface mode between 11 to 13 weeks of gestation. Arms and hands are often in front of the face.

in 3D. The nose and mouth regions are often different from one fetus to another, and the eyeballs are still very prominent at this stage, which surprises many parents. Movements are not fluid enough and are of short duration to ensure a good 4D live session. We prefer to focus on a static 3D acquisition with good resolution at this gestational age.

3D face in the third trimester: After 26 weeks of gestation, subcutaneous tissue increases and the images of the face start resembling the face of a baby after birth. Facial movements become more realistic and coordinated. Figures 15.12 and 15.13 show several 3D faces after 28 weeks of gestation and illustrate the differences between various fetal physiognomies. Figure 15.14 shows the similarities between two fetal faces and their respective neonatal appearance.

3D Faces in Second Trimester

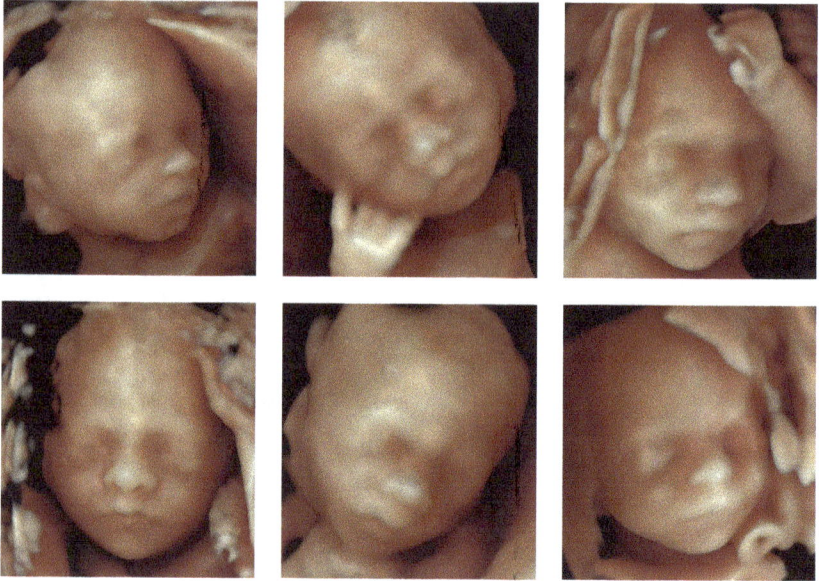

Fig. 15.11: Collection of 3D face images in surface mode around 20 to 25 weeks. Different facial expressions are evident, and at this gestational age the orbit region frequently appears prominent, which is normal. The eyes are always closed.

3D Faces in Third Trimester

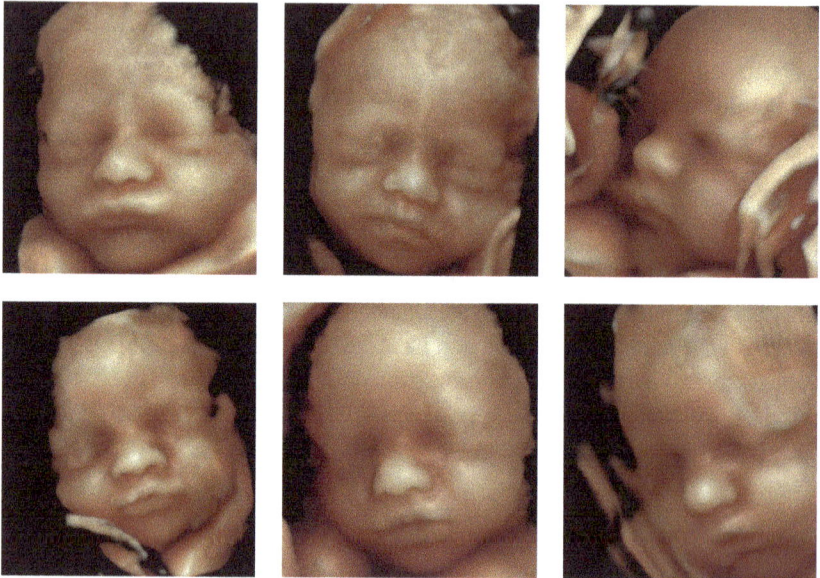

Fig. 15.12: While first and second trimester fetuses may be similar (see Figures 15.10, 15.11), third trimester fetuses already have their individual features and often resemble the postnatal portraits.

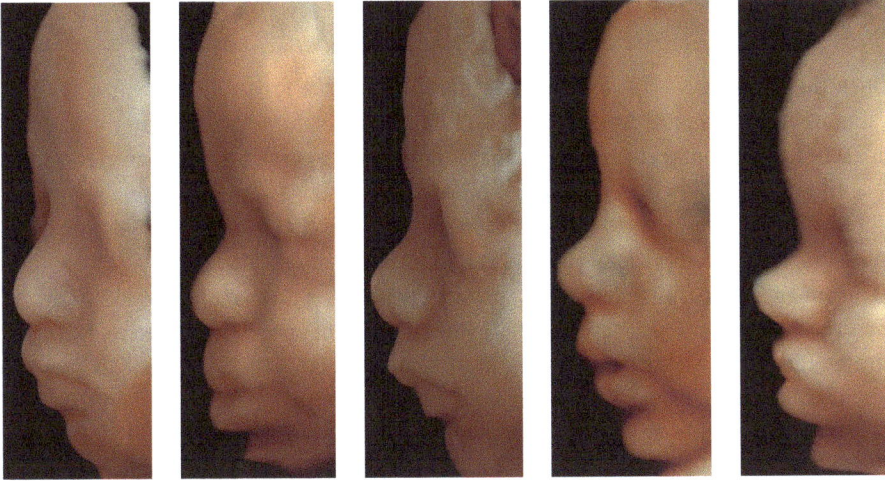

Fig. 15.13: In the third trimester after 28 weeks' gestation, the fetus begins to develop its personal facial features. The shape of the nose and mouth, the facial proportions and the thickness of the cheeks give the face its typical features. Here we can observe the profile of five fetuses with different appearances.

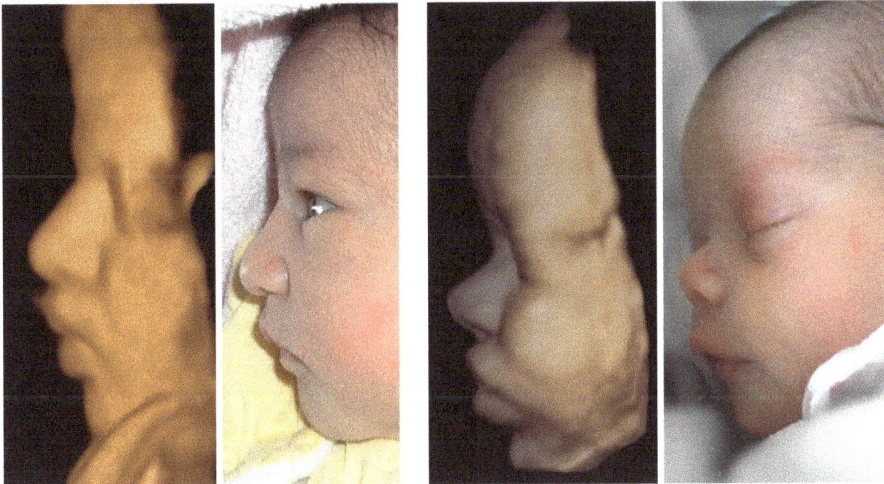

Fig. 15.14: Comparison of a profile in 3D of two fetuses in the third trimester with the postnatal profile. The forehead, nose and mouth are often identical pre- and postnatally.

15.5 The abnormal face in 3D/4D

Since the early days of 3D ultrasound, there has been a great interest and a clinical value in imaging a fetal dysmorphic face. While some features can be better visualized in 2D (e. g., prefrontal edema, absent nasal bone, and others), a 3D surface view of the face can be of great help in obtaining a more complete image. In this mode, the proportions of the face and its various regions, such as the forehead, eyes, nose, mouth, chin, and ears, can be well visualized. Abnormal proportions of face to forehead ratio, such as in anencephaly, microcephaly or macrocephaly, as shown in Figure 15.15, can be well recognized. The spectrum of cleft lip and palate can be well identified and demonstrated (Fig. 15.16) and make its extent more understandable for the patient and professional colleagues. Dysmorphic facial features, such as in trisomy 21, 13 and 18 (Fig. 15.17), the flat profile in Binder syndrome, or in holoprosencephaly (Fig. 15.18) can be clearly visualized. One should not rely solely on the 3D image, as the appearance can sometimes be much milder than in the 2D profile view. We consider the 3D face image an important complement to the 2D assessment, but not a substitute for it. Examples of faces in fetuses with syndromes are shown in Figures 15.15 to 15.20.

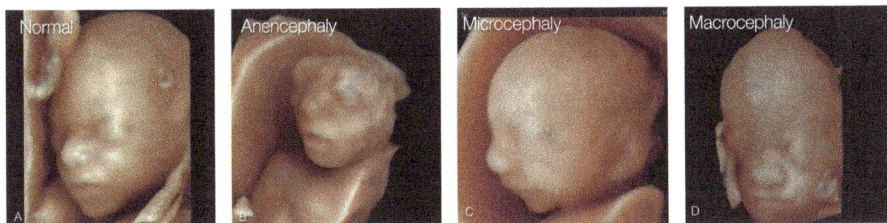

Fig. 15.15: Fetuses with normal (A) and abnormal face and head shape (B, C and D) at 22 to 25 weeks. The fetus in (A) is normal with normal face and forehead ratio. The fetus in (B) is anencephalic with no forehead and skull. Fetus (C) has microcephaly with a small skull, and fetus (D) has a high forehead as turricephaly along with macrocephaly in Apert syndrome.

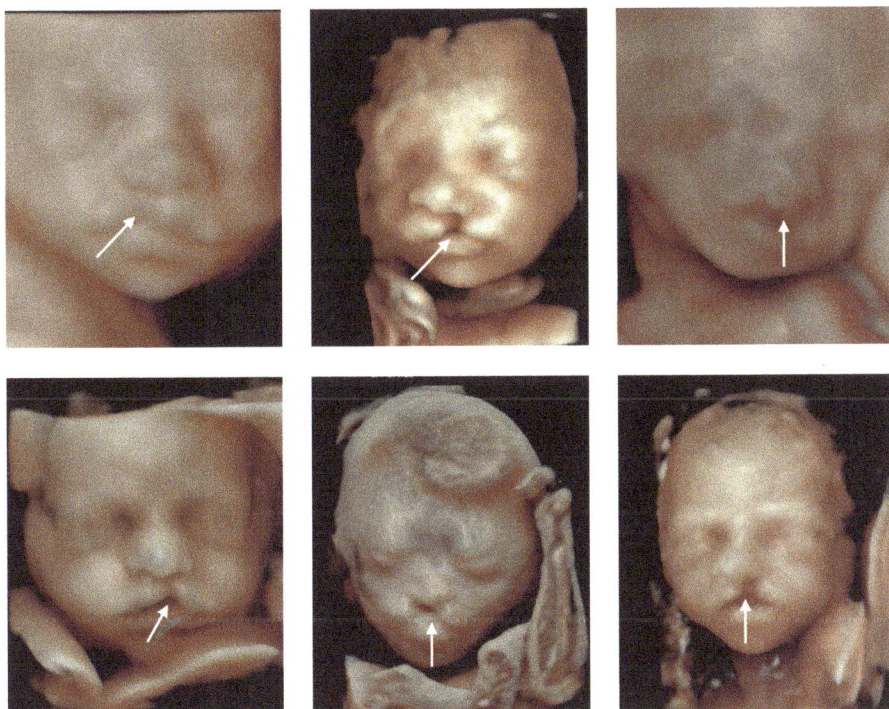

Fig. 15.16: Fetuses with various facial clefts (arrows) including isolated cleft lip, mediolateral cleft lip and palate, and median cleft lip and palate.

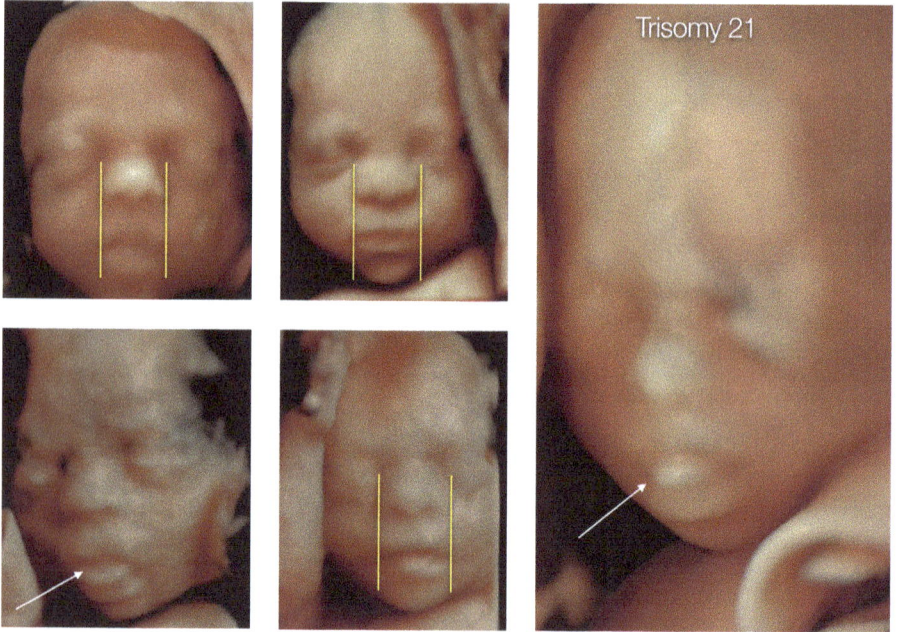

Fig. 15.17: Faces in 3D surface mode in fetuses with trisomy 21. In such cases, some fetuses may be suspicious, showing an open mouth with occasional protruding tongue (arrow). One of the interesting features is the nose to mouth ratio with a small nose and microstomia. Nose and mouth in trisomy 21 show the same width compared to normal fetuses, where the mouth is usually larger than the nose.

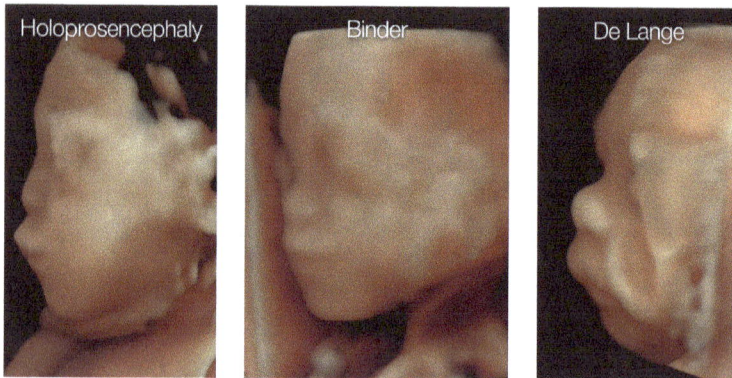

Fig. 15.18: Abnormal profile in three fetuses with midline anomaly and holoprosencephaly (left), in Binder's face (middle) and in Cornelia de Lange syndrome with suspicious philtrum (right).

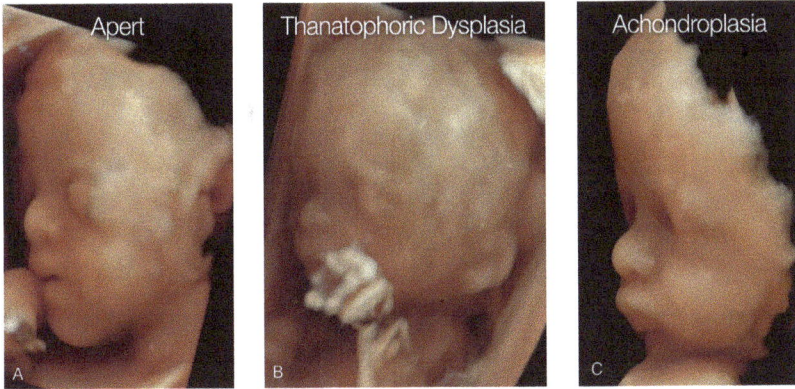

Fig. 15.19: Abnormal profile in three fetuses with skeletal dysplasia, all of which have a prominent forehead as a frontal bossing. In (A) the fetus has Apert syndrome, in (B) thanatophoric dysplasia, and in (C) achondroplasia.

15.6 The normal and abnormal ear

Compared to 2D ultrasound, the ear is better visualized with 3D surface mode. Ideal insonation of the ear is best achieved from a frontal-lateral angle. Figure 15.21 shows examples of normal and abnormal findings of the ears, including microtia of varying degrees, abnormal ear shape or position in syndromes (Figs. 15.20, 15.21). With 3D ultrasound, the ability to include the ears in the workup of detecting fetal syndromes has evolved significantly.

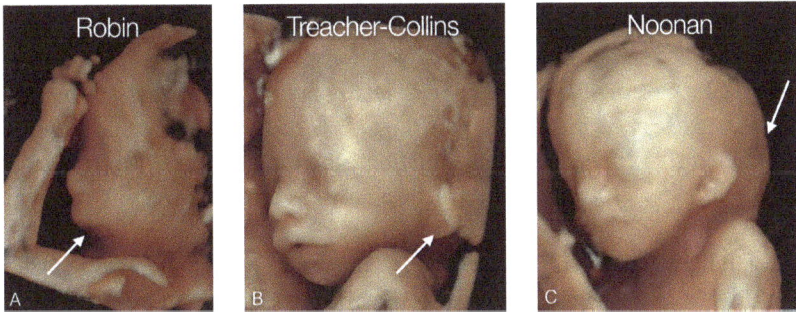

Fig. 15.20: Abnormal face in three fetuses with syndromic disorders. In (A) the fetus has Robin sequence with underdeveloped mandible (arrow), in (B) Treacher-Collins syndrome with large mouth, slanted eyes and ear dysplasia (arrow), and in (C) with Noonan syndrome with down-slanting eyes, ear rotation and thickened neck (arrow).

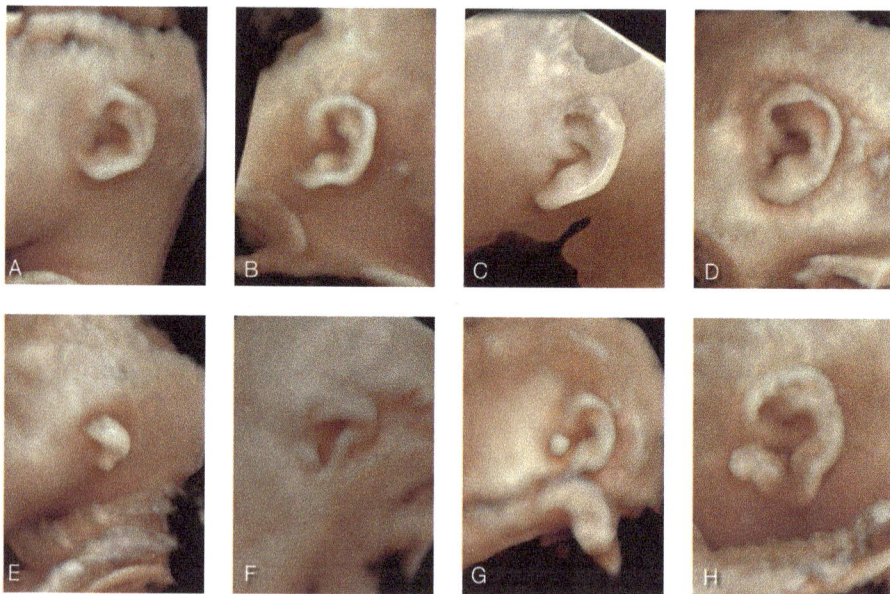

Fig. 15.21: The ears can be better visualized with 3D than with 2D alone and may play an important role in syndromic disorders. The upper images (A) through (D) display normal ears; the images (E) through (H) display small and dysplastic ears as well as ear tags that occur in syndromic conditions but can also be isolated.

15.7 The face in multiplanar display

For the multiplanar imaging of the face, the volume is best acquired from cranial to caudal or from left to right. In the former case, both orbits or the nose should be visible in the initial plane; in the latter case, the insonation begins in the profile plane. By navigating through the volume in either multiplanar orthogonal (Fig. 15.22) or tomographic (Fig. 15.23) mode, the face can then be visualized with all the necessary details, such as forehead, eyes, nose, mouth, and jaw (Figs. 15.22–15.24). One can take the eyes as good orientation structures. In certain situations, the examiner can use the Omniview mode to selectively visualize some structures such as the hard and soft palate in normal fetuses (Fig. 15.25) and use this approach or another multiplanar mode in fetuses with a cleft lip and palate (Figs. 15.26, 15.27). For specific focus on the hard palate, acquisition is ideally performed in an axial view starting at the level of the mandible, as shown in Figures 15.24 and 5.7 in Chapter 5. Figure 15.28 shows the face of a fetus with microphthalmia in tomography mode. Figure 15.29 shows the multiplanar rendering of a normal lens and, in comparison, an opaque lens in a fetus with cataract.

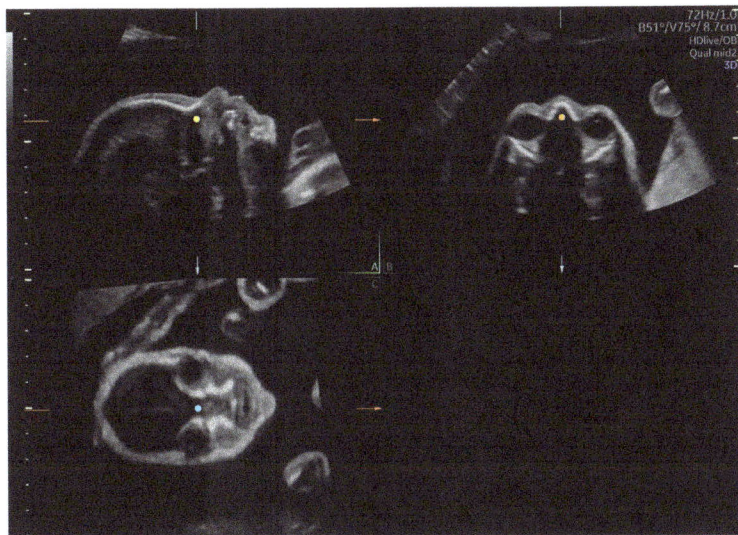

Fig. 15.22: Face in multiplanar display in orthogonal mode. The intersection point (navigation point) was placed on the nose and the images were rotated and adjusted accordingly.

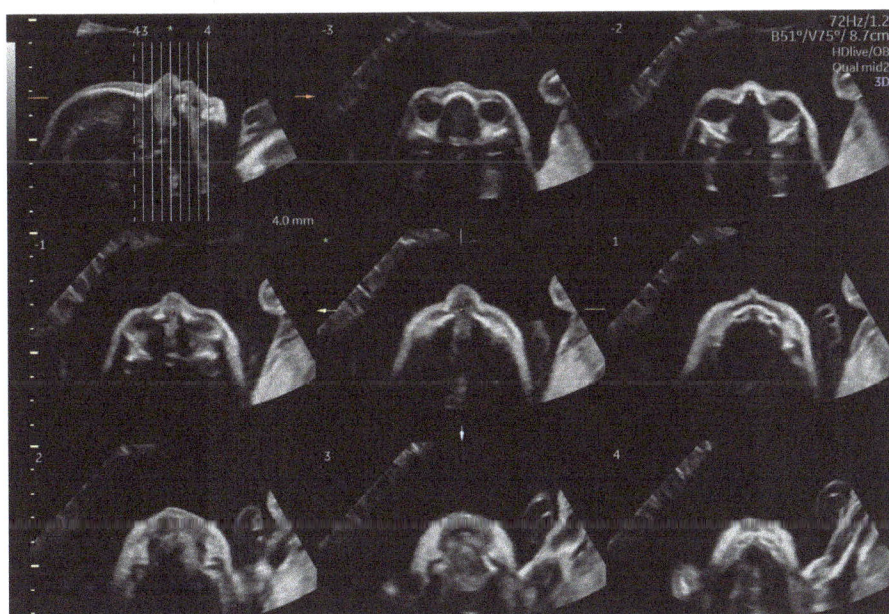

Fig. 15.23: Face in multiplanar display in tomography mode. The reference plane in the upper left corner shows the profile, while the tomographic images show axial parallel slices of the face from the eyes (upper center) to the lower jaw (bottom right).

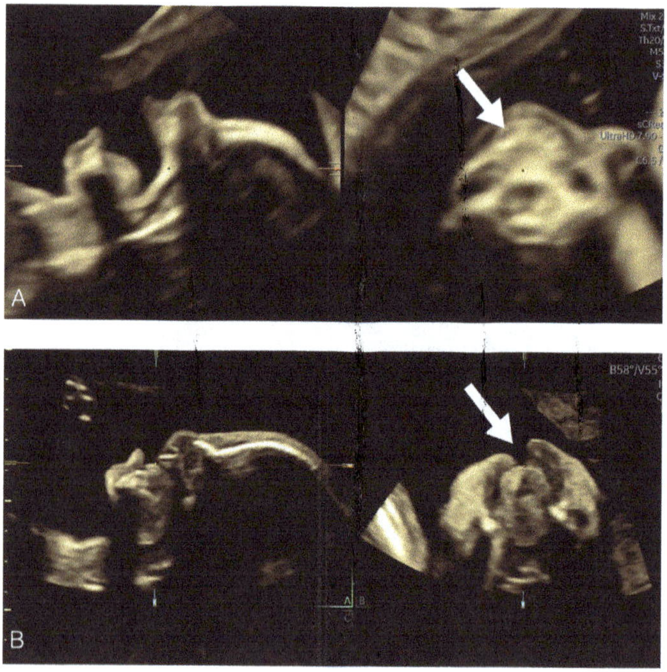

Fig. 15.24: Representation of the hard palate (arrow) in orthogonal mode in a normal fetus (A) and in a fetus with mediolateral cleft lip and palate (arrow) (B).

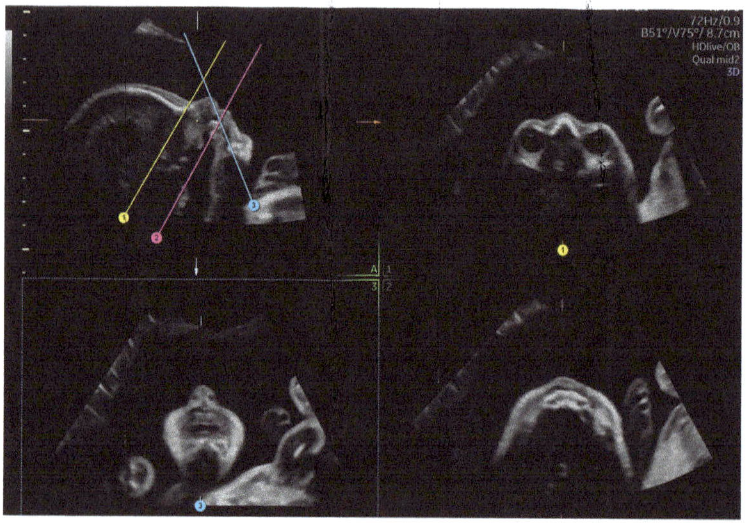

Fig. 15.25: Selective planes in multiplanar mode shown as Omniview planes. Three cross-sectional planes shown in yellow (1), magenta (2), and cyan (3) were placed in the reference plane in the upper left image to show the typical landmarks. The upper right plane shows the orbits, the lower left plane shows the nose-mouth triangle, and the lower right plane shows an axial view of the maxilla.

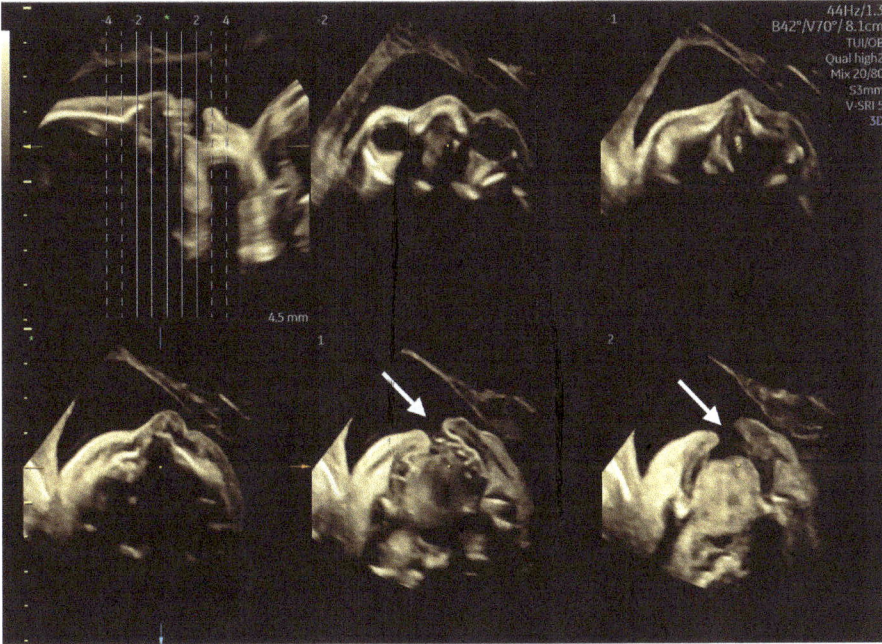

Fig. 15.26: Fetus with a mediolateral cleft lip and palate (arrow) shown in tomography mode. The two orbits appear normal, and the defect is shown in a lower plane axial view (arrow).

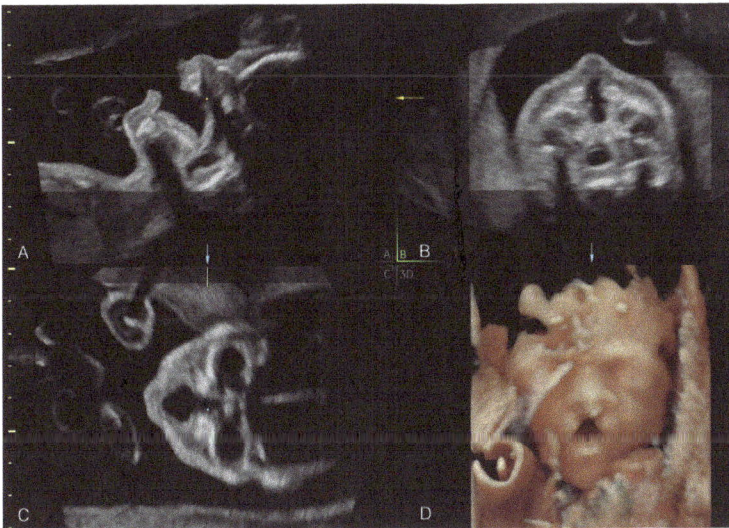

Fig. 15.27: Fetus with bilateral cleft lip and palate shown in multiplanar mode (A, B and C) and rendered with 3D surface mode in (D).

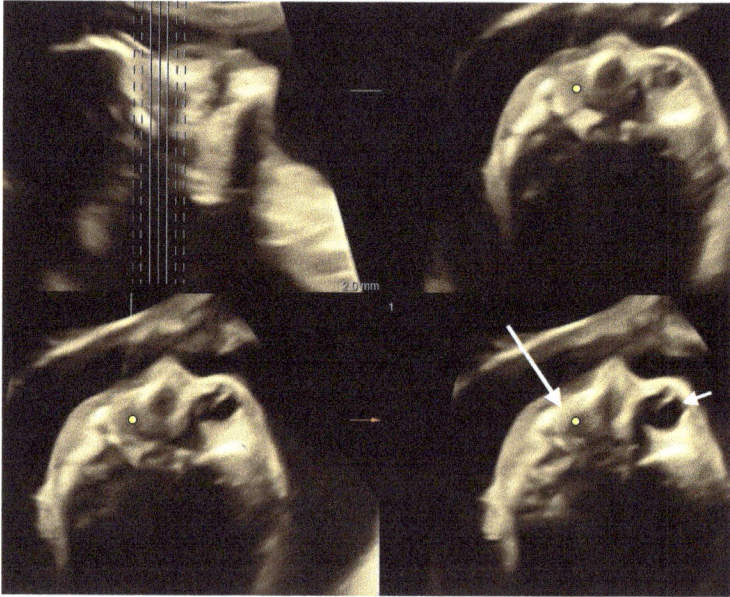

Fig. 15.28: Face in multiplanar rendering in tomographic mode in a fetus with unilateral microphthalmia (long arrow). The different planes show the difference between the normal eye (short arrow) and the abnormal eye (long arrow).

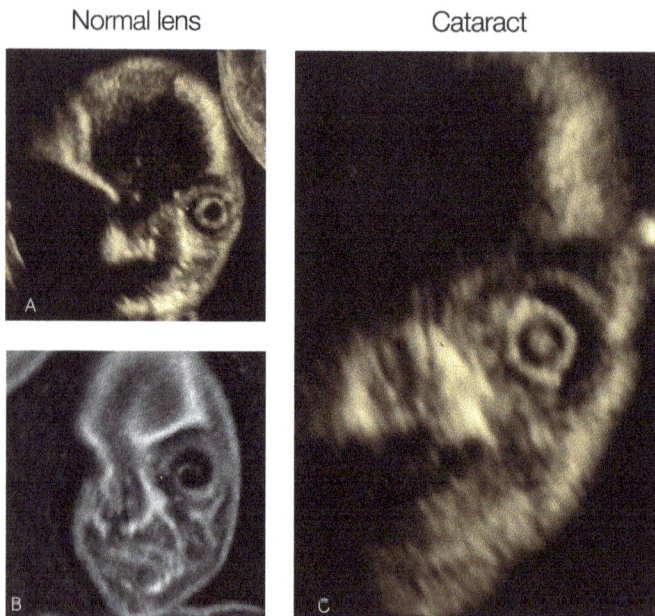

Fig. 15.29: Multiplanar reconstruction of the fetal eye with the normal translucent lens (A and B) and in a fetus with cataract with an opaque lens (C).

15.8 Conclusions

The fetal face is still the most often performed examination and the first 3D visualization an operator learns, despite the variety of visualization options and organs accessible to volume ultrasound. Facial abnormalities can be visualized quite well in multiplanar mode, but 3D surface rendering provides a spatial view of the face that is often very similar to the postnatal image. Some prerequisites for a good 3D image are the use of a good preset in 2D grayscale before acquisition, a large box that includes adjacent structures such as limbs, and good lateral insonation of the face rather than from the front. A step by step manipulation of the 3D image with Magicut, with different surface modes and smooth skin then allows demonstration of a very realistic image. Facial features and grimaces become more apparent in the third trimester and are best visualized with 4D ultrasound. Facial anomalies such as facial clefts or anomalies of the eyes, nose, lips, and ears, or some syndromic disorders can be visualized quite well in 3D and are generally an important supplement to the information provided in 2D.

16 3D Fetal Neurosonography

16.1 Introduction

Interest in the fetal brain has increased in the last two decades thanks to the introduction of new imaging technologies and the increasing growth of knowledge. Nowadays, the brain can be examined with ultrasound as early as the seventh week of the developing embryo, and this development can be followed with ultrasound until birth around 40 weeks of gestation. The goal of the examination varies, depending on the gestational age and the information needed. From the 11th week of gestation, the usual approach is to visualize typical axial planes of the head showing the symmetry of the different brain areas, and this can be completed with sagittal and coronal planes if needed. It is now recognized that 3D imaging has contributed significantly to the radical development of modern fetal neurosonography and is used in both screening and targeted examinations.

From a clinical point of view, the most important aspects of the use of 3D in fetal neurosonography are the different multiplanar modes (see Chapters 2, 4, 5 and 6) that allow either the reconstruction of a selected view (corpus callosum, vermis) or the display of the tomographic view. Volume rendering has great potential for use in the embryonic brain, but also in fetuses with increased fluid content in the ventricular system. In addition, the 3D glass-body mode can be used to visualize the course of normal and abnormal arterial and venous vessels. In this chapter, various aspects of 3D use in fetal brain examination are discussed and illustrated.

16.2 Transabdominal 3D examination of the brain and multiplanar reconstruction

Routine transabdominal ultrasound screening of the fetal brain performed after the 15th week of gestation focuses primarily on imaging the axial planes, which are typically used to measure biparietal and transcerebellar diameters. If an abnormality is suspected or if fetuses are at high risk for CNS anomalies, additional sagittal and coronal sectional planes are required as part of a comprehensive fetal neurosonogram. Additional planes are often difficult to obtain, especially in unfavorable fetal positions such as in a vertex presentation. This can be solved either by transvaginal examination or by acquisition of a 3D volume with reconstruction of the plane of interest.

With 3D neurosonography, the examiner can acquire a volume and store it digitally on a hard drive. For a later evaluation such a volume can be restored on the ultrasound system for display and manipulation as explained in Chapter 2. The 3D volume acquisition can be performed from different insonation angles as an axial, coronal, or sagittal approach. The two main advantages of the multiplanar 3D mode are:

https://doi.org/10.1515/9783111249513-016

1. The ability to use the tomography mode to visualize any region of the brain along with adjacent structures in a single image. This provides an overview of the brain as known from CT- or MR studies of the infant brain (Figs. 16.1, 16.2).
2. The possibility to virtually reconstruct any brain structure from a 3D volume data set, e. g., typical midline structures like the corpus callosum or the cerebellar vermis (Figs. 16.3, 16.4).

Some technical aspects are discussed in the following section.

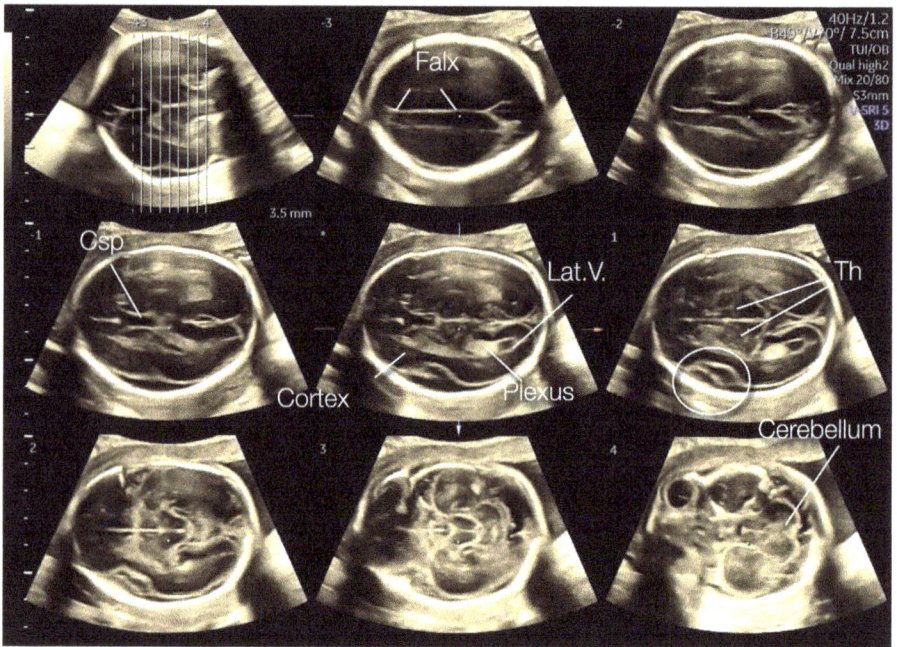

Fig. 16.1: 3D volume data set of an axial acquisition of a fetal brain in tomography mode. The different planes give an overview of the main structures of a normal brain, such as the falx cerebri (Falx), the lateral ventricles (Lat.V.), the choroid plexus (Plexus), the thalami (Th), the cavum septi pellucidi (Csp), the Sylvian fissure (Circle), the cerebral cortex, and the cerebellum with the cisterna magna.

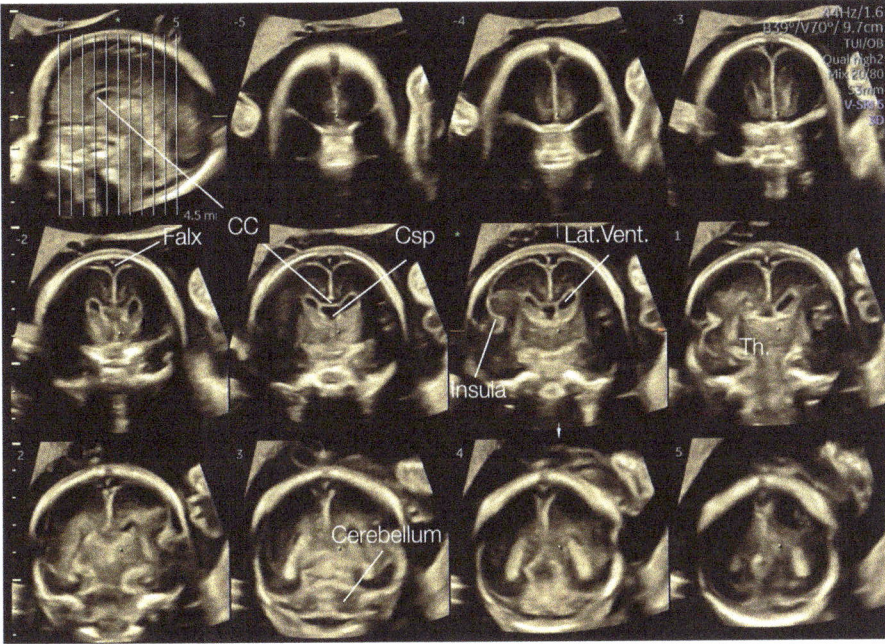

Fig. 16.2: Coronal sectional planes in tomography mode after transabdominal volume acquisition through the fontanelle. At one glance, an overview is provided and the following structures can be identified: the falx cerebri (Falx), the corpus callosum (CC), the cavum septi pellucidi (Csp), the thalami (Th), the insula and the anterior horns with the lateral ventricles (Lat.Vent.).

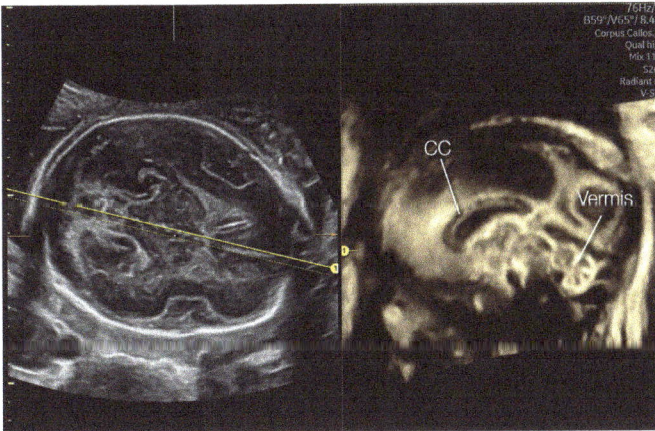

Fig. 16.3: Omniview with VCI along the midline showing the corpus callosum (CC) and vermis. The falx cerebri and cavum septi pellucidi were used as landmarks.

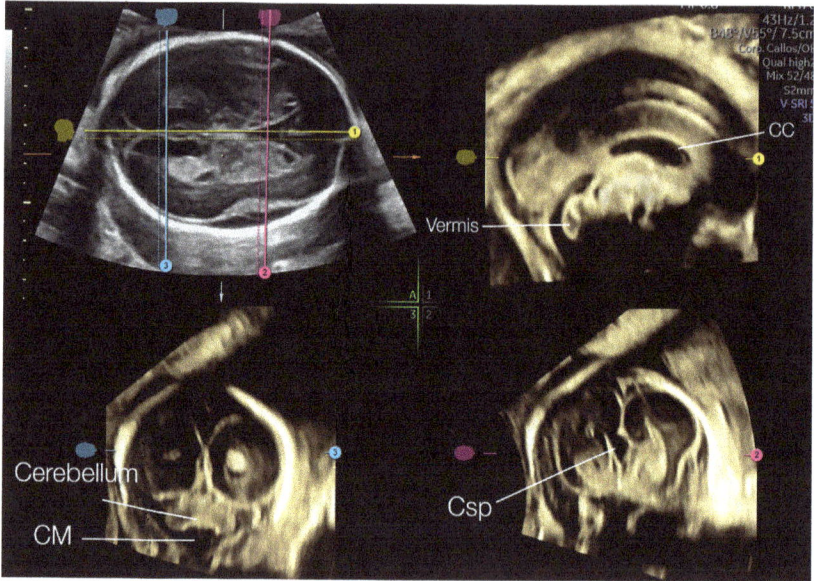

Fig. 16.4: After a lateral static 3D acquisition of a fetal head, three Omniview lines were drawn to visualize the corpus callosum (CC) in a sagittal plane, a coronal plane to visualize the cavum septi pellucidi (Csp), and another posterior coronal plane to visualize the cerebellum and cisterna magna (CM).

16.2.1 3D acquisition of a brain volume

The most often performed 3D acquisition is from an axial view of the head, in most cases when the fetus is in a vertex presentation (Fig. 16.1) but other fetal positions are also possible (Fig. 16.2). Before acquiring a volume, care should be taken to minimize shadowing of the cranial bones. We perform a virtual manual sweep and adjust the transducer position accordingly before pressing the 3D acquisition button. The examiner should have the final picture in mind before acquiring a volume and adapt the acquisition presets correspondingly. If the goal is to document brain structures on the tomography display, the acquisition angle should be large enough to capture the entire brain and the resolution should be high (High-1 to Max). In our experience, there is no "perfect" volume that should be acquired; rather, one should have a series of multiple volumes acquired from adjacent insonations and select the best one after post-processing. This "trial and error" approach is also quite common among experts who use 3D prenatally.

16.2.2 Multiplanar reconstruction and display

In fetal neurosonography, some structures such as the corpus callosum or the cerebellar vermis are often the two most important regions of interest that need to be visualized and reconstructed in 3D using orthogonal or Omniview imaging; they are explained below.

3D reconstruction of the corpus callosum: For the experienced examiner, visualization of the corpus callosum is part of a comprehensive ultrasound examination. This structure is visualized either directly or with a rapid reconstruction of a sagittal plane after a 3D volume acquisition from an axial plane. The cavum septi pellucidi is an important landmark in both volume acquisition and 3D imaging. Figures 16.5 to 16.7 explain the 3D reconstruction of the corpus callosum step by step. Based on the authors' experience, the following is recommended: (1) try to lighten the 2D image before acquisition, as the additional use of VCI obscures the 3D image; (2) perform a virtual manual sweep of the region of interest before volume acquisition to ensure that the corpus callosum is not in the shadow of a skull bone. A good result is obtained when the corpus callosum is clearly visible as a hypoechoic structure, as shown in Figures 16.3 and 16.7.

3D reconstruction of the cerebellar vermis: The anatomy of the cerebellum is generally assessed in the axial view. This shows the normal shape of the two hemispheres with the vermis between them and the cisterna cerebello-medullaris is of normal size, while the inferior part of the vermis is visible and separates the fourth ventricle from the cisterna. If the posterior fossa shows suspicious findings in the axial plane, imaging a midsagittal view of the vermis may be of great importance in distinguishing between the different entities. This can be well accomplished with an axial acquisition of a 3D volume of the posterior fossa. In this view, the shape, size, and position of the cerebellar vermis can be objectively assessed. Figures 16.8 to 16.10 explain the 3D reconstruction of the cerebellar vermis. After volume acquisition, the images are rotated so that both the brain axis and vermis are aligned. The vermis can then be seen in plane C, particularly in its relationship to the cisterna magna and brainstem (Fig. 16.9). If possible, not only the cisterna magna and cerebellum but also the fourth ventricle and brainstem should be included in the 3D volume data set. This can be difficult due to ossification of the adjacent occipital bone, as shown in Figure 16.10. Conditions such as a mega-cisterna magna can also be easily differentiated from a Blake's pouch cyst, partial or complete agenesis of the vermis, or a true Dandy-Walker malformation, as shown in Figure 16.11.

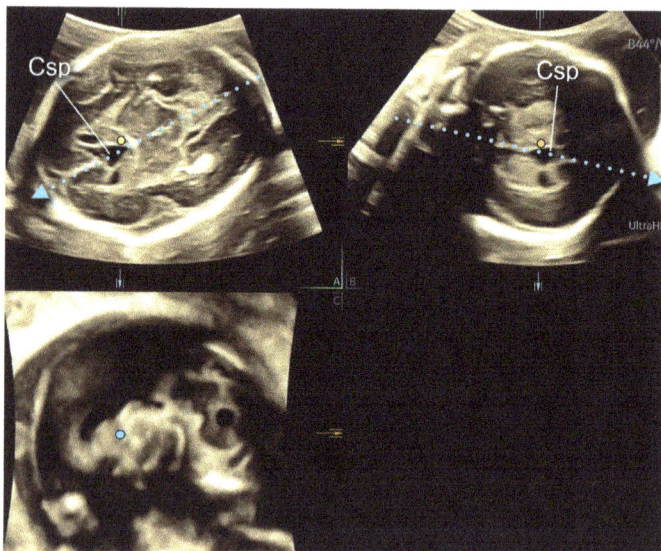

Fig. 16.5: Despite the vertex position in this fetus, the corpus callosum, which cannot be seen, can be re-constructed here using 3D in combination with VCI. Step 1: Orientation is best achieved by locating the ca-vum septi pellucidi (Csp) and placing the intersection point there. The axes of the head (dashed arrows) are still oblique but should be aligned with the horizontal line. See Figure 16.6.

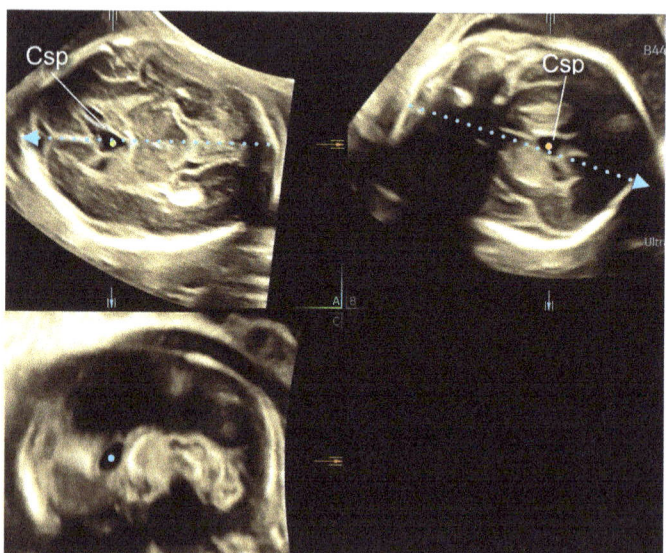

Fig. 16.6: After placing the intersection point on the cavum septi pellucidi (Csp), plane A was rotated so that the axis of the falx cerebri is aligned with the horizontal axis (dashed arrow). In plane B, the axis is still ob-lique. See Figure 16.7.

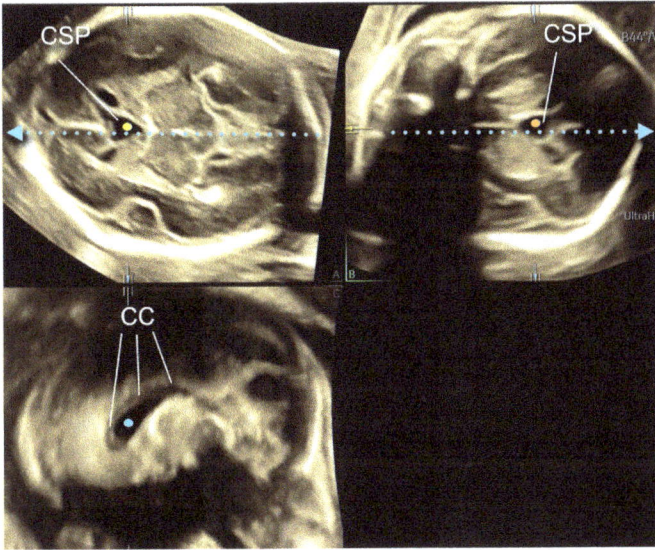

Fig. 16.7: Completing the process in the previous figure, now both axes in planes A and B are aligned horizontally (dashed arrows) and the corpus callosum (CC) appears in plane C. Note that the intersection point is in the cavum septi pellucidi (Csp), which can be seen in all three planes.

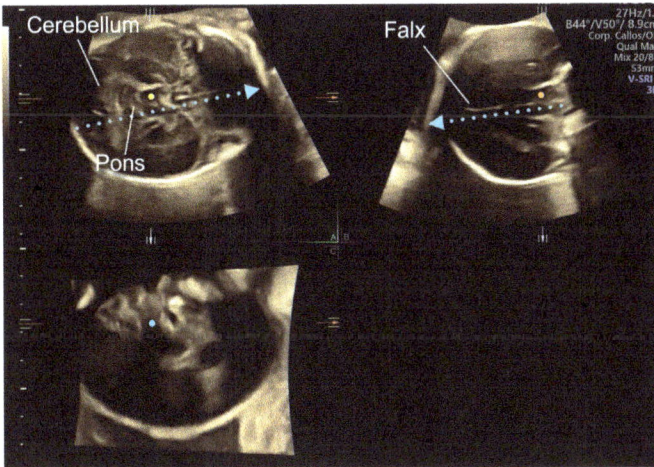

Fig. 16.8: In this fetus in a vertex presentation the cerebellar vermis needed to be visualized. Care has been taken to capture a volume that includes the cerebellum and pons. Note that the axes are oblique in both planes A and B (dashed arrows). Place the intersection point in the 4th ventricle and planes A and B so that the axes are horizontal. See Figure 16.9.

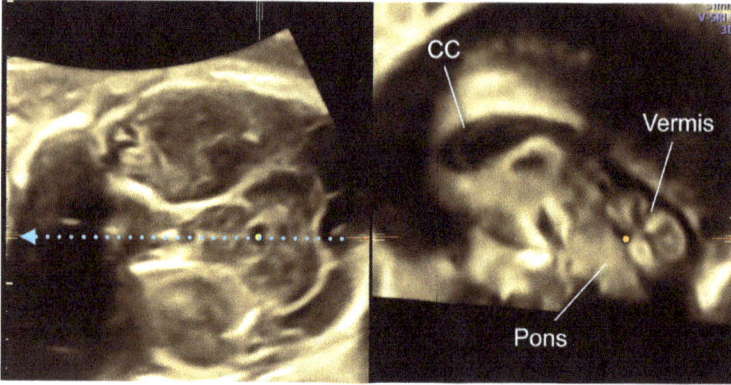

Fig. 16.9: Completion of Figure 16.8. With the axes now aligned horizontally (dashed arrow), the sagittal view of the cerebellum can be readily identified with the pons. The intersection point is in the region of the fourth ventricle and fastigium. Corpus callosum (CC). Compare with Figure 16.10.

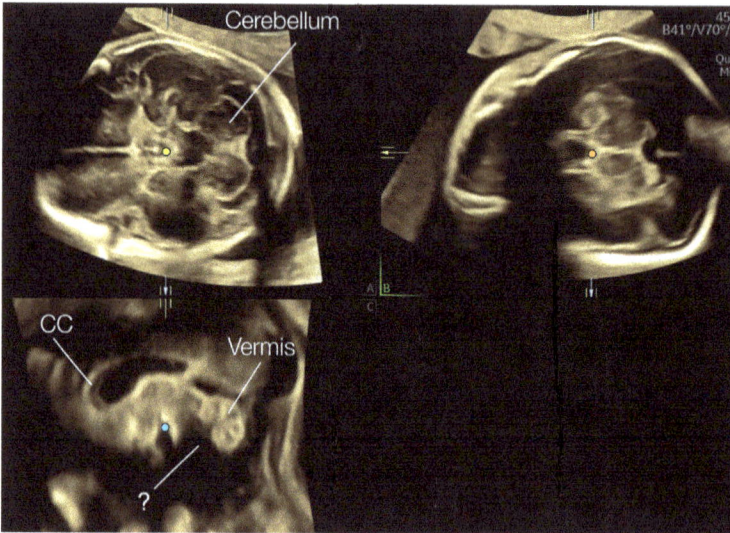

Fig. 16.10: In this good 3D volume of the brain, the cerebellum is well contained, but the pons region was in the shadow of the skull bones and not visible (?). After the 3D reconstruction, the vermis and corpus callosum (CC) can be well assessed though the pons cannot.

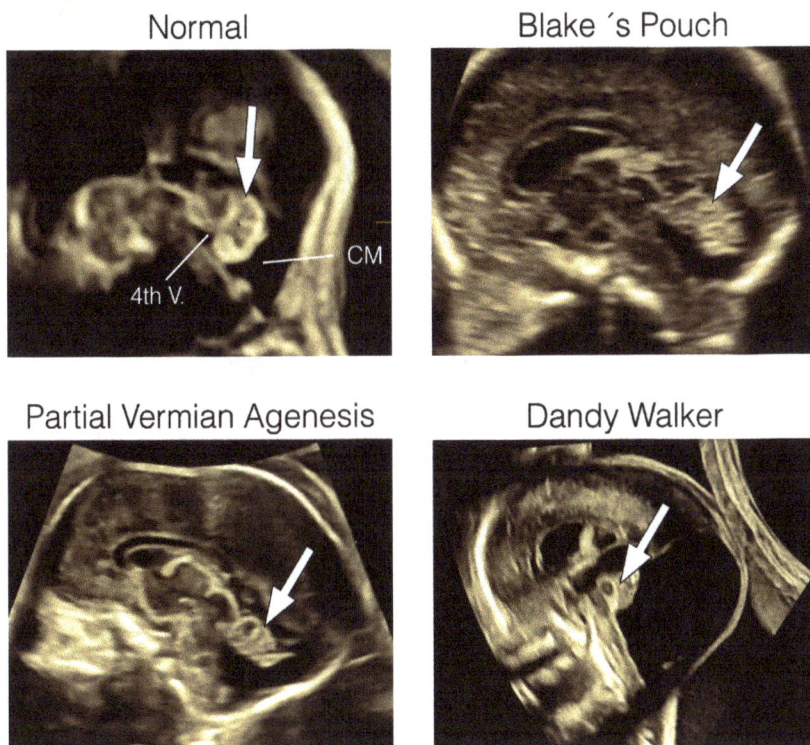

Fig. 16.11: Midsagittal plane of the posterior fossa with vermis in a normal fetus (upper left). The vermis size is normal and there is no connection between the fourth ventricle (4th V.) and the cisterna magna (CM). The other three images display three fetuses with an abnormal posterior fossa. The fetus in the upper right image has a Blake's pouch with a normal height of the vermis but a connection between the 4th ventricle and CM as an upward rotation of the vermis. The fetus in the bottom left image has a smaller vermis due to partial vermian agenesis, and the fetus in the bottom right image has vermian hypoplasia with severe dilatation of the fossa and elevation of the tentorium cerebelli as Dandy Walker malformation.

Tomography mode display of the normal and abnormal brain: The most used 3D imaging of intracranial structures is multiplanar reconstruction such as orthogonal, tomographic, or Omniview mode, often in combination with VCI to improve contrast and detail (see Chapter 4). For documentation of a normal and suspicious brain, we recommend using the tomography mode (Fig. 16.1), which allows demonstration and documentation of a series of parallel planes with a good overview of the brain anatomy. As shown in Figure 16.1, landmarks such as cerebellum with cisterna magna, cortex parenchyma, posterior and anterior horns of the lateral ventricle, and falx cerebri with cavum septi pellucidi can be combined into a single image as an overview. Figures 16.12 to 16.15 show 3D volume images in tomography mode of some typical brain anomalies, such as holoprosencephaly (Fig. 16.12), spina bifida (Fig. 16.13) and agenesis of the corpus callosum (Figs. 16.14, 16.15).

Holoprosencephaly

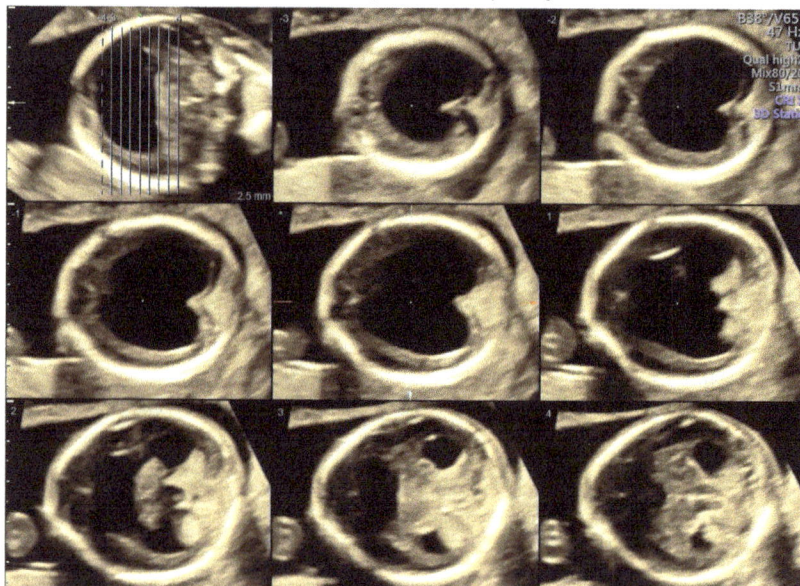

Fig. 16.12: A fetus at 18 weeks of gestation with alobar holoprosencephaly shown in tomography mode.

Spina Bifida

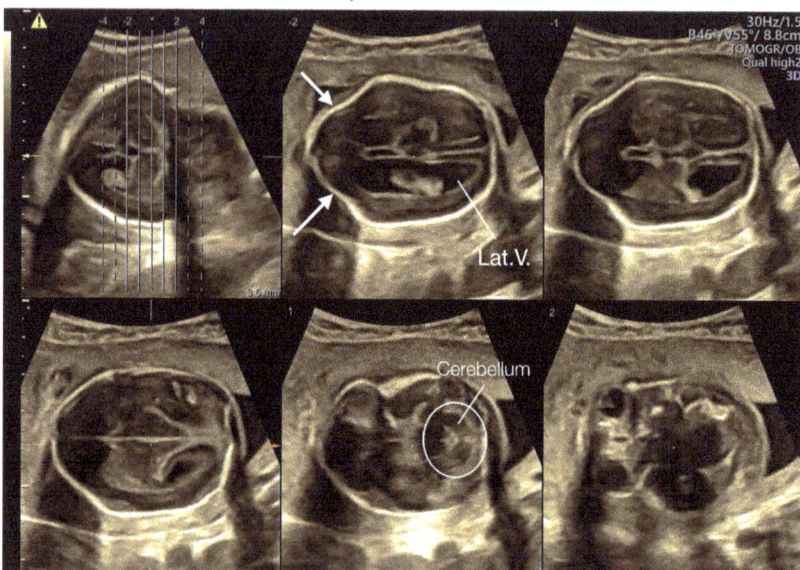

Fig. 16.13: Fetus with open spina bifida showing in one tomography plane all typical cerebral features, such as the scalloping of the frontal bones (arrows) ("lemon sign"), the cerebellum compressed in the posterior fossa ("banana sign") (circle), and the ventriculomegaly with dilated lateral ventricles (Lat.V.).

Agenesis Corpus Callosum

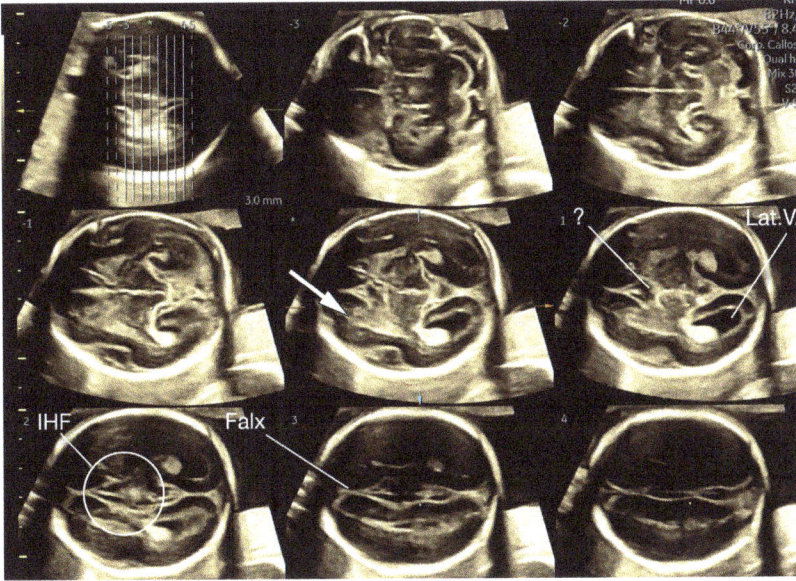

Fig. 16.14: Fetus with agenesis of the corpus callosum shown in the axial planes in tomography mode. The cavum septi pellucidi is absent (?) and there is a dilated interhemispheric fissure (IHF) in the midline (circle). The shape of the lateral ventricles (Lat.V.) shows typical colpocephaly (arrow); falx cerebri (Falx).

Agenesis Corpus Callosum with Schizencephaly

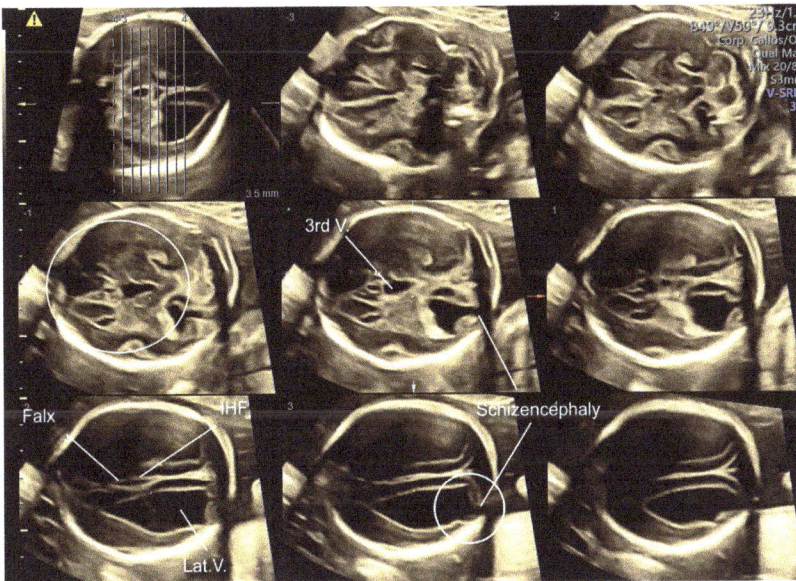

Fig. 16.15: Fetus with agenesis of the corpus callosum associated with schizencephaly (small circle). The third ventricle (3rd V.) is dilated, and the typical features are found (large circle) as described in Figure 16.14. Tomography provides a more complete image of the brain compared to a single image.

16.3 Transvaginal 3D examination of the brain and multiplanar reconstruction

For years, it has been agreed that the best resolution in brain imaging is achieved by transvaginal examination with the fetus in vertex presentation. Some examiners manipulate even the fetus to place it in a vertex position and perform a transvaginal neurosonogram. The three reasons for the better visibility and higher image quality are:

1. The close distance to the brain without an interposed maternal layer as in the transabdominal examination;
2. the high-resolution frequency of the transvaginal transducers, and
3. scanning the brain through the fontanelle or larger open sutures.

The fetus is not always in a perfect position for the exact midline view in the 2D scan. Especially in such scan situations of a few seconds of good fetal head position, it may be difficult to quietly analyze all cerebral structures during a live scan, especially if a brain abnormality is suspected. Therefore, acquisition of multiple 3D volumes has become a requirement, as it allows for subsequent offline examination and reconstruction of the planes of interest. Good 3D images of the brain become more difficult in late gestation after 28 weeks (Figs. 16.16, 16.17), but the period between 20 and 27 weeks is ideal. Between 14 and 20 weeks of gestation, transvaginal examination of the brain is incomparably better than transabdominal views. Transvaginal 3D examinations of the developing brain between 7 and 13 weeks are presented at the end of the chapter.

The approach to 3D reconstruction is similar to that described in the section on transabdominal views, and imaging in tomography mode provides the best overview, as shown in Figures 16.16 and 16.17. Occasionally, an axial view of the brain can be acquired (Fig. 16.18), but when possible, scanning through the anterior or posterior fontanelle is preferred. For this reason, most transvaginally imaged 3D tomographic views are shown in either the coronal or sagittal/parasagittal planes. Figures 16.16 to 16.21 show examples of normal and abnormal brains in 3D tomography mode.

Normal: Sagittal /Parasagittal Views

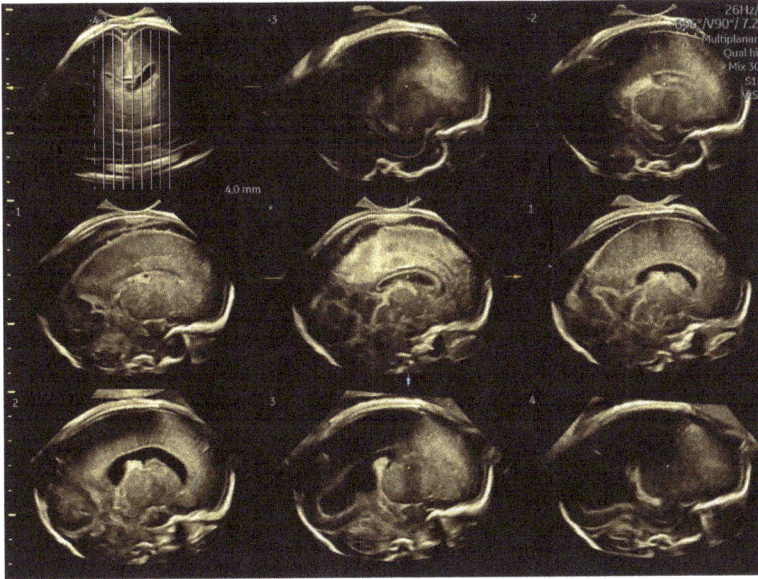

Fig. 16.16: Sagittal and parasagittal sectional planes in tomography mode after transvaginal volume acquisition through the fontanelle. At one glance, the corpus callosum, cerebellar vermis, and lateral ventricles with posterior horns are clearly visible.

Normal: Coronal Views

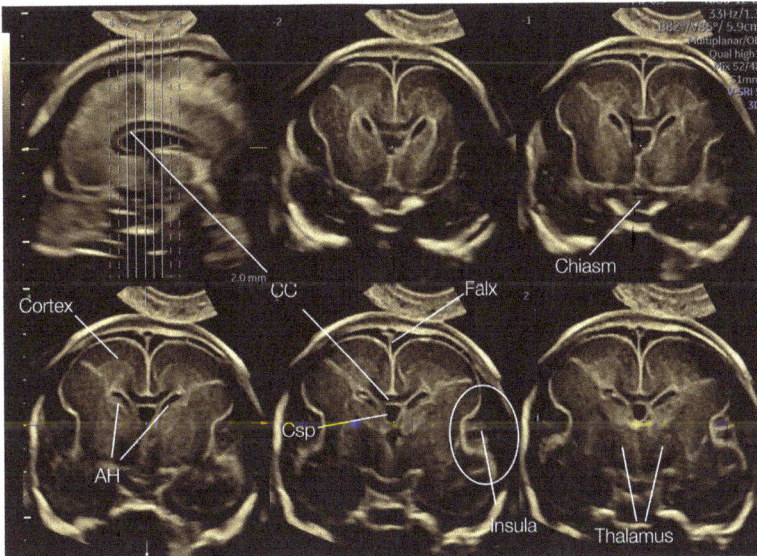

Fig. 16.17: Coronal slice planes in tomographic mode after transvaginal volume acquisition through the fontanelle. At one glance, an overview is given and the following structures can be seen: Cortex, cerebral falx (Falx), corpus callosum (CC), cavum septi pellucidi (Csp), thalami, insula (circle), and anterior horns (AH).

Rhombencephalosynapsis with Aqueductal Stenosis

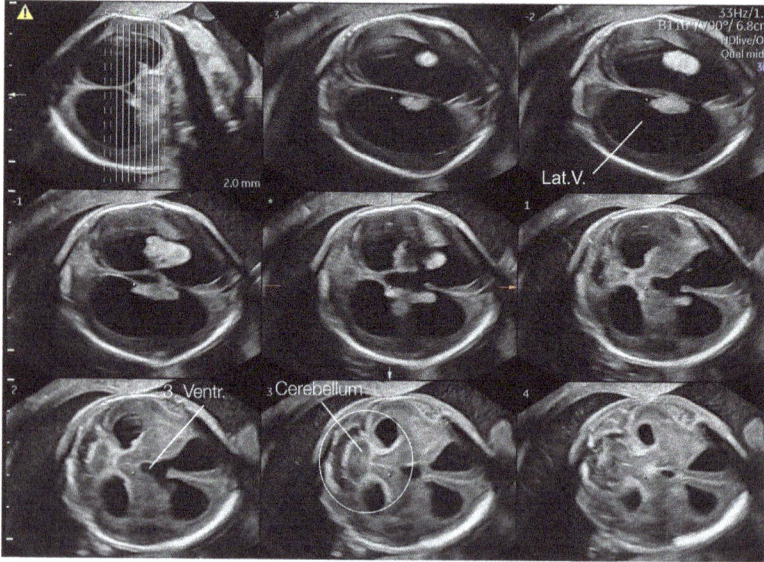

Fig. 16.18: Transvaginal neurosonography and tomography mode in a fetus with ventriculomegaly. The lateral ventricles (Lat.V.) and third ventricle (3. Ventr.) are dilated, suggestive of aqueductal stenosis. This is due to the abnormal cerebellum, which has the features of rhombencephalosynapsis (circle).

Agenesis Corpus Callosum

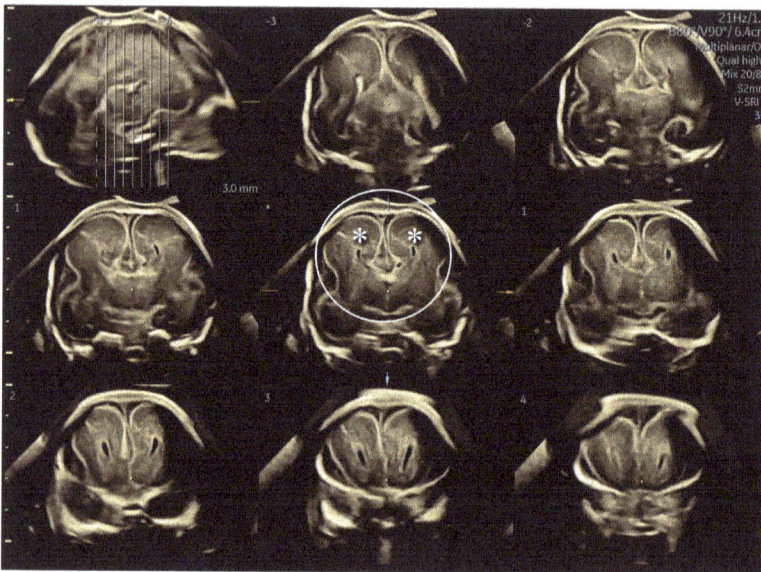

Fig. 16.19: Coronal sections after transvaginal 3D volume acquisition across the fontanelle in a fetus with agenesis of the corpus callosum. No corpus callosum is seen in this view, but the typical "steer horns" shape (circle) is seen. The frontal anterior horns (*) are compressed and lateralized in this anomaly.

Absent Septum Pellucidum

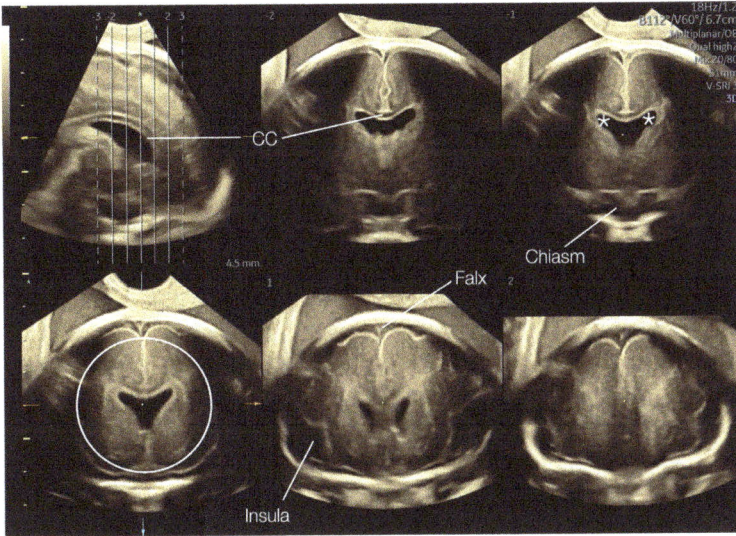

Fig. 16.20: Coronal sections after transvaginal 3D volume acquisition through the fontanelle in a fetus with absent septum pellucidum (circle) in tomography mode. In this view, both anterior horns (*) are fused, but a falx cerebri (Falx) and corpus callosum (CC) are present, ruling out lobar holoprosencephaly. Assessment of the optic chiasm and gyration (insula) is important in such cases.

Lissencephaly, Polymicrogyria, Thick Corpus Callosum

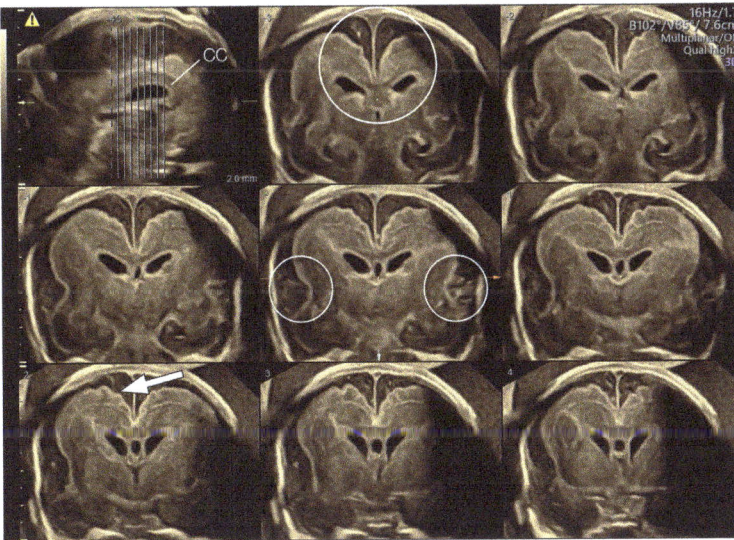

Fig. 16.21: Coronal sections after transvaginal 3D volume acquisition through the fontanelle in a fetus with trisomy 21 and abnormal brain anatomy in tomography mode. Tomography provides a good overview of most findings, such as an enlarged pericerebral space (large circle), shallow Sylvian fissure (small circles), polymicrogyria (arrow), and thickened corpus callosum (CC).

16.4 Fetal brain visualized with 3D volume rendering

The use of 3D in neurosonography focuses mainly on the multiplanar mode, as explained in detail in the previous sections. However, there are still some situations and cases where 3D volume rendering is possible using the different modes presented in this book. In many of these cases, the rendering completes the information provided by the 2D- and multiplanar 3D images (Figs. 16.22, 16.23). In general, we often use the surface mode of the area of interest and occasionally complete it with the silhouette mode. The introduction of the silhouette mode has opened a new window to visualize intracerebral brain structures (Figs. 16.24, 16.25). In cases of increased fluid accumulation, the surface mode and the inversion or silhouette mode can be used. In early pregnancy, the not yet ossified cranial bones allow the use of silhouette mode to visualize the ventricular system, as discussed in Section 16.6. Figures 16.22 to 16.25 show some examples of different 3D surface modes. In a recent study, Chen and Li from China used the inversion mode to visualize the Sylvian fissure and gyration in the distal hemisphere, a technique that shows promise (Fig. 16.26).

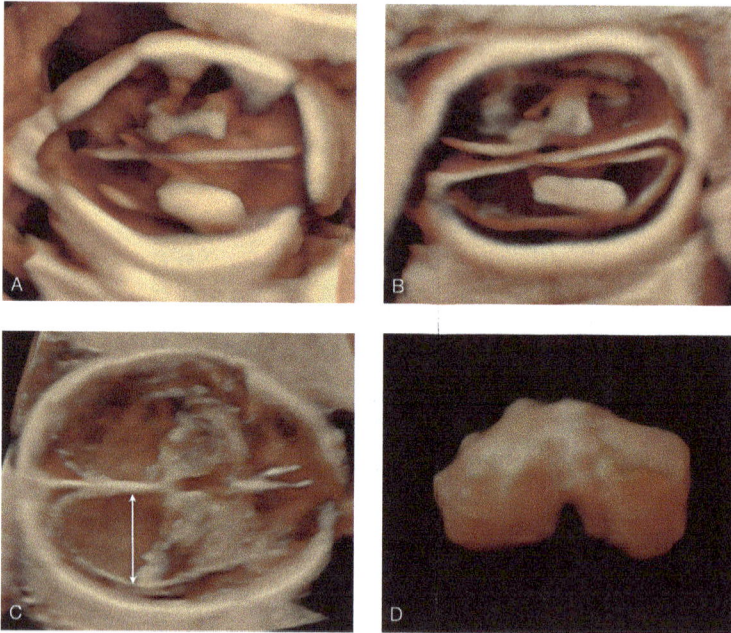

Fig. 16.22: Surface mode looking into the brain of two fetuses with spina bifida (A and B), one fetus with ventriculomegaly (double arrow) (C), and the reconstruction of a normal cerebellum in (D).

Cephaloceles

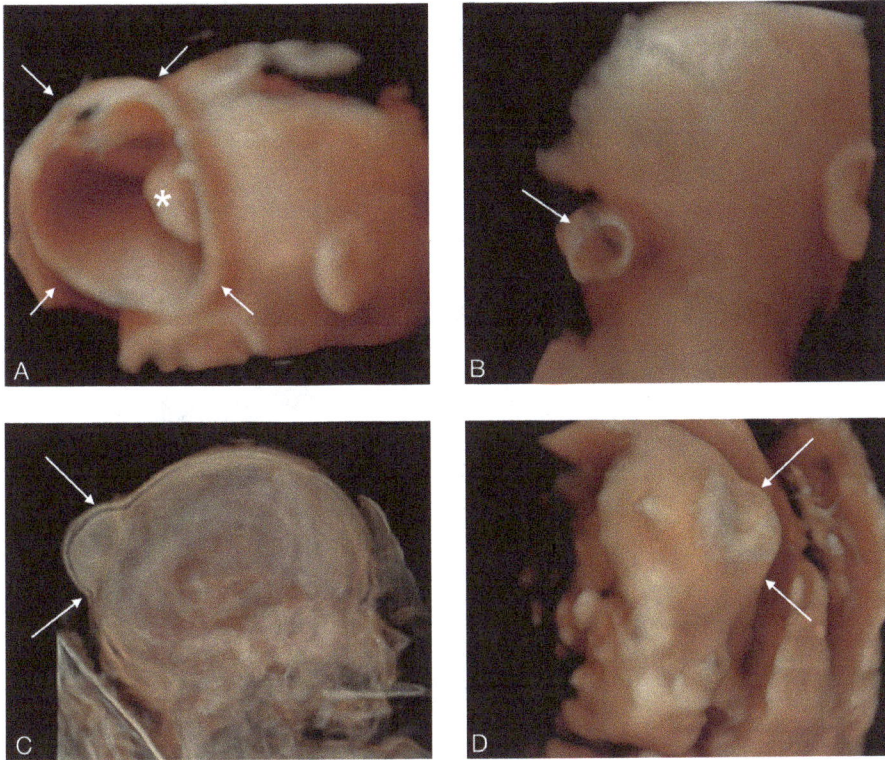

Fig. 16.23: Surface mode rendering in fetuses with various cephaloceles (arrows): (A) encephalocele, (B) suboccipital meningocele, (C) atretic parietal cephalocele, (D) frontal meningocele.

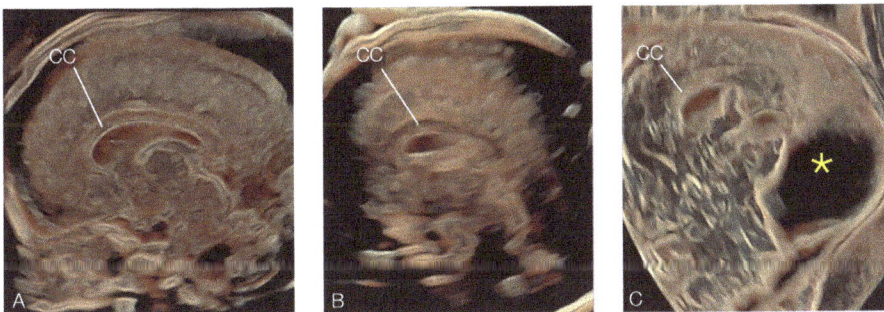

Fig. 16.24: Rendering with silhouette mode of the midline in a normal fetus with normal corpus callosum (CC) in (A), a fetus with thickened CC in (B), and a fetus with short CC and a Dandy-Walker malformation (*) in (C).

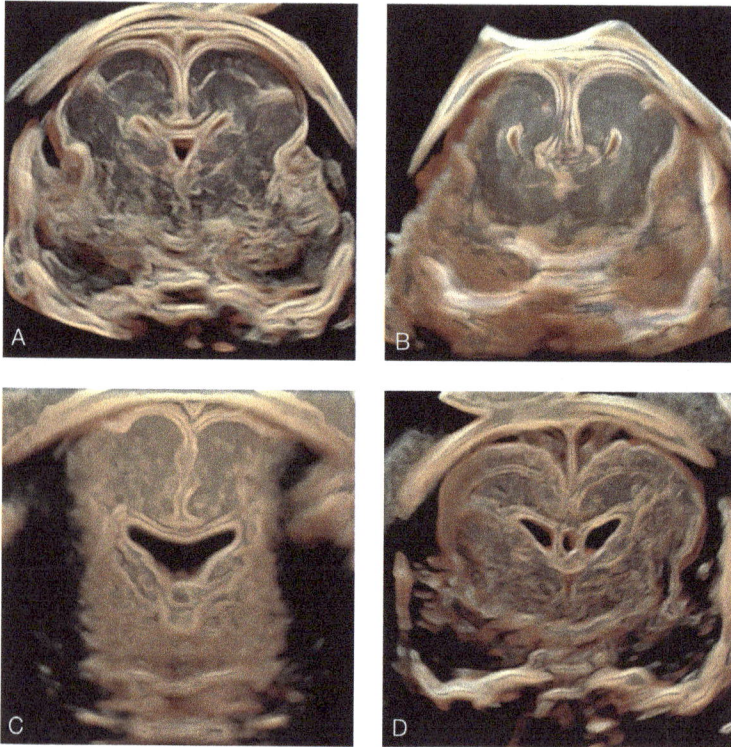

Fig. 16.25: Rendering with silhouette mode of the coronal plane in a normal fetus (A), a fetus with agenesis of the corpus callosum (B), a fetus with absent septum pellucidum (C), and a fetus with lissencephaly and polymicrogyria (D).

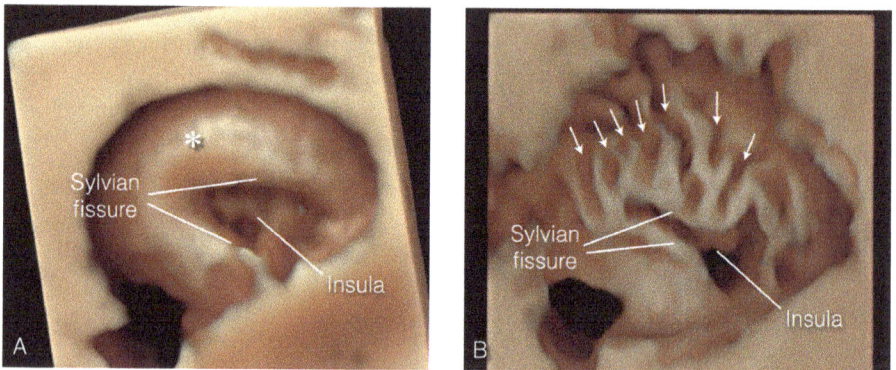

Fig. 16.26: Inversion mode of the convex surface of the distal cerebral hemispheres in one fetus at 23 weeks (A) and 31 weeks of gestation (B). The fetal brain surface in (A) is smooth (*), the Sylvian fissure is wide and the insula is well seen. In (B), maturation of the brain at 31 weeks shows the cortex gyration (arrows), the narrowing of the Sylvian fissure, and the covering of the insula called operculisation (see also Fig. 10.12).

16.5 The intracerebral vascular system in 3D glass-body mode

The major intracerebral arteries and veins can be well visualized with both axial and sagittal approaches (Fig. 16.27). The left and right internal carotid arteries and basilar artery enter at the base of the skull and soon form the circle of Willis. Latter can be easily visualized with color Doppler and 3D glass-body mode in an axial plane (Fig. 16.27A). In the midsagittal view, one of the major arteries that is easily seen is the anterior cerebral artery which runs along the corpus callosum and forms the pericallosal and callosomarginal arteries (Fig. 16.27B). In fetuses with partial or complete agenesis of the corpus callosum, these arteries have an abnormal course, as shown in Figures 16.27 and 16.28. Recently, the intracranial venous system has been the subject of intense research. Interest has focused not only on the superior and inferior sagittal sinus, the straight sinus, and the transverse sinus (Fig. 16.27B), but also on other veins such as the vein of Galen, the internal cerebral veins, and the deep medullary veins, thus detecting anomalies such as the arteriovenous malformation of the vein of Galen (Fig. 16.29) and others. Of interest is the new ability to combine the 3D glass-body mode with silhouette mode in grayscale, making the brain structures slightly transparent and thus improving the visualization of the vessels (Fig. 16.27). Glass-body mode can also be combined with monochrome color and special light rendering (Fig. 16.28). Another tool, which is easier to use clinically, is the addition of volume contrast VCI to the color Doppler image; this enhances the area of interest by a few millimeters and produces an image like the glass-body mode (Fig. 16.28B). Figures 16.27 to 16.30 show some typical anomalies involving the intracerebral vasculature.

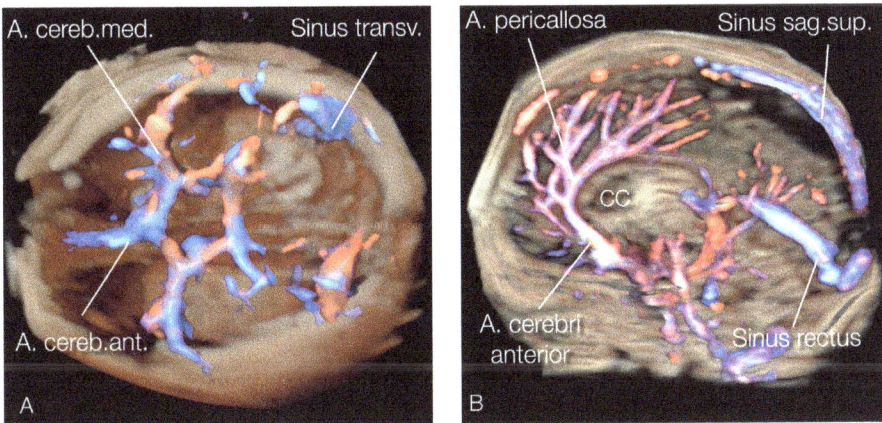

Fig. 16.27: Intracranial arteries and veins in 3D glass-body mode in axial view (A) and sagittal view (B) in two normal fetuses. In (A), the Circle of Willis is clearly visible with the middle and anterior cerebral arteries and the transverse sinus. In (B), the anterior cerebral arteries and pericallosal arteries are well seen anteriorly, and the superior sagittal sinus and straight sinus are well seen posteriorly. Below the pericallosal artery, the corpus callosum (CC) can be seen.

Agenesis Corpus Callosum

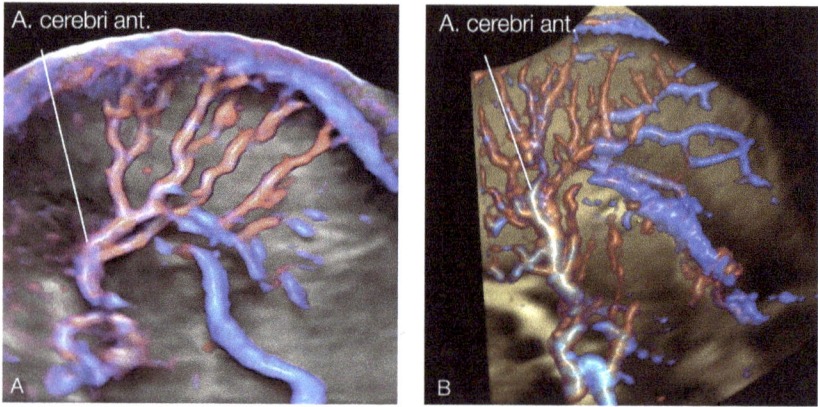

Fig. 16.28: Intracranial arteries and veins in 3D glass-body sagittal section in two fetuses with complete agenesis of the corpus callosum. The anterior cerebral artery shows an abnormal course in both cases. Compare with Figure 16.27B.

Vein of Galen Aneurysmal Malformation

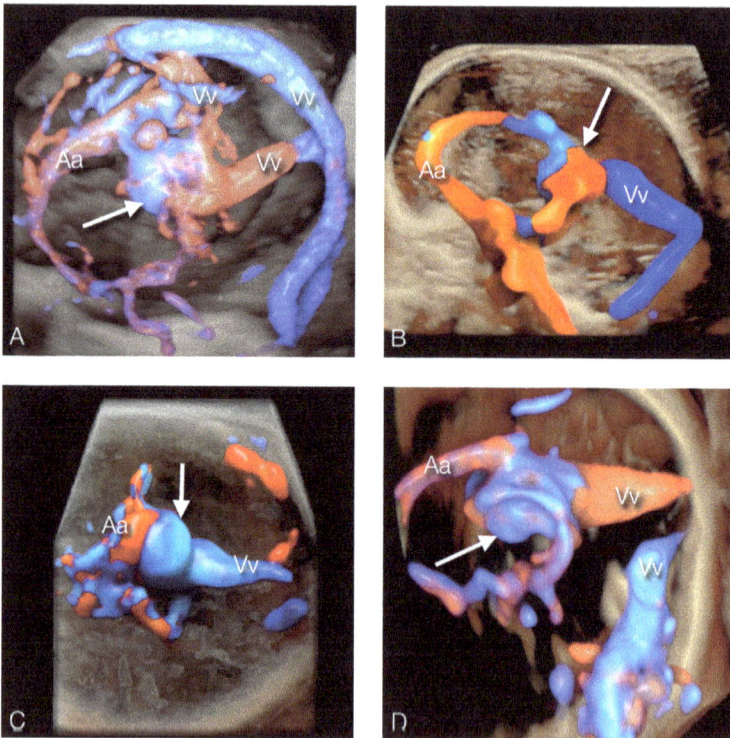

Fig. 16.29: 3D glass-body mode of the intracerebral vasculature in four fetuses with Vein of Galen aneurysmal malformation with enormous dilatation of the vein of Galen (arrow) including the feeding arteries (Aa) and draining veins (Vv).

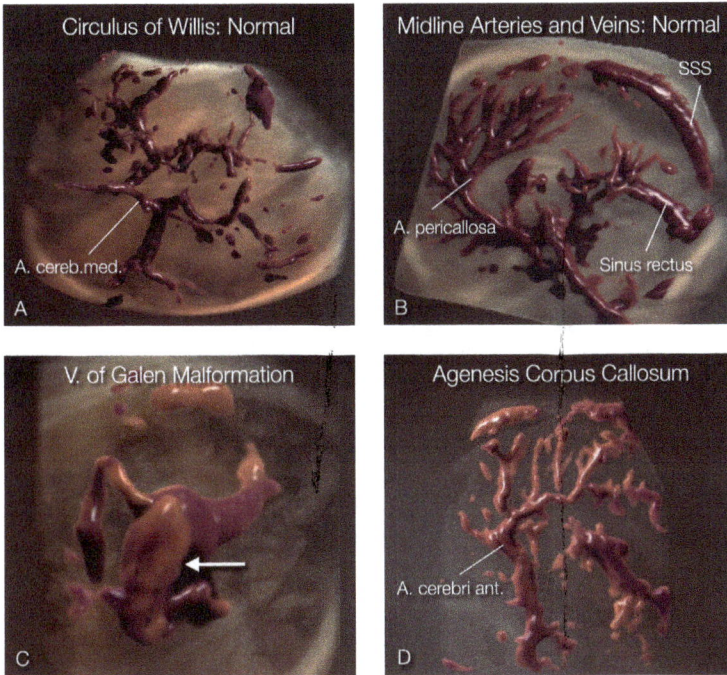

Fig. 16.30: Intracranial arteries and veins in 3D glass-body mode with monochrome imaging in axial view (A) and sagittal view (B) in two normal fetuses. In (C), a fetus with vein of Galen aneurysmal malformation and in (D) with complete agenesis of the corpus callosum. Superior sagittal sinus (SSS).

16.6 3D of the fetal brain before 14 gestational weeks

Interest in normal fetal anatomy and anomalies in the first 14 weeks of gestation has increased with the introduction and routine use of nuchal translucency screening. For many years, brain assessment at this gestational age was limited to visualization of the skull to rule out anencephaly and visualization of the falx cerebri to rule out holoprosencephaly. With the advent of intracranial translucency assessment and the ability to detect spina bifida early in pregnancy, interest in understanding brain development and anatomy in the first trimester has grown. In many conditions, a 3D volume with tomographic imaging (Figs. 16.31, 16.32) provides a good overview of intracranial anatomy and allows discrimination between normal and abnormal findings (Figs. 16.33–16.35). Figures 16.33 and 16.34 show intracerebral changes in the brain of 12- and 13-week-old fetuses with open spina bifida, and Figures 16.35 and 16.36 show the use of 3D in fetuses with holoprosencephaly.

Few scientists have used 3D ultrasound to study the embryonic development of the human brain before 11 weeks of gestation (Figs. 16.37, 16.38). This can be readily accomplished by using the multiplanar views discussed previously to visualize the ventricular system and adjacent structures. Interestingly, a few volume rendering modes such as silhouette or inversion mode are also capable of visualizing the developing ventricular system (Fig. 16.38). With the increasing resolution of 2D and 3D, it is expected that more insights will be available at this early stage of brain development and that high-risk patients can be offered earlier examination.

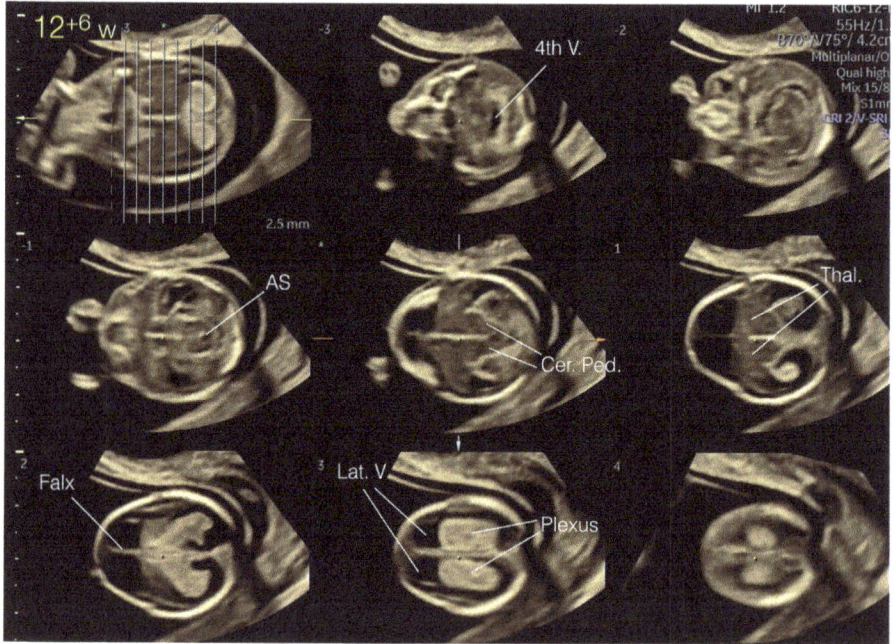

Fig. 16.31: Tomography mode of an axial view of the fetal brain at 12 weeks of gestation, giving an overview of the major landmarks of the brain at this stage of development. These include the large choroid plexus, the falx cerebri (Falx), the two lateral ventricles (Lat.V.), the thalami (Thal.), the Sylvian aqueduct (AS), the cerebral peduncles (Cer. Ped.), and the fourth ventricle (4th V.).

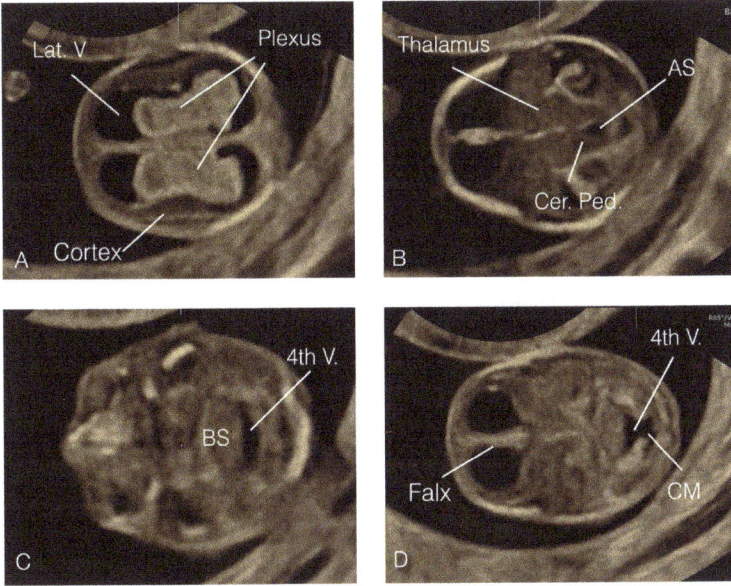

Fig. 16.32: Single essential planes extracted from a 3D volume of the fetal brain at 12 weeks of gestation showing following structures: (A) Transventricular plane with lateral ventricles (Lat.V.), cortex and both choroid plexuses; (B) transthalamic plane with thalami, cerebral peduncles (Cer.Ped.) and Sylvian aqueduct (AS); (C) plane with brainstem (BS) and fourth ventricle (4th V.); (D) the fourth ventricle connecting to the cisterna magna (CM) at the level of the inferior posterior fossa.

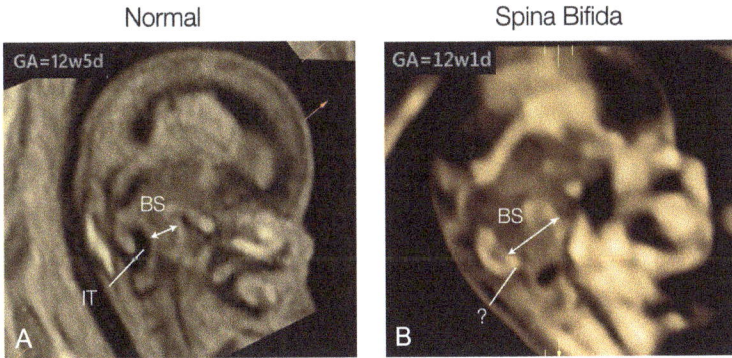

Fig. 16.33: Reconstruction of the posterior fossa from two volumes of a normal fetus (A) and a fetus with spina bifida (B) at 12 weeks of gestation. The intracranial translucency (IT) representing the fourth ventricle is clearly visible in (A), while it is absent (?) in (B). The brainstem (BS) (double arrow) is thin in (A) and thickened and compressed in (B).

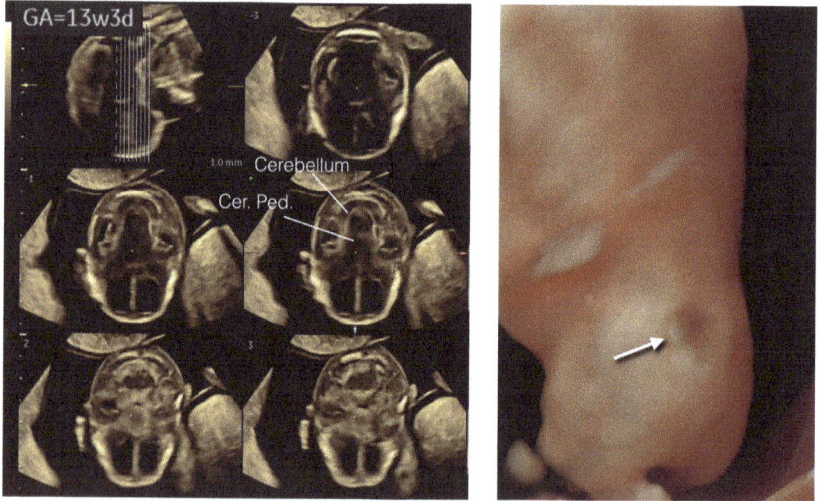

Fig. 16.34: Tomography mode of an axial view of the brain in a 13-week-old fetus (left) with spina bifida (right). Note that the cerebellum already obliterates the posterior fossa (left), and the surface view of the lower spine (right) shows the spinal lesion (arrow).

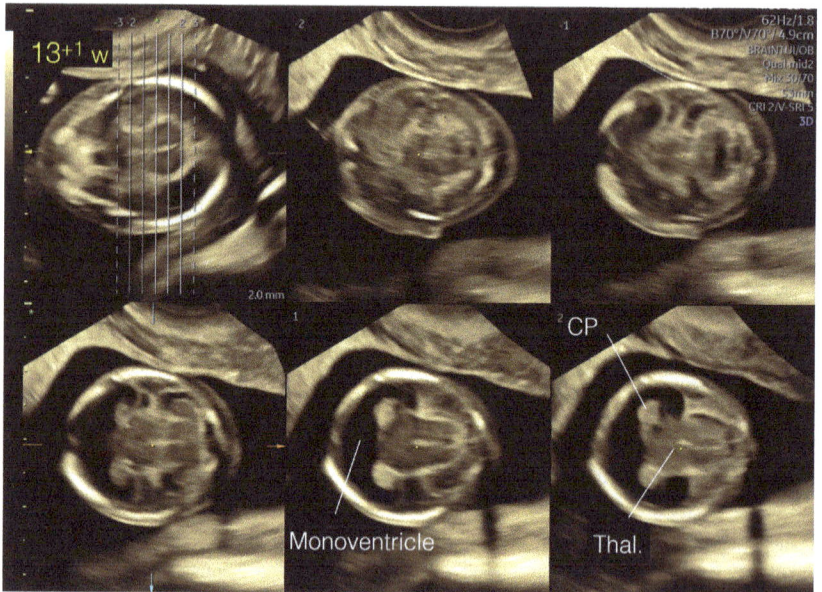

Fig. 16.35: Tomography mode in a fetus at 12 weeks of gestation with alobar holoprosencephaly showing the fused thalami (Thal.) and choroid plexus (CP) and the absence of a falx cerebri with a monoventricle.

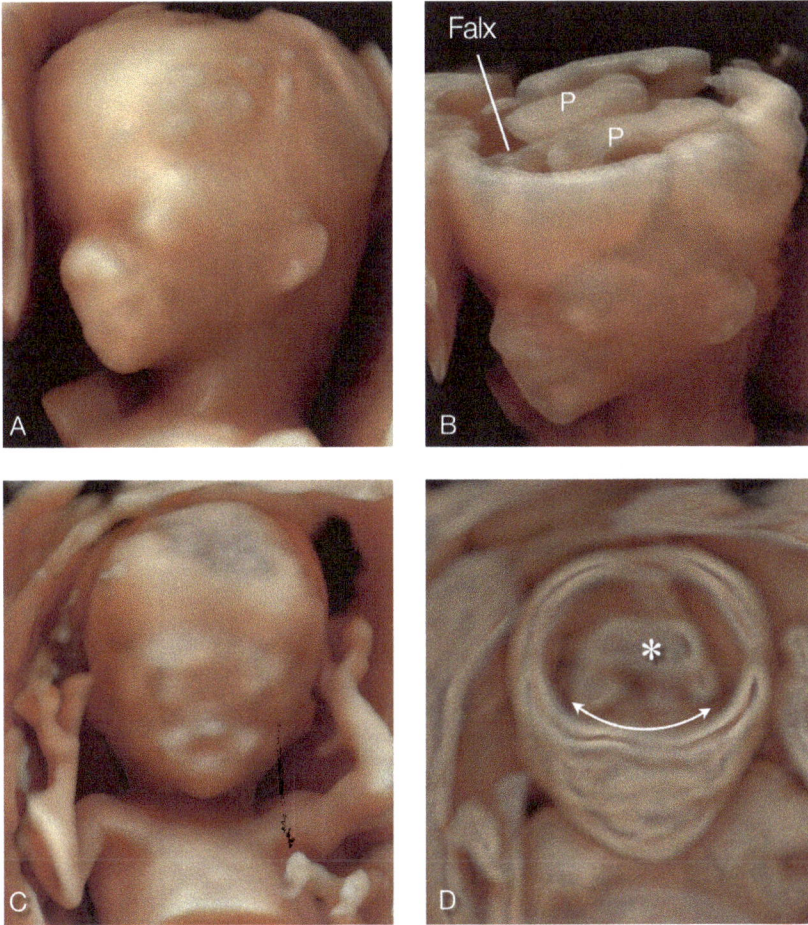

Fig. 16.36: 3D surface mode at 12 weeks of gestation of the face and underlying brain in a normal fetus (A and B) and a fetus with trisomy 13 with median cleft and holoprosencephaly (C and D). The faces are obviously different; the brain in (B) shows the clear separation of the two hemispheres and the choroid plexus (P) by the cerebral falx, while in (D) the holoprosencephaly is obvious with fused ventricles (double arrow) and fused choroid plexus (*).

Normal

Exencephaly

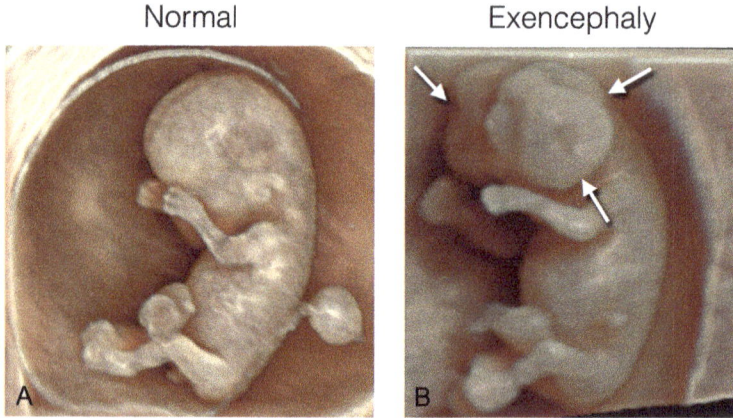

Fig. 16.37: 3D surface mode of two embryos at 10 weeks of gestation: (A) with normal head and (B) with exencephaly (arrows). The 3D surface mode illustrates well the severity of the findings in (B).

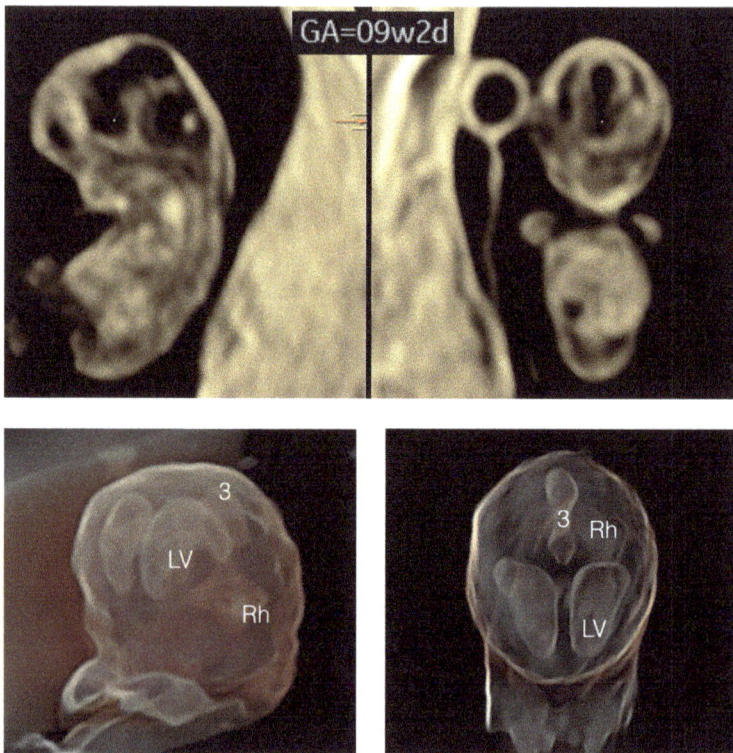

Fig. 16.38: 3D volume in orthogonal view of skull and brain at 9 weeks of gestation. The ventricular system can be well assessed in multiplanar mode (upper panel), but silhouette mode (bottom panel) allows clear visualization of the two lateral ventricles (LV), the third ventricle (3), and the rhombencephalon (Rh).

16.7 Conclusions

Fetal neurosonography is an important component of a comprehensive ultrasound to exclude fetal brain malformations, especially in the second half of pregnancy. The combination of 3D and 2D ultrasound facilitates assessment of the fetal brain and provides the opportunity to reconstruct planes that are inaccessible on routine scans. Reconstruction as well as offline analysis and detailed visualization of structures in multiplanar mode are the main advantages of 3D examinations. Tomographic imaging of slice planes also provides a reliable tool for comparison with other diagnostic modalities such as MR examination of the fetal brain. The study of early embryonic brain development with 3D ultrasound under normal and abnormal conditions offers significant future potential.

17 3D of Skull, Spine, and Limbs

17.1 Examination of the fetal skeleton with 2D ultrasound

Examination of the fetal skeleton, including the skull, spine, and limbs by 2D ultrasound is often limited to those bones that are readily accessible. Routine screening involves measuring the long bones, visualizing the spine, and imaging the hands and feet as best as possible. Skull bones, ribs, and some other structures can only be assessed to a limited extent with 2D ultrasound. A better approach for visualizing the skeletal system is the combined examination of 2D and 3D ultrasound using maximum, surface, or silhouette mode. The acquisition of static 3D volumes combined with the subsequent display in the different multiplanar modalities or 3D rendering modes, such as surface or transparency modes, can help in obtaining images of the typical bones of interest. This chapter briefly discusses the study of the different parts of the skeletal system, such as the skull, spine, and extremities under normal and abnormal conditions.

17.2 3D imaging of the facial and cranial bones

The facial and cranial bones with their corresponding sutures are best rendered in maximum mode or with the silhouette mode with the presets for bones (see Chapter 8 and Chapter 11). Volume acquisition can be performed in either static 3D, 4D, VCI-A or VCI Omniview mode. A prerequisite for optimal bone rendering in 3D is the reduction of gain and increase of contrast in 2D prior to volume acquisition. The volume is acquired from either a sagittal view of the face or a lateral insonation of the skull and jaw, depending on the region to be imaged. To better highlight the bones in maximum mode, VCI-Omniview with a thick slice thickness (15–20 mm) can also be selected.

Facial bones and cranial bones: The frontal view of the bony face shows the two frontal bones with the metopic suture, the two orbits, the nasal bone, the maxilla, and the mandible (Figs. 17.1, 17.2A). Figure 17.1 shows the progression of ossification of the metopic suture between the first and second trimesters of pregnancy. Evaluation of this view can aid in the assessment of the metopic (or frontal) suture, orbital cavities, nasal bone, maxilla, and mandible. Figures 17.1 through 17.6 show normal and various abnormal findings in this frontal view. The skull bones and sutures are best seen in these planes. Abnormal findings include the wide metopic suture typically found in Apert syndrome (Fig. 17.2B) or other conditions associated with craniosynostosis of the coronal suture. The presence of additional bones, so-called Wormian bones, may occasionally be found in the metopic suture or in the fontanelles. They are commonly found in syndromic midline diseases, but their true clinical significance is not yet known (Fig. 17.2C). In addition, the metopic suture may be fused in fetuses with alobar holoprosencephaly (Fig. 17.3). In frontal view, an absent nasal bone is readily apparent (Fig. 17.4),

https://doi.org/10.1515/9783111249513-017

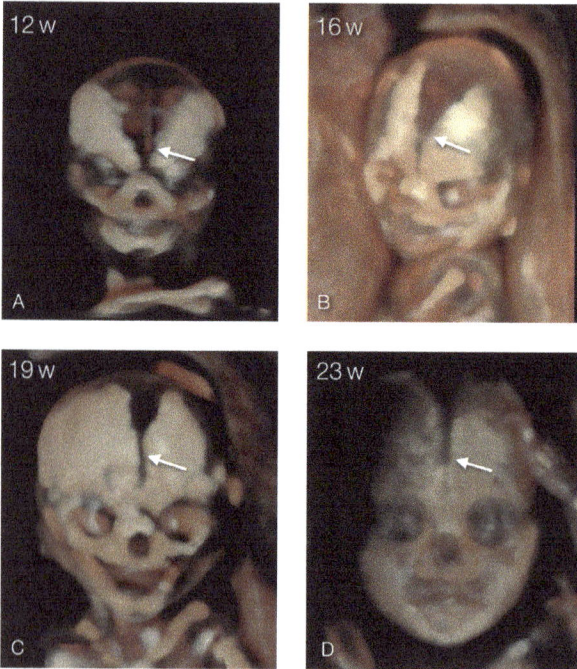

Fig. 17.1: Development of the metopic suture (arrow), displayed in silhouette mode and showing four fetuses at 12 weeks (A), 16 weeks (B), 19 weeks (C), and 23 weeks of gestation (D). Note the successive narrowing of the suture margins from the nose toward the fontanelle.

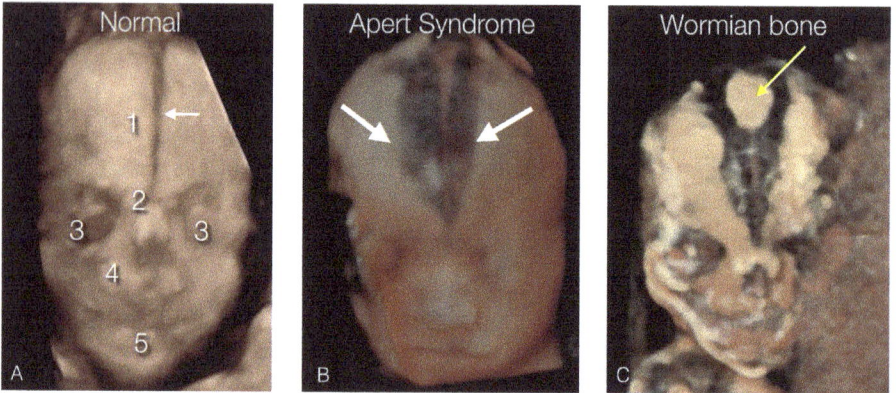

Fig. 17.2: Visualization of the bony face in maximal and silhouette mode in three fetuses at 23 weeks of gestation: in (A) a normal fetus with the typical landmarks, such as the metopic suture (1), the nasal bone (2), the orbits (3), the maxilla (4), and the mandible (5). Note the metopic suture in (A) (short arrow); in comparison, two anomalies including a fetus with craniosynostosis (here in Apert syndrome) in (B) with a wide metopic suture (two arrows), and another fetus in (C) with a Wormian bone (yellow arrow) as an additional bone in the fontanelle with a wide metopic suture in a severe facial syndrome of unknown etiology.

as is the presence of facial clefts involving the anterior alveolar ridge (Figs. 17.5, 17.6). Lateral or cranial insonation of the head allows visualization of the various cranial bones with their corresponding sutures (see also Chapter 8), and 3D imaging can visualize fused sutures in craniosynostosis (Fig. 17.7B) better than 2D ultrasound alone. Decreased ossification of the cranial bones is seen in both osteogenesis imperfecta and cleidocranial dysplasia (Fig. 17.8B).

Maxilla and mandible: The jaw can be well imaged in the frontal view, but a better assessment is obtained with a lateral 3D acquisition. With a lateral insonation and acquisition, the skull bones can be visualized with the upper and lower jaw (Fig. 17.8).

Holoprosencephaly

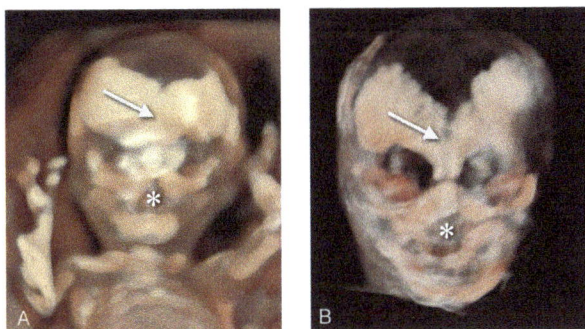

Fig. 17.3: Two fetuses with holoprosencephaly, in (A) at 12 weeks and in (B) at 17 weeks, both showing the early synostosis of the metopic suture (arrows) characteristic of this midline anomaly. Compare with Figure 17.1 for the normal metopic suture. Note the median cleft (*) in both fetuses and the hypotelorism in (B).

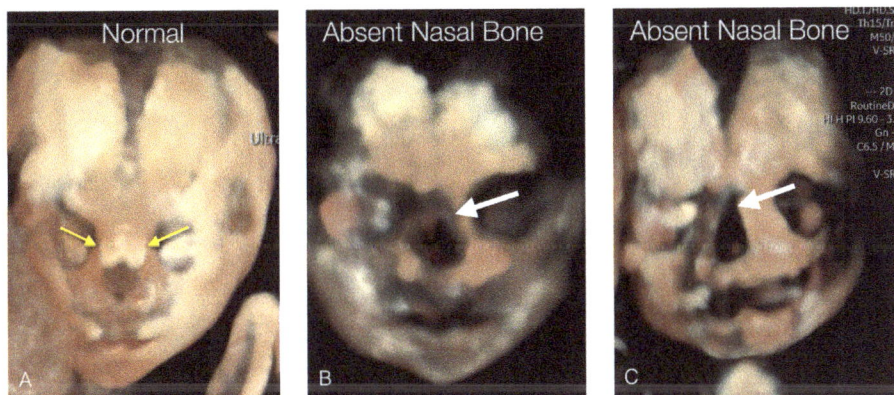

Fig. 17.4: In (A) a fetus with normal ossification of the nasal bone and in (B) and (C) with absent ossification, as shown in 3D silhouette mode with the bones viewed from the front. The fetus in (B) has trisomy 21, while the fetus in (C) has Cornelia de Lange syndrome.

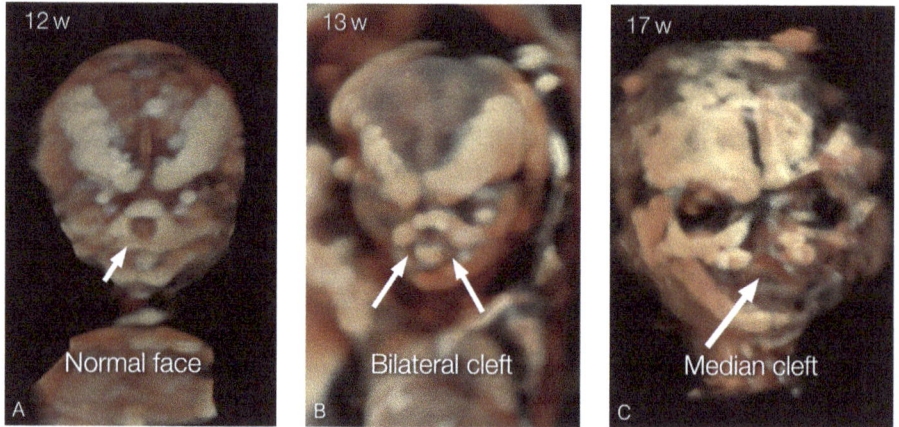

Fig. 17.5: Three fetal faces at 12, 13 and 17 weeks of gestation, shown in silhouette mode with highlighted facial bones. In (A) a normal fetus with intact maxilla (short arrow), in (B) with bilateral cleft (two arrows), and in (C) with median cleft (long arrow).

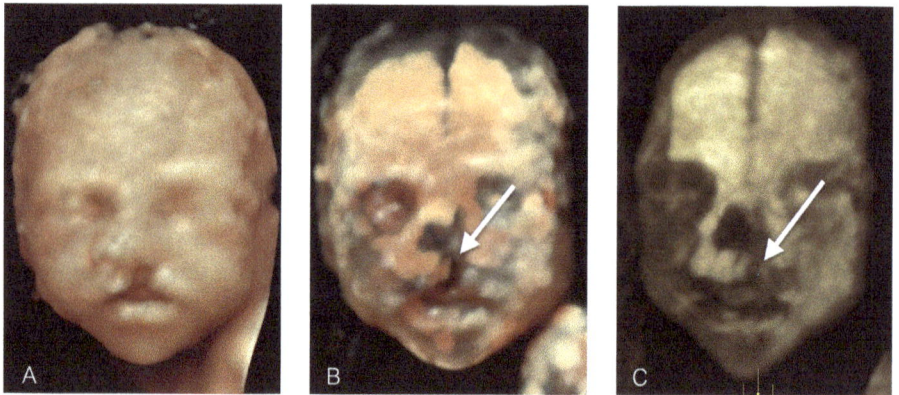

Fig. 17.6: Fetus with mediolateral cleft lip and palate shown in surface mode (A), silhouette mode (B) and maximum mode (C).

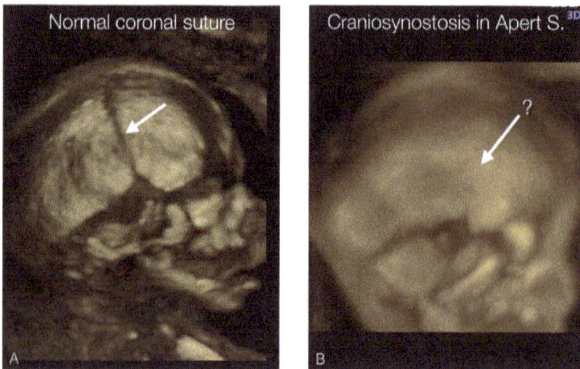

Fig. 17.7: Maximum mode of a lateral view of the cranial bones in a normal fetus (A) and in a fetus with Apert syndrome and coronal suture synostosis (B). The coronal suture can be seen in the fetus in (A) (arrow), while it appears fused (?) in the fetus in (B).

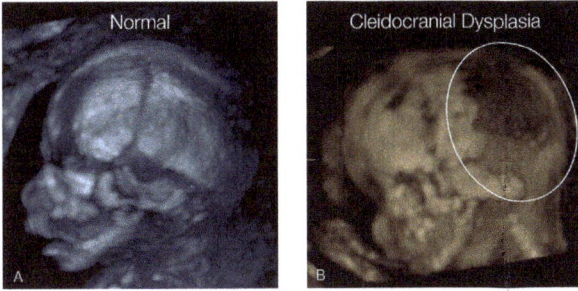

Fig. 17.8: Fetus with normal ossification of the cranial bones in (A); in (B), a fetus with skeletal dysplasia from the cleidocranial dysplasia family with the typical abnormal ossification of the parietal bone (circle).

17.3 3D imaging of the fetal spine and ribs

The fetal spine can be imaged using various 3D methods, shown in Figures 17.9 to 17.11 and discussed in Chapter 8. These tools provide good visualization of the bony spine with the vertebral bodies and arches in various stages of ossification. Navigation through the volume also provides an overview of the spine with all vertebral bodies and associated intervertebral disks in both maximum and silhouette modes (Figs. 17.10, 17.11). Individual vertebral bodies can also be visualized with Magicut or with navigation in multiplanar mode (Fig. 17.12). In the frontal projection of the spine, the ribs can be well visualized, allowing assessment of symmetry and number of ribs. Typical anomalies that can be visualized with this procedure include the various forms of open spina bifida (Figs. 17.13–17.17), hemivertebrae (Fig. 17.18) or other spinal deformities (Figs. 17.19, 17.20). In open spina bifida, the surface mode can be used first to assess the size and type of defect as myelomeningocele (Fig. 17.15) or myeloschisis (Fig. 17.16). In addition, the bone defect and the height of the lesion can be better visualized with a transparency mode that highlights the bones (Fig. 17.17). Severe findings such as kyphoscoliosis, sacral agenesis, or segmental spinal dysgenesis are detected in 2D ultrasound, but the full extent of the lesion can be better visualized in 3D mode with transparency, as shown in Figures 17.19 and 17.20.

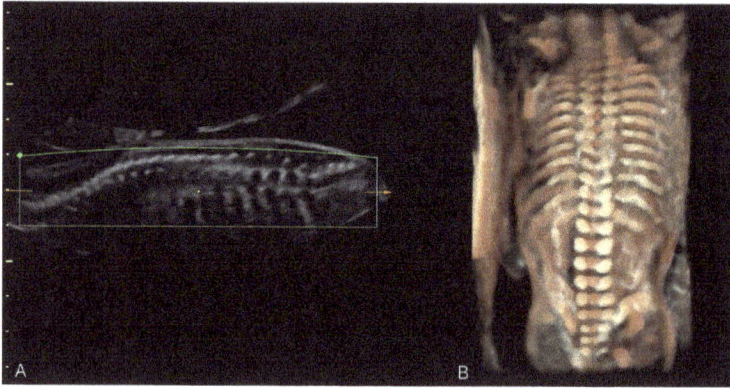

Fig. 17.9: 3D volume data set of a spine with ribs shown in silhouette rendering mode with highlighted bones (B). Note the shallow depth of the volume box in (A).

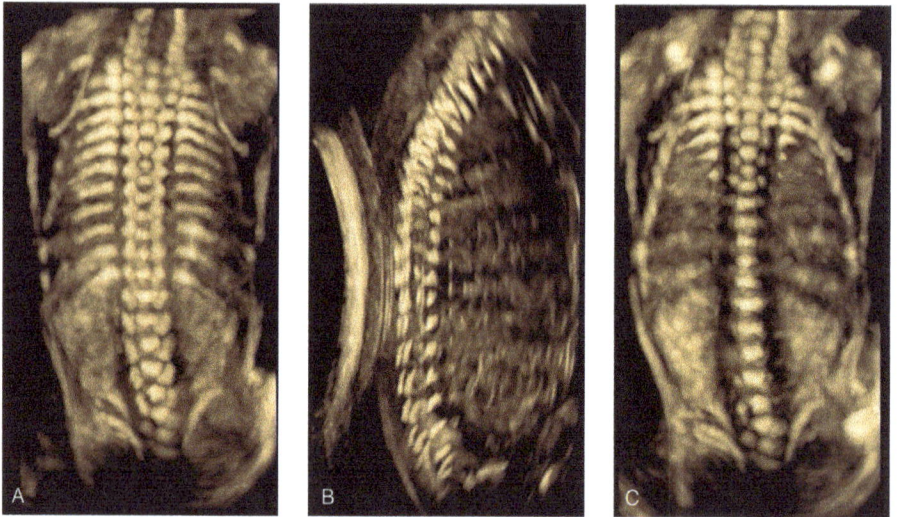

Fig. 17.10: In a 3D volume data set with maximum mode rendering, the image can be rotated or the perspective changed. (A) Dorsal view of spine and ribs, (B) lateral view of the spine with intact skin covering the spine, and (C) view in a deeper layer from dorsal with direct view of the vertebral bodies.

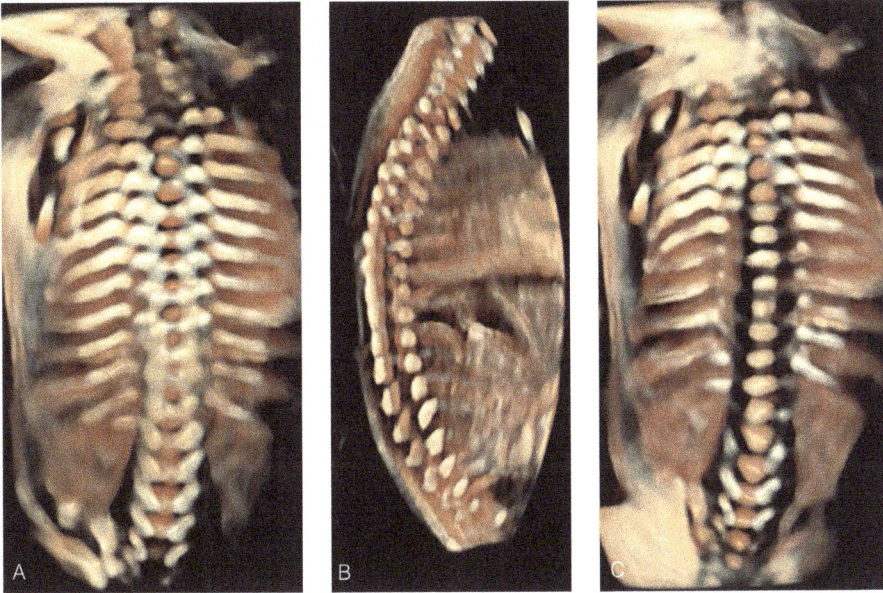

Fig. 17.11: In this 3D volume, similar to Figure 17.10, the silhouette mode has been activated to show the bones. It shows in (A) a dorsal view of the spine and ribs, in (B) a lateral view of the spine with the intact skin covering the spine, and in (C) a view in a deeper layer from dorsal with a direct view of the vertebral bodies.

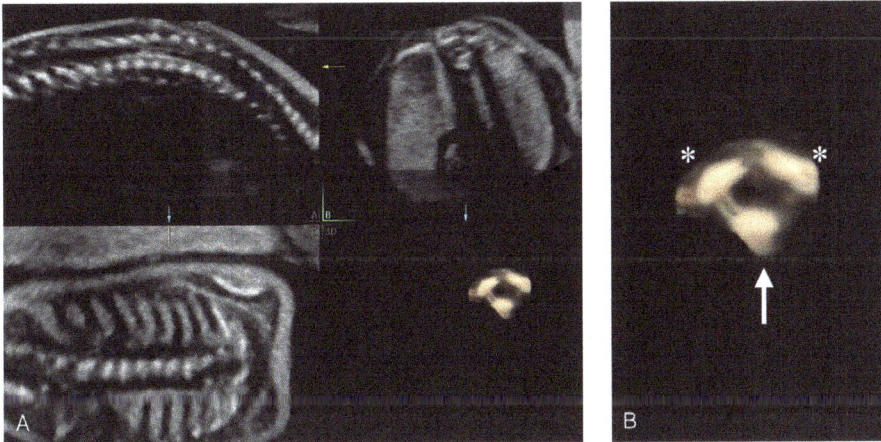

Fig. 17.12: The user can also selectively cut out anatomical structures from a volume. In this example, a vertebra has been cut out (A) and enlarged (B). In cross-section, the vertebral body (arrow) and the two vertebral arches (*) can be seen. Compare with Figure 17.13.

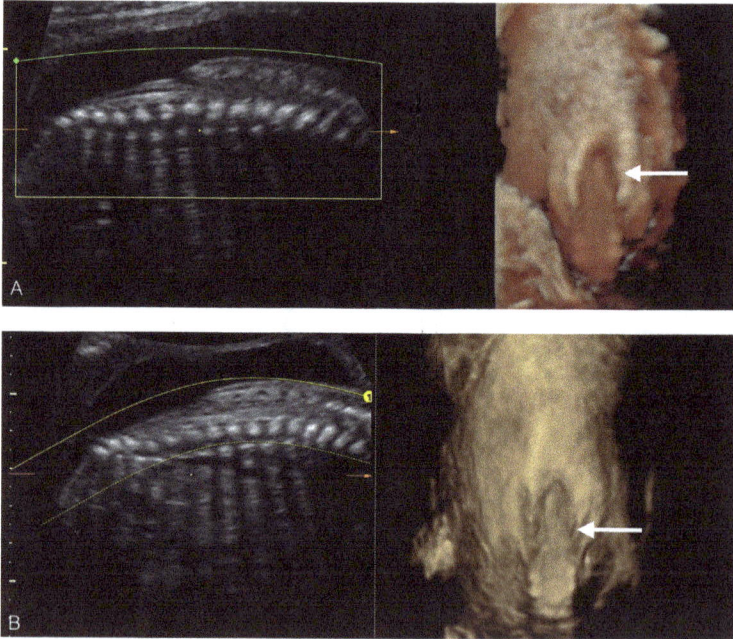

Fig. 17.13: Fetus with spina bifida as myeloschisis shown in 3D surface mode in (A) and in Omniview mode in (B) with a 17 mm slice and surface mode showing a direct view of the defect in both cases (arrows).

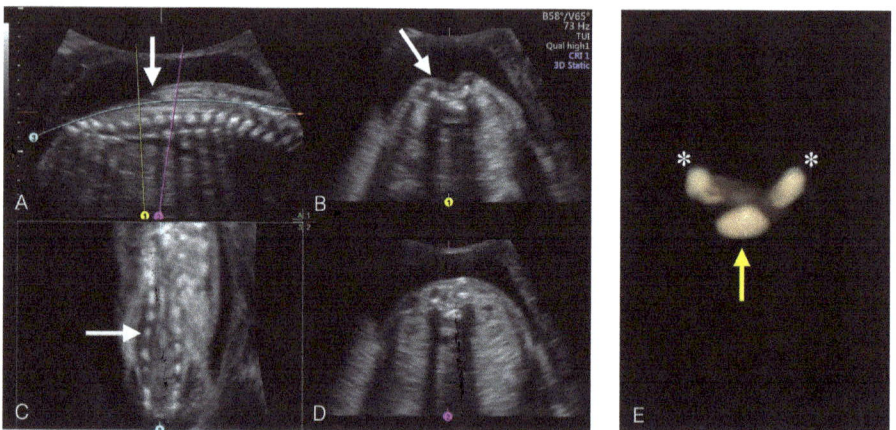

Fig. 17.14: Omniview planes (A) in a fetus with myeloschisis (arrow) showing an axial cross-section at the level of the defect (B), at a level of a few vertebrae higher than the defect (D), and in a coronal direct view on the defect (arrow) (C). In addition, similar to Figure 17.13, (E) shows the extraction of a single vertebra from the volume, revealing a vertebra with the dorsal defect with the vertebral body (yellow arrow) and the open vertebral arches (*).

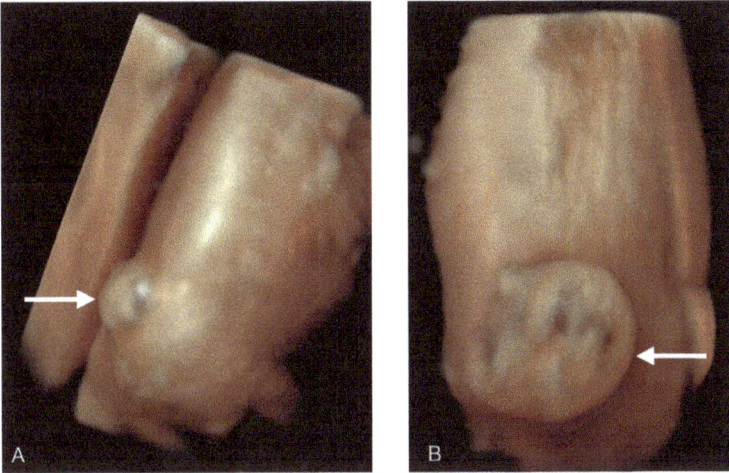

Fig. 17.15: Lateral view (A) and frontal view (B) of the back of two fetuses with a small (A) and large (B) lumbosacral myelomeningocele (arrow) in surface mode.

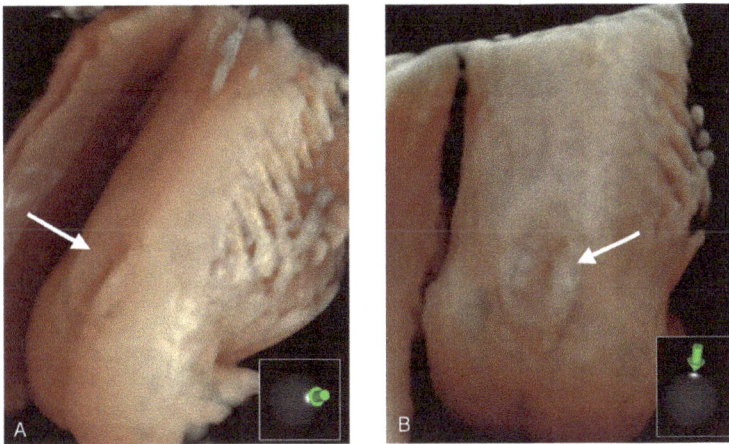

Fig. 17.16: Lateral view (A) and frontal view (B) of the back of one fetus with a lumbosacral myelomeningocele (arrow) in surface mode. Such findings are more difficult to visualize with 3D and changing the position of the light source (at the bottom right corner) can be helpful in such cases.

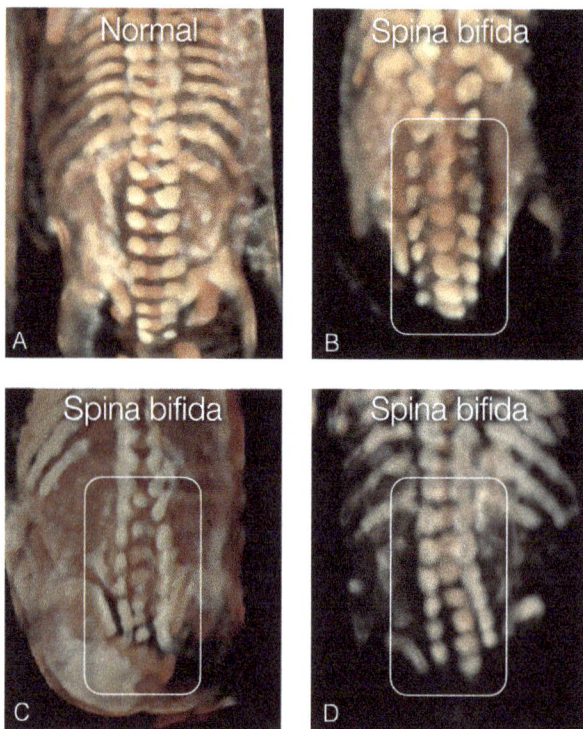

Fig. 17.17: 3D volumes of the back of a normal fetus (A) and three fetuses (B, C and D) with open spina bifida (boxes), all rendered using silhouette mode for bones. While in (A) the vertebral arches are closed and aligned parallel, the fetuses in (B), (C) and (D) show open arches and widening of the vertebrae.

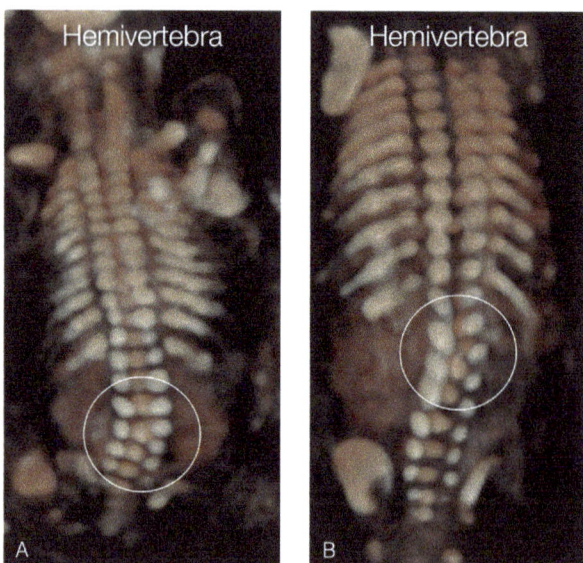

Fig. 17.18: Two fetuses with hemivertebrae (circle) in silhouette mode showing a deviation of the spine. The extent of the deviation can be better seen and illustrated in the 3D transparency mode.

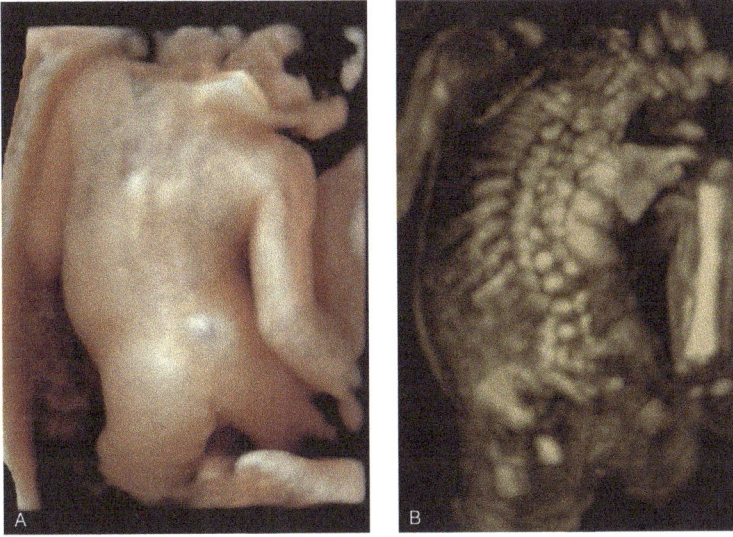

Fig. 17.19: Fetus with closed spina bifida and severe spinal and ribs anomalies in a case of spondylocostal dysostosis. The findings can be better assessed by switching from surface mode (A) to maximum mode (B).

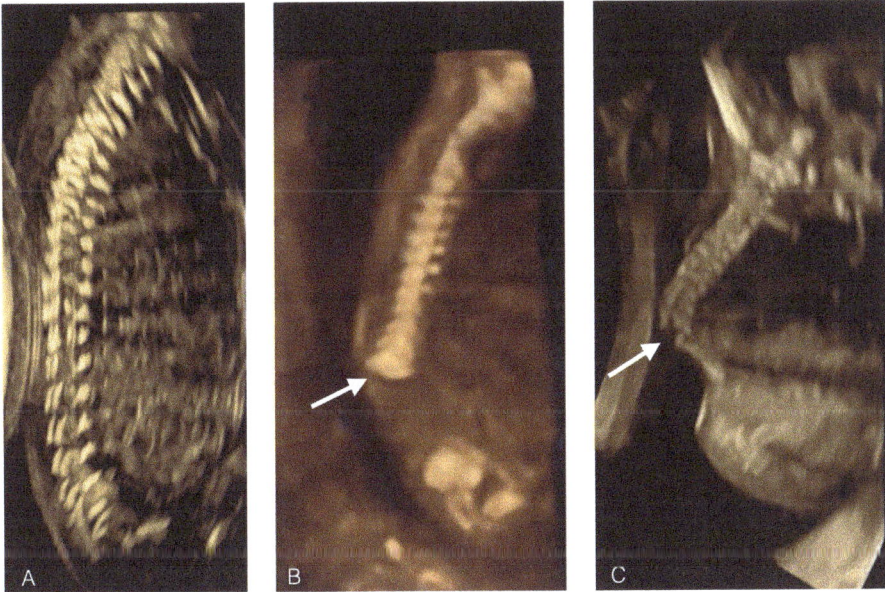

Fig. 17.20: Lateral view of the bony spine in maximum mode in a normal fetus (A) and in two fetuses with severe spinal anomalies. In (B), there is segmental spinal dysgenesis with disruption of the lumbosacral spine, while in (C) the fetus has severe caudal regression syndrome caused by maternal diabetes mellitus.

17.4 3D imaging of the fetal limbs

Ultrasound examination of the limbs, including arms with hands and legs with feet, is often expected by parents and is part of a screening examination. 3D imaging of the limbs can be performed either with the surface mode or by highlighting the bony parts with the maximum or silhouette mode (Fig. 17.21). For a good result, the acquisition plane should be a perpendicular insonation of the arm or leg to obtain a good perspective of the limb under examination. Ideally, the entire limb to be examined should be horizontal during volume acquisition (see Chapter 7), often making good volume acquisition a challenge. However, when this approach is successful, visualization of the limb reliably confirms normal anatomy; when abnormal conditions are present, the extent of the lesion can be well documented. Upper and lower limb abnormalities can be complex and have a wide spectrum, so a good 3D image can provide an excellent overview of the underlying lesion. Figure 17.22 shows various hands in 3D surface mode, and Figure 17.23 documents limb development in the first trimester. Anomalies involving the forearm, hand, and fingers are shown in Figures 17.24 through 17.29 in both surface and transparency modes. Anomalies may include abnormal hands in aneuploidies (Fig. 17.24), in syndromic conditions (Figs. 17.25–17.29), or isolated anomalies. Legs and feet can be visualized from the side or from below, with the toes visible. Figures 17.30 and 17.31 show some examples of 3D images of legs and feet displayed with surface mode and with silhouette mode when needed. The typical anomalies often reported and displayed with 3D are clubfeet (Fig. 17.32), either as an isolated finding or in association with a complex fetal malformation including spina bifida. Other lower extremity anomalies are rare, and some are shown in Figures 17.33 to 17.35.

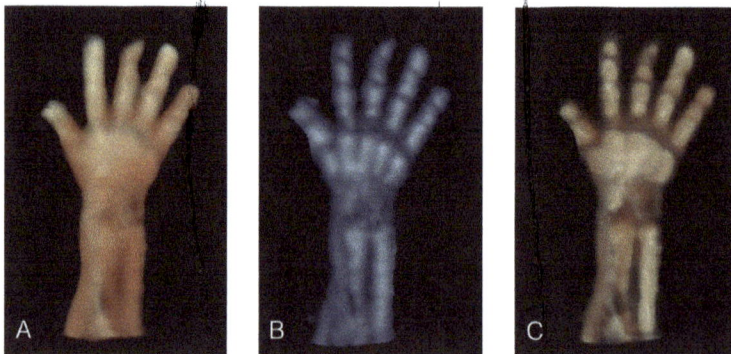

Fig. 17.21: Visualization of the arm and hand can be achieved in surface mode, maximum mode, or silhouette mode, as shown in these cases.

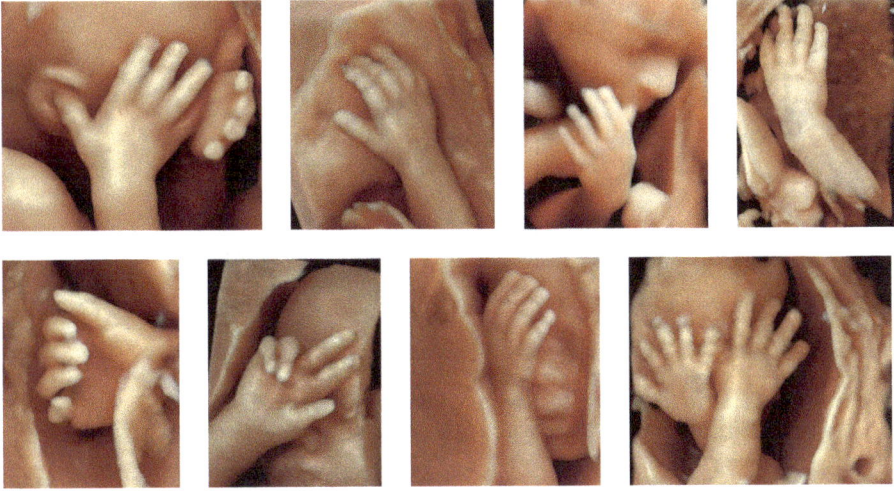

Fig. 17.22: Fetal hands are best visualized using surface mode, as shown in these examples.

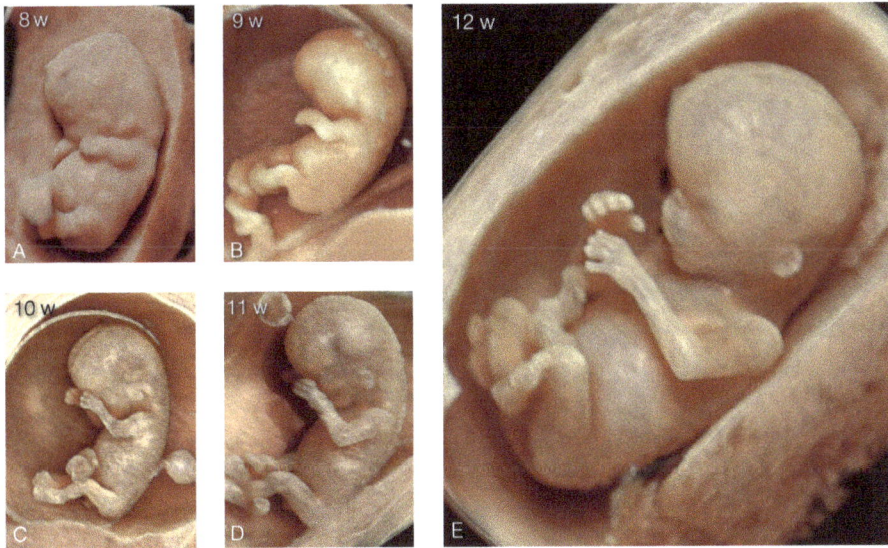

Fig. 17.23: The development of the limbs between weeks 8 and 12, especially the arms, shown in 3D surface mode. From the small bud and the two-segment arm (A) to the development of the three-segment arm (B), on to an arm with fingers (C, D and E), the embryology of the limbs can now be followed in vivo with 3D.

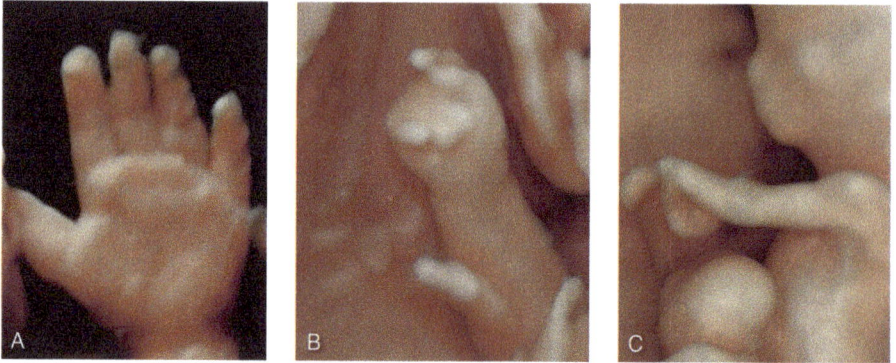

Fig. 17.24: Hands in fetal aneuploidies showing in (A) a hand with short fingers in trisomy 21, in (B) a hand with overlapping fingers in trisomy 18, and in (C) a hand with radius aplasia in trisomy 18.

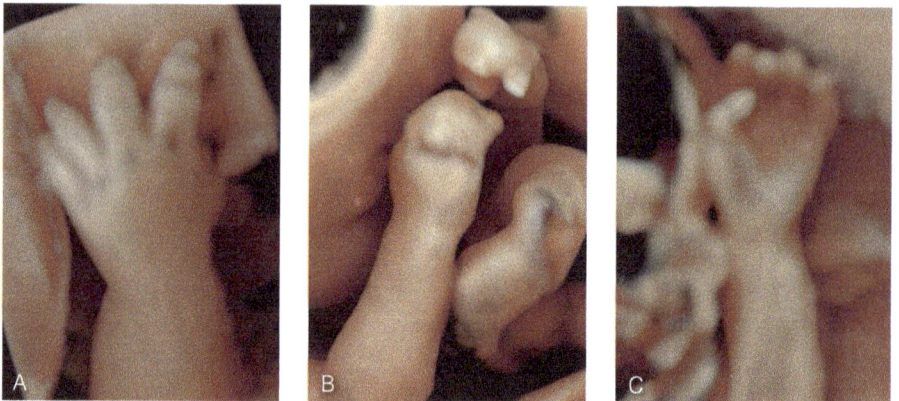

Fig. 17.25: Hands in syndromic disorders: (A) shows a so-called trident hand in a fetus with achondroplasia, (B) shows a hand with syndactyly in a fetus with Apert syndrome, and (C) shows a hand with adducted thumb in a neurological syndrome.

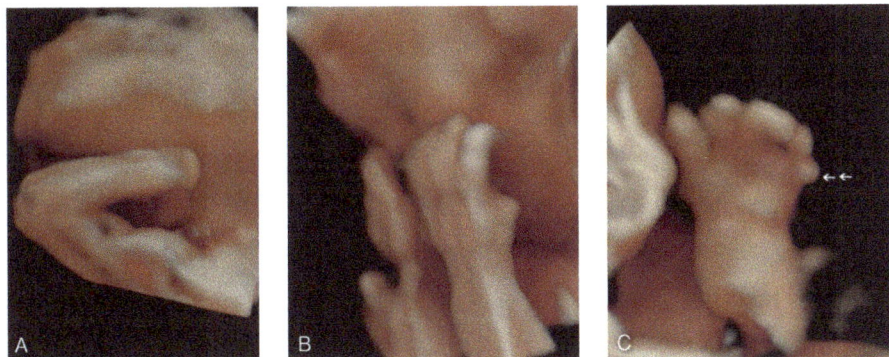

Fig. 17.26: Fetal hand anomalies showing a missing hand in (A), a missing thumb in (B), and postaxial poly-dactyly in (C).

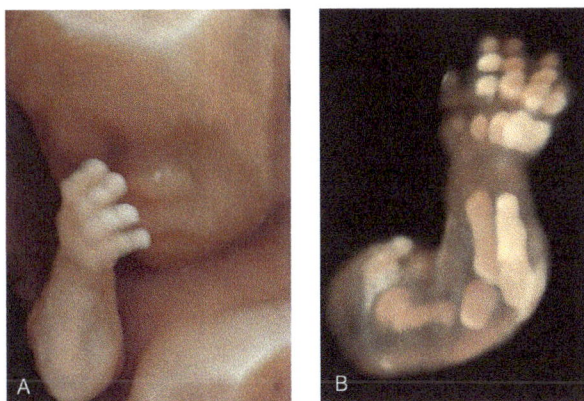

Fig. 17.27: Fetus with thanato-phoric dysplasia showing the ty-pical short hands and fingers as brachydactyly, visualized in sur-face 3D (A) and in silhouette mode of the bones (B).

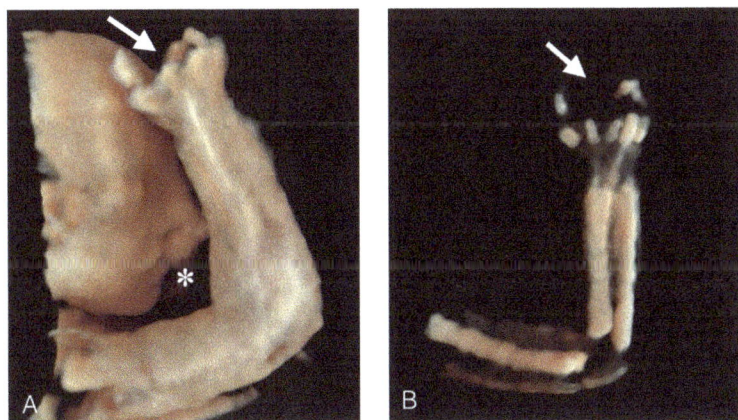

Fig. 17.28: Fetus with ectrodactyly and ectodermal dysplasia (EEC) syndrome with the typical features such as split hands (arrows) and facial clefts (*).

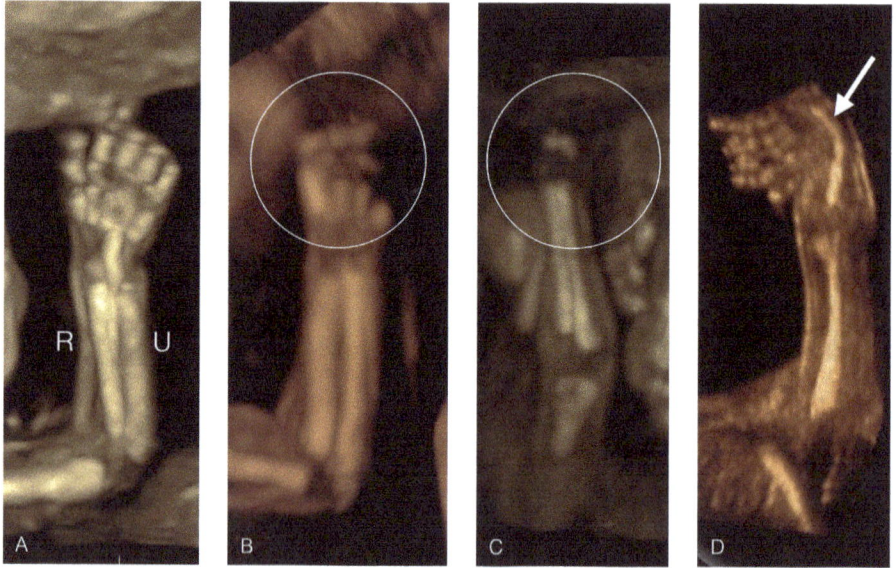

Fig. 17.29: Maximum mode showing forearm with radius (R), ulna (U) and hand; (A) normal fetus, (B) fetus with syndactyly in Apert syndrome, (C) fetus with missing hand, (D) fetus with radius aplasia, short ulna (arrow) and typical hand position.

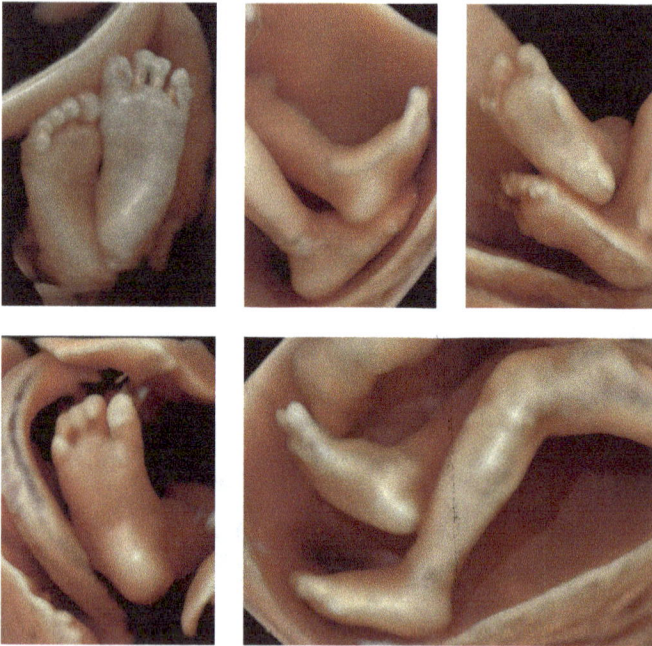

Fig. 17.30: Legs and feet can be easily displayed in surface mode from the side or from below with the single toes visible.

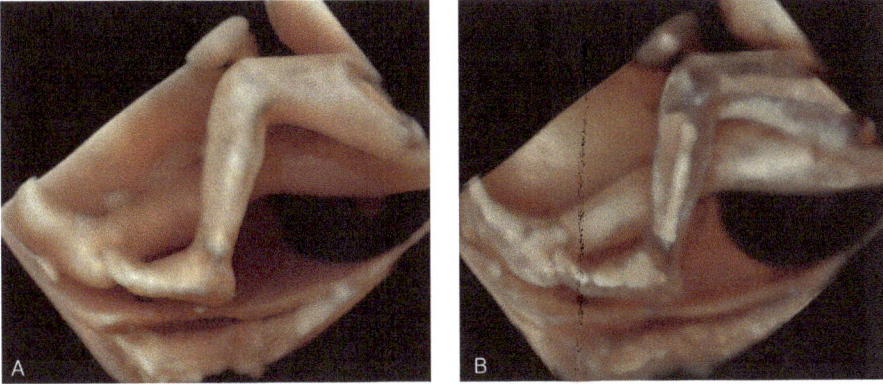

Fig. 17.31: Legs and feet can be displayed well with the 3D surface (A) and the silhouette mode for bones (B).

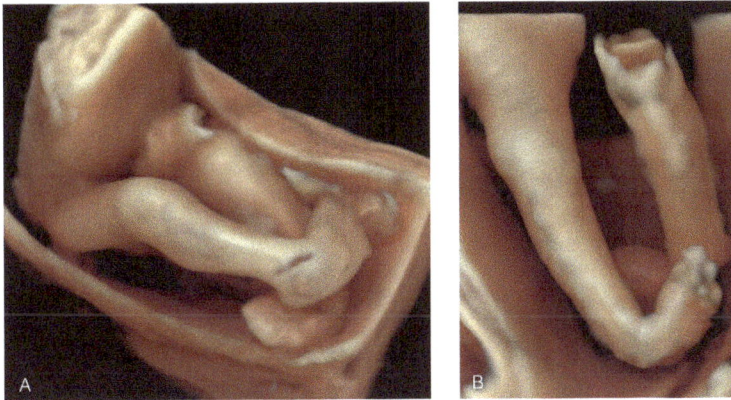

Fig. 17.32: Clubfeet in two fetuses shown in surface mode. In (A), the bilateral clubfeet were an isolated finding, while in (B) the bilateral clubfeet were a complication of open spina bifida.

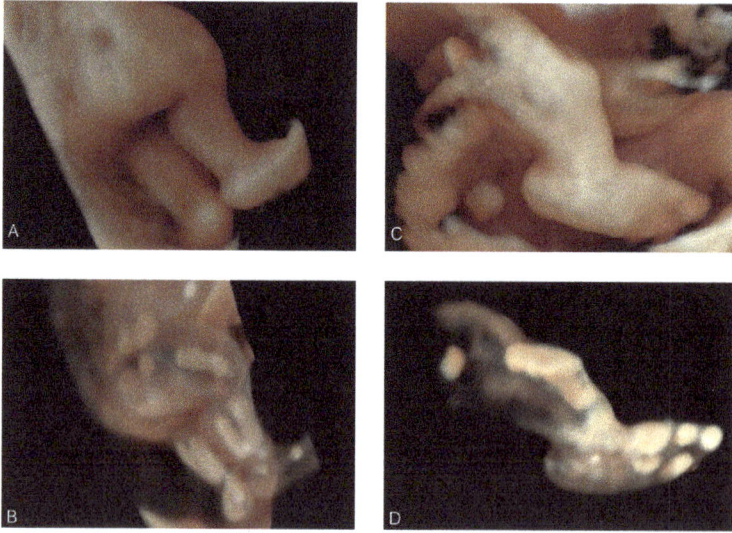

Fig. 17.33: 3D Surface mode (upper panel) and silhouette mode (lower panel) of a short leg in a fetus with thanatophoric dysplasia (A and B) and another short and abnormal leg in a fetus with a proximal femoral focal deficiency (C and D).

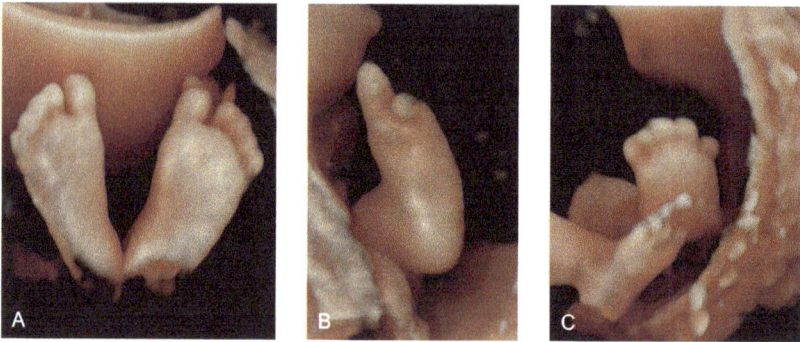

Fig. 17.34: 3D surface mode of a normal foot and toes in (A) and anomalies in (B) and (C). In (B), a foot with oligodactyly and in (C) an abducted toe with short digits in a fetal syndrome (otopalatodigital syndrome).

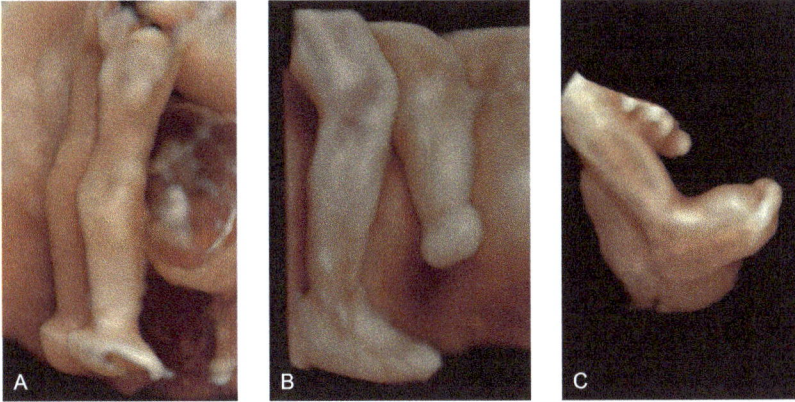

Fig. 17.35: 3D surface mode of leg and foot anomalies, such as permanently stretched legs in (A), absent foot in (B), and foot edema in (C) in a fetus with Turner syndrome.

17.5 Conclusions

Maximum mode and, more recently, silhouette mode are good tools for the accurate examination of the fetal skeleton with 3D ultrasound. Because of their curved shape, most bones of the body can be examined better in a 3D volume than in 2D ultrasound. Normal anatomy can be well distinguished from abnormal conditions involving areas of interest, such as the spine and ribs, upper and lower limbs, and the bony face and skull. An important prerequisite is a good angle of insonation and a high-contrast image. Anomalies of the limbs and spine, either isolated or as part of skeletal dysplasias, can be clearly visualized and identified with the maximum mode. Assessment of the bony face and skull can be of great help in evaluating syndromes, but a learning curve is required to obtain reliable images.

18 3D of Intrathoracic and Abdominal Organs

18.1 Introduction

A comprehensive examination of the fetal thorax and abdomen with 2D ultrasound includes a series of parallel axial planes to visualize the lungs, heart, diaphragm, stomach, liver, gallbladder, bowel, anterior abdominal wall, urinary bladder, and kidneys, among others. In addition, sagittal and parasagittal planes can show the diaphragm and other organs from a different perspective. The presence, location, and integrity of these organs can thus be assessed, and fetal abnormalities can be ruled out step by step. This purpose can be easily achieved by using different 3D modes, as described in this book. It is generally agreed that a finding shown in tomography display mode, as in Figure 18.1, provides better documentation than a single image or a collection of single images. Such overview of a finding can be well complemented by a transparent 3D projection of the thoracic and abdominal organs, which can provide a better picture of the extent of the findings compared with a 2D plane. In this chapter, the potential application of different 3D tools in anomalies of the intrathoracic (excl. heart) and intraabdominal organs is discussed with reference to individual cases that are summarized in tables and illustrated with examples. The tools used, such as tomography mode,

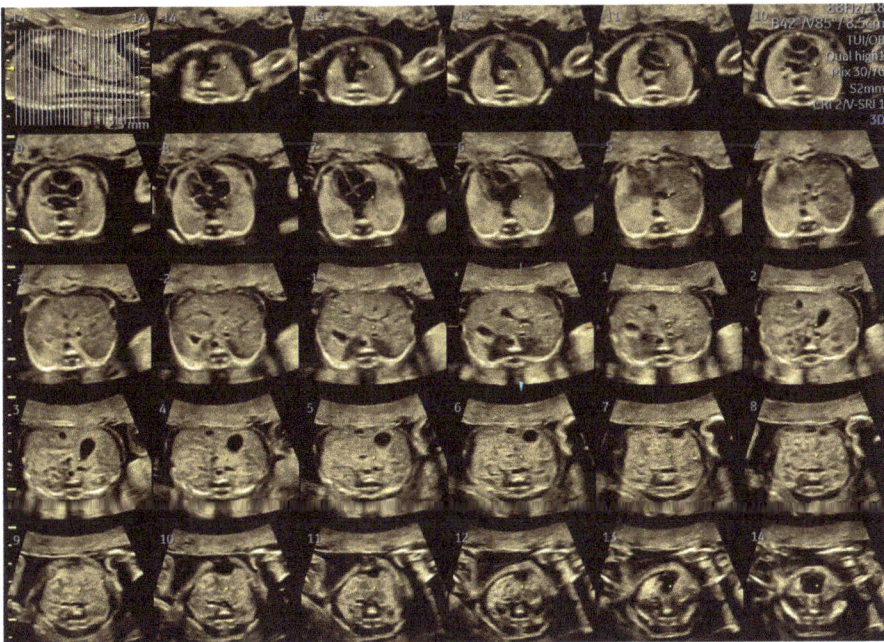

Fig. 18.1: A 3D volume of the thorax and abdomen displayed in tomography mode. In this case, a total of 30 images was selected. This overview shows all the required details from the thorax and heart in the top two rows to the middle abdomen in the third and fourth rows and the lower abdomen in the bottom row.

https://doi.org/10.1515/9783111249513-018

VCI, or silhouette mode, have been discussed in the respective chapters. The examination of the heart and great vessels is discussed separately in Chapter 19.

18.2 The intrathoracic organs

Typical anomalies involving the organs within the chest include congenital diaphragmatic hernia, where one can mainly focus on the documentation of the displacement of the intrathoracic organs (Fig. 18.2) and the demonstration of different lung sizes with the hypoplastic lung on the ipsilateral side. Lung anomalies such as congenital pulmonary airway malformation (CPAM) (Fig. 18.3), bronchopulmonary sequestration (Fig. 18.4), and other cystic lesions can also be well visualized in 3D, demonstrating the extent of the lesion and the distinction between normal and abnormal lung tissue. In hydrothorax, the extent of the fluid collection can be better assessed and documented with 3D ultrasound (Figs. 18.5, 18.6) and fluid volume can be calculated if needed. Tomography mode is the best 3D tool for documenting a lesion with its neighboring organs. The recently developed new tools of the silhouette mode allow an image-based 3D projection of all findings. Table 18.1 summarizes common diagnoses involving the intrathoracic organs with suggestions for applicable 3D tools. Figures 18.2 to 18.6 show examples of 3D imaging of intrathoracic lesions in both tomography and rendering modes.

Congenital Diaphragmatic Hernia

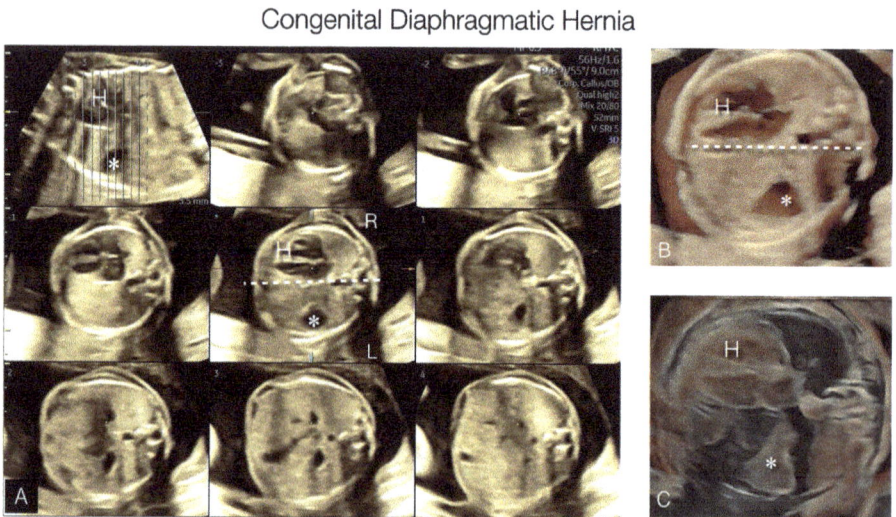

Fig. 18.2: Left-sided congenital diaphragmatic hernia shown in 3D tomography mode (A), with surface mode (B), and silhouette mode (C). The stomach (*) is seen on the left side (I) next to the heart (H). In (A), the line in the middle plane divides the chest into two halves and shows that the heart is completely displaced to the right chest (R). This is easily seen in (B), but in (C) it is more difficult to assess the spatial position of the stomach in this view due to transparency.

Congenital Pulmonary Airway Malformation

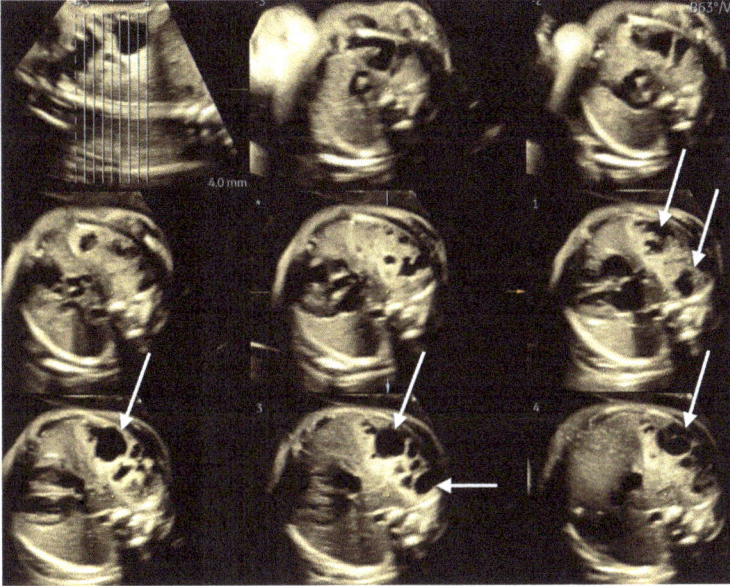

Fig. 18.3: Tomography mode in a fetus with a congenital pulmonary airway malformation (CPAM). The arrows indicate the multiple medium-sized cysts in a right lobe of the lung.

Bronchopulmonary Sequestration

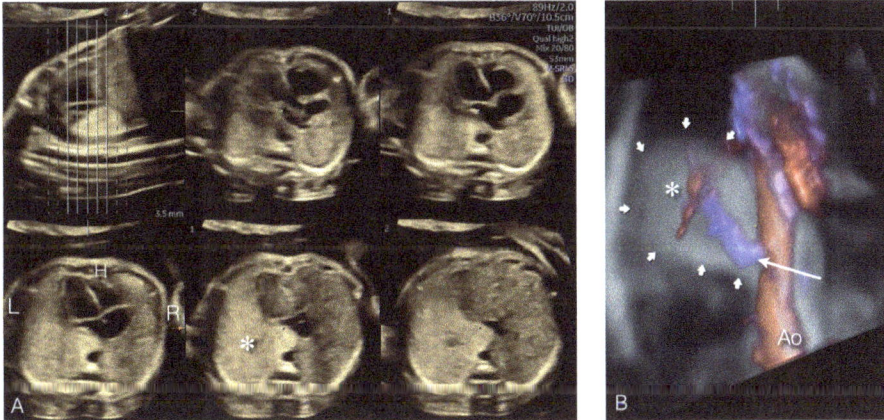

Fig. 18.4: (A) shows a tomography mode of the thorax in a fetus with a left hyperechogenic lung (*) in suspected bronchopulmonary sequestration with the heart (H) shifted to the right (R). In (B), color Doppler tomography with VCI shows the lung lesion (short arrows) and the presence of a feeding artery (long arrow) arising from the descending aorta (Ao), which is a typical finding in pulmonary sequestration; left (L).

Hydrothorax

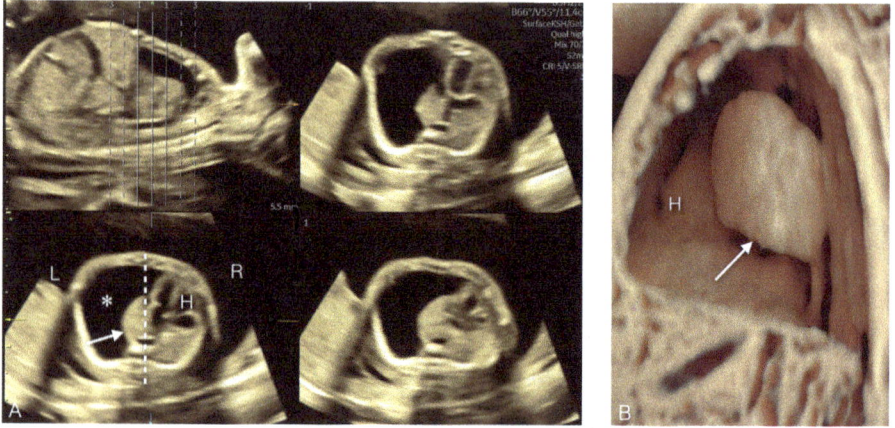

Fig. 18.5: Left-sided hydrothorax (*) with heart (H) displaced to the right (R) and compression of the left lung (arrow) in tomography mode (A). In (B), a view from the left side into the thorax with surface mode showing the lung (arrow) with the heart in the background.

Hydrothorax

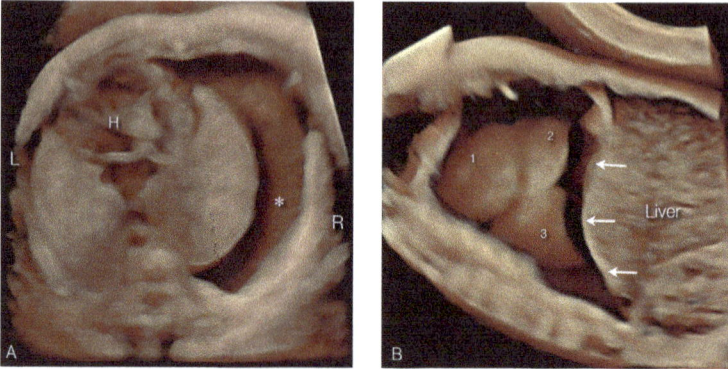

Fig. 18.6: Right-sided hydrothorax (*) with heart (H) shifted to the left (L) from cranial view in (A) and right-sided view in (B) in surface mode. Note the three lobes (1, 2, and 3) of the right lung. The arrows in (B) point to the diaphragm; right (R).

Tab. 18.1: Typical intrathoracic anomalies with the potential use of different 3D render modes.

Anomalies	3D Techniques
Congenital diaphragmatic hernia	Tomography mode Minimum mode Silhouette mode Surface mode VOCAL for lung volume calculation
CPAM: Congenital Pulmonary Airway Malformation	Tomography mode Minimum mode Silhouette mode Sono-AVC (cysts volume calculation)
Bronchopulmonary sequestration	Tomography mode Minimum mode Silhouette mode Glass-body mode for visualization of feeding artery
Hydrothorax	Tomography mode Minimum mode Silhouette mode Surface mode Sono-AVC (fluid volume calculation)

18.3 The gastrointestinal organs

Anomalies of the gastrointestinal tract (GIT) include abnormal position of the stomach (e. g., situs inversus), obstruction of the GIT as duodenal atresia (Fig. 18.7), ileus (Fig. 18.8), and abdominal wall defects such as omphalocele (Fig. 18.9) or gastroschisis (Fig. 18.10). Intrahepatic anomalies mainly involve the intrahepatic vessels, such as agenesis of the ductus venosus or interruption of the intrahepatic inferior vena cava with azygos continuation; however, these are better visualized with glass-body mode, as discussed in Chapter 12. The presence of ascites, either isolated or as part of a generalized fetal hydrops, can be well documented with 3D in either tomography or surface mode (Figs. 18.11, 18.12). The surface mode for ascites, as shown in Figs. 18.11 B and 18.12, reminds of a "virtual laparoscopy." The presence of cystic lesions can also be well documented with 3D tools (Fig. 18.13), as discussed in the section 18.2 on intrathoracic lesions. Table 18.2 summarizes common diagnoses involving GIT with suggestions for applicable 3D tools. Figures 18.7 to 18.13 show examples of 3D visualization of anomalies of the GIT.

Tab. 18.2: Typical anomalies of the gastrointestinal system with the potential use of different 3D render modes.

Anomalies	3D Techniques
Situs inversus	Tomography mode Silhouette mode Minimum mode
Duodenal atresia	Tomography mode Silhouette mode Minimum mode Inversion mode Surface mode Sono-AVC (stomach-duodenum-volume)
Omphalocele / Gastroschisis	Tomography mode Surface mode
Ileus	Tomography mode Silhouette mode Minimum mode
Intrahepatic vessels	Glass-body mode Silhouette mode Minimum mode
Ascites	Tomography mode Silhouette mode Minimum mode Surface mode

Double Bubble in Duodenal Atresia

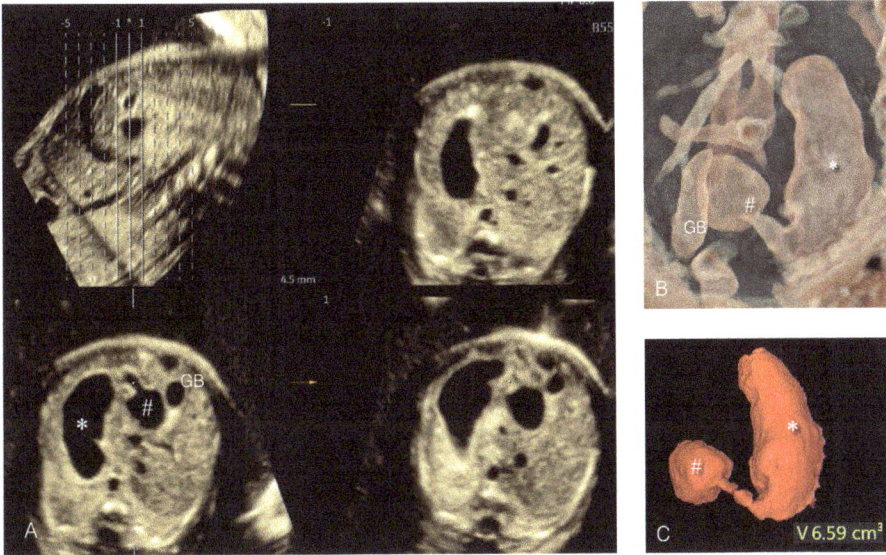

Fig. 18.7: In (A) tomography mode of the upper abdomen in a fetus with trisomy 21 and double bubble with suspected duodenal atresia. In (B), an anteroposterior view of the abdomen (arrow) is shown with a dilated stomach (*) and duodenum (#) in silhouette mode, and in (C) with Sono-AVC. The latter allows calculation of fluid volume. Gallbladder (GB).

Ileus

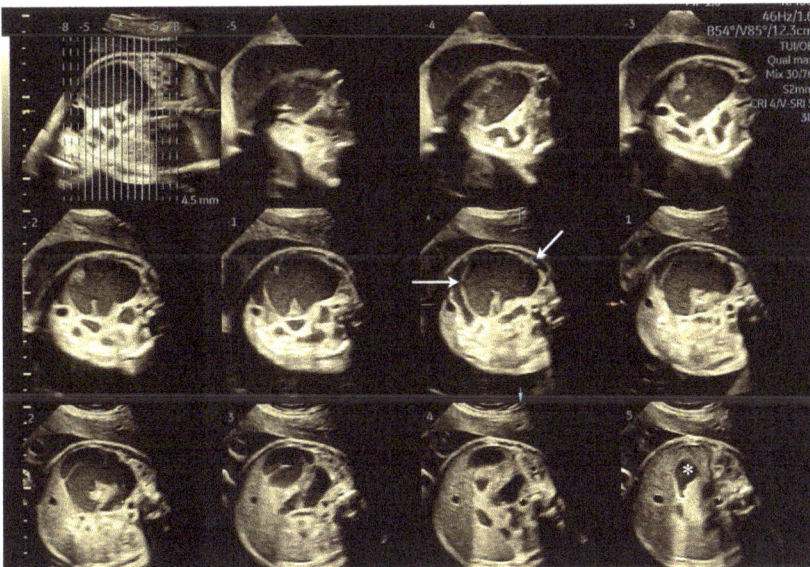

Fig. 18.8: Tomography of the abdomen in a fetus with ileus and bowel perforation. The stomach (*) is seen in the bottom right plane; the echogenic contents of the cyst (arrows) are typical of bowel perforation.

Omphalocele

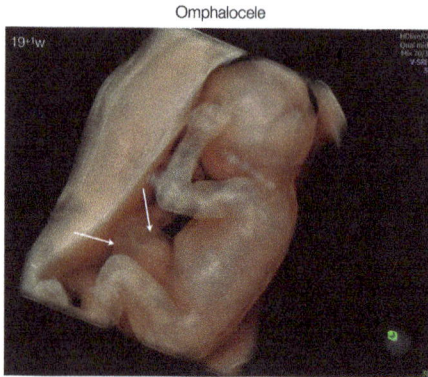

Fig. 18.9: Small omphalocele with bowel content (arrows) in a fetus at 19 weeks of gestation in surface and silhouette mode. This fetus has Beckwith-Wiedemann syndrome.

Gastroschisis

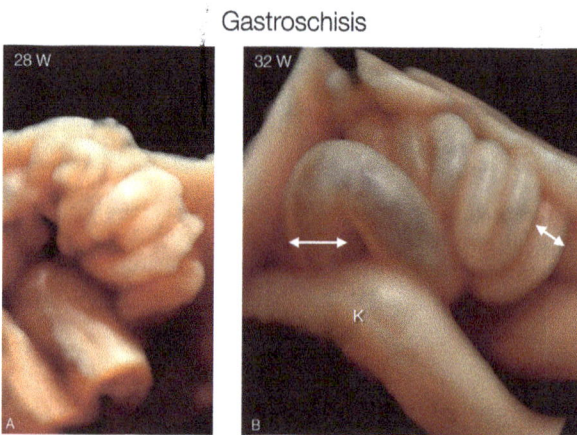

Fig. 18.10: Gastroschisis in a fetus at 28 and 32 weeks of gestation in surface mode. In late gestation, the intestines are often dilated. In the third trimester (B), the difference between the small intestine (short arrow) and the large intestine (long arrow) is easily seen, especially when highlighted with the silhouette mode; knee (K).

Ascites

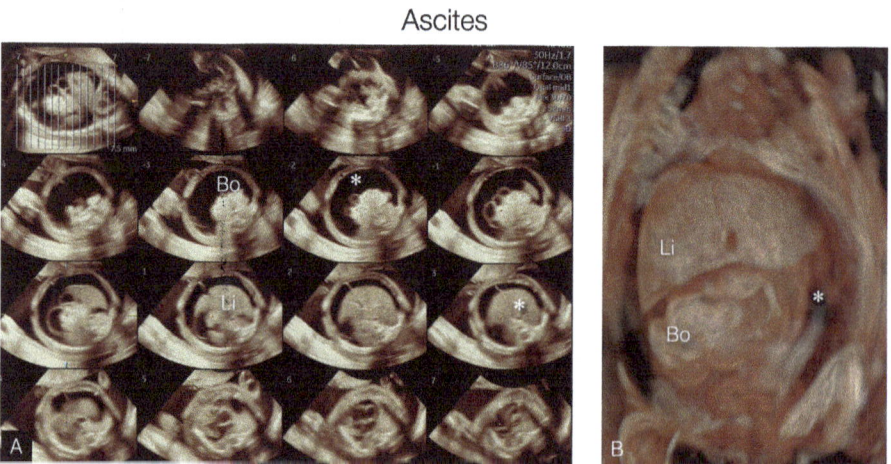

Fig. 18.11: In (A), tomography mode of the abdomen in a fetus (27 weeks) with ascites (*) and in (B) in surface mode with silhouette mode from a frontal projection reminding of a "virtual laparoscopy". One can see the liver (Li) and the intestine (Bo). Tomography gives an overview of the extent of ascites and can be used well for follow-up.

Ascites

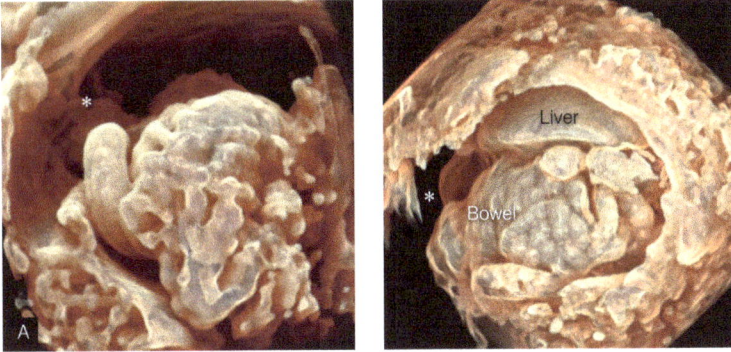

Fig. 18.12: 3D surface mode with silhouette of the (open) abdomen in a fetus (32 weeks) with ascites (*) in a frontal projection reminiscent of a "virtual laparoscopy", similar to the case in Figure 18.11. Liver and bowel can be seen.

Splenic Cyst

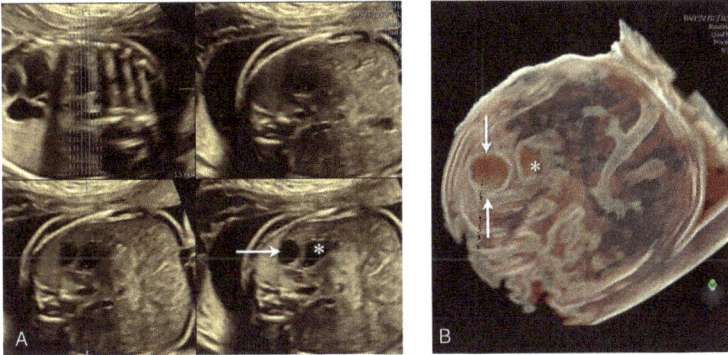

Fig. 18.13: Cystic structure (arrows) in the upper abdomen behind the stomach (*) as a splenic cyst, shown in tomography mode (A) and in silhouette mode (B).

18.4 The urogenital system

Congenital anomalies of the kidneys and urinary tract (CAKUT) can be demonstrated with different 3D tools and include renal anomalies such as pelvic kidney, horseshoe kidney, and unilateral or bilateral renal agenesis and diverse increased fluid collections in the renal pelvis (Fig. 18.14) as found in vesicoureteral reflux (Fig. 18.15), duplex kidneys with ureterocele, and obstruction of the uretero-pelvic junction and hydronephrosis (Figs. 18.14–18.16). Cystic kidney diseases may be unilateral in multicystic renal dysplasia (Fig. 18.17) or bilateral, typically in genetic polycystic kidney disease. In addition, enlarged hyperechogenic kidneys may be also present and tomographic mode enables the demonstration of the extent of the lesion (Fig. 18.18).

Intrapelvic cystic lesions including ovarian cysts may be found as large cystic areas in the lower abdomen in female fetuses after 30 weeks of gestation (Fig. 18.19). The external genitalia are well assessed with the surface mode, often allowing good differentiation between normal and abnormal findings (Fig. 18.20).

In summary, findings involving the kidneys can be well visualized in an overview in tomography mode. On the other hand, in the presence of intra-abdominal fluid collections, 3D rendering modes such as surface, inversion, silhouette, or Sono-AVC can be then used. Table 18.3 summarizes common anomalies with suggestions for applicable 3D tools.

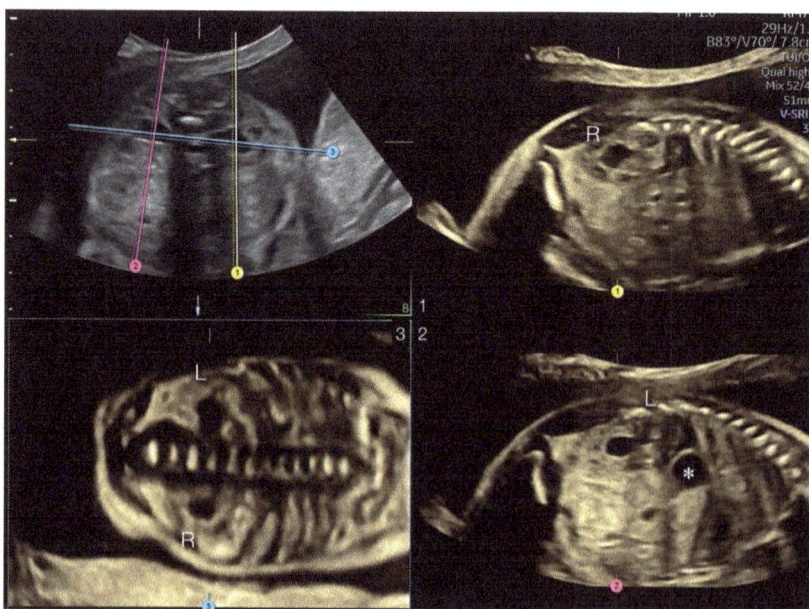

Fig. 18.14: Bilateral pyelectasia visualized using the Omniview planes. The three lines have been placed to show the right (R) and left (L) kidneys in anterior-posterior view and in coronal view (Panel 3). The asterisk indicates the stomach.

2D	Tomography	Minimum
Inversion	Silhouette	Sono-AVC

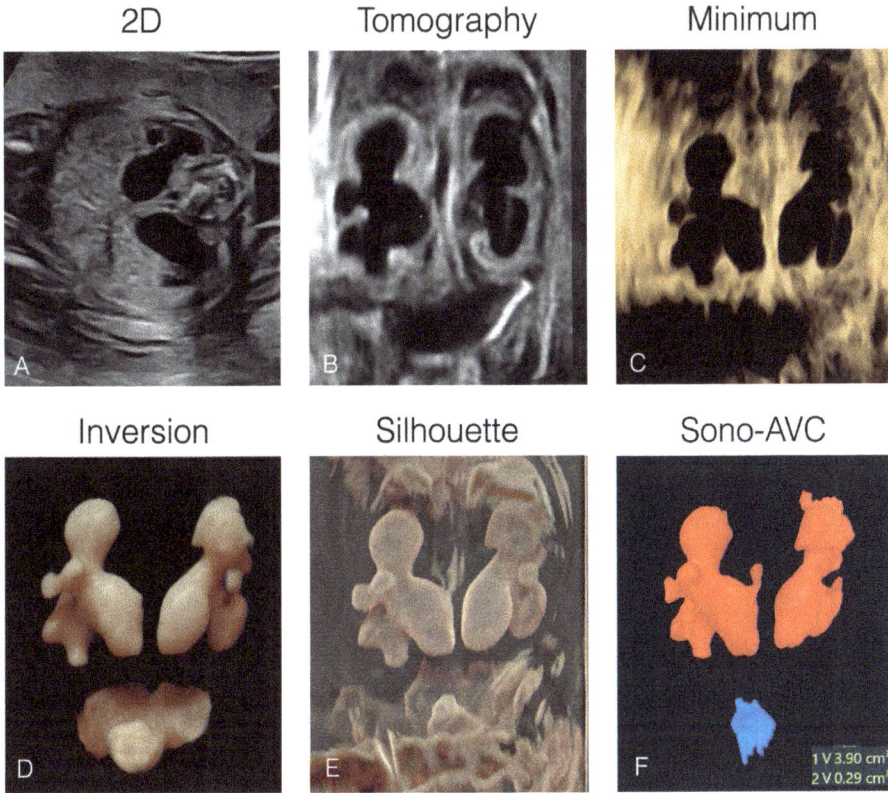

Fig. 18.15: A fetus with vesicoureteral reflux and hydronephrosis visualized with different imaging modalities. In (A) the usual 2D image, in (B) with tomography showing an anterior-posterior view of the pyelectasia. With the same view, (C) is shown in minimum mode, (D) in inversion mode, (E) in silhouette mode, and (F) in Sono-AVC with volume calculation of both renal filling and urinary bladder.

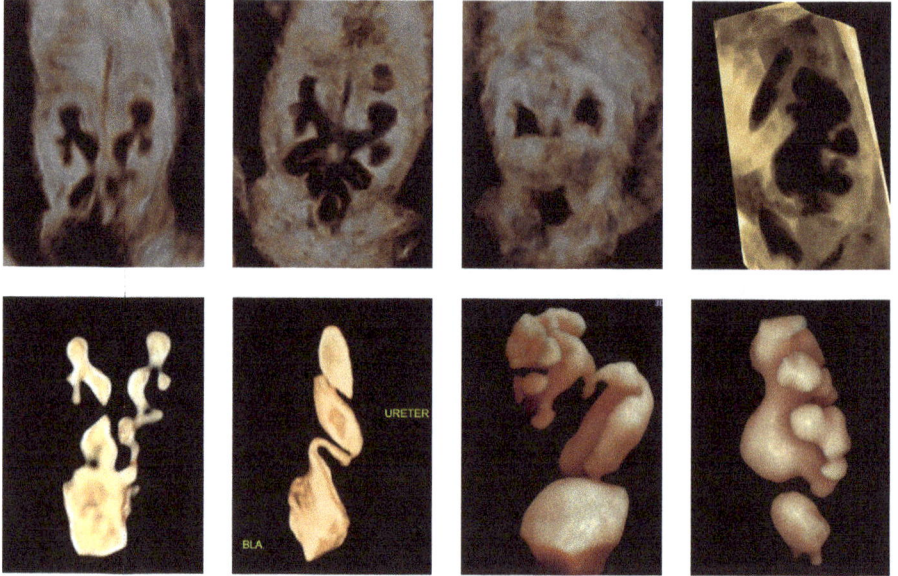

Fig. 18.16: Different fetuses with mild to severely dilated renal pelvis and ureters with an antero-posterior view displayed in minimum mode (upper row) and inversion mode (lower row).

Multicystic Renal Dysplasia

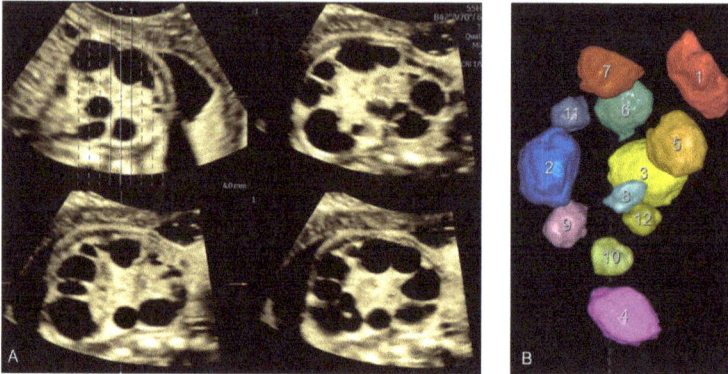

Fig. 18.17: In (A), tomography mode in a fetus with multicystic renal dysplasia at 29 weeks of gestation. In (B), the individual cysts were visualized with Sono-AVC and calculated separately (see also Chapter 13).

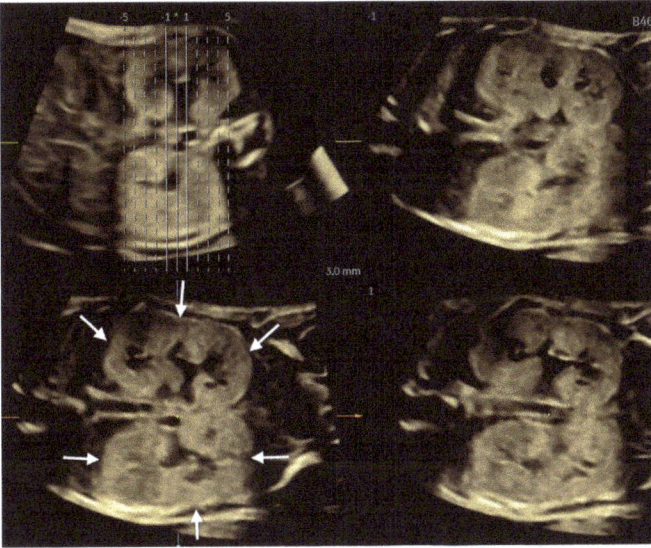

Fig. 18.18: A fetus with bilaterally enlarged hyperechogenic kidneys (arrows) in an autosomal recessive Bardet-Biedl syndrome, shown in tomography mode. Tomography display provides a good overview of the extent of the findings.

Ovarian Cyst

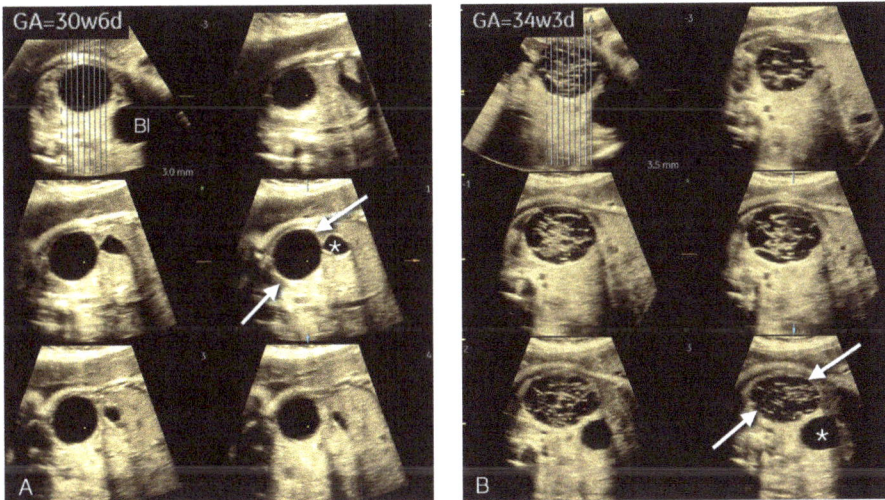

Fig. 18.19: A fetus at 30 weeks of gestation with an isolated cyst (arrows) in the left lower abdomen below the stomach (*). The likely diagnosis in the female fetus is an ovarian cyst, shown here in tomographic mode. The cyst is typically echolucent. In (B), four weeks later, a hemorrhage has occurred in the cyst, which is readily distinguishable from the findings in (A).

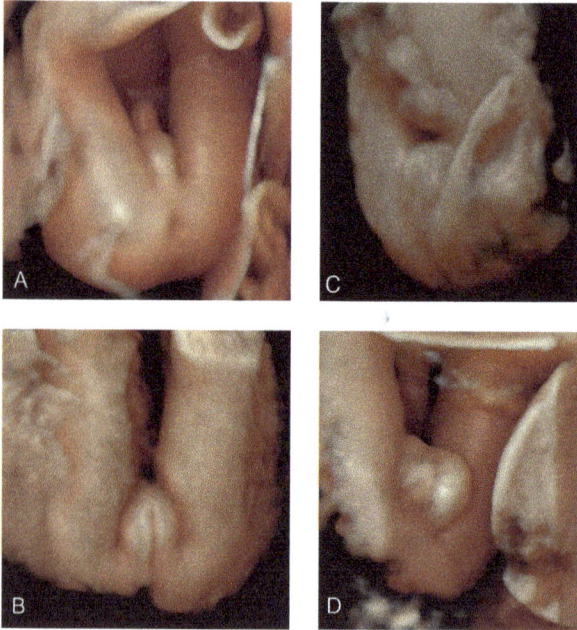

Fig. 18.20: 3D surface mode in a male (A) and female fetus (B) and in two fetuses with abnormal genitalia in (C) and (D).

Tab. 18.3: Typical anomalies of the urogenital system with the potential use of different 3D render modes.

Anomalies	3D Techniques
Pyelectasia, hydronephrosis, pelvic ureteric junction obstruction, vesicoureteral reflux, duplex kidney with ureterocele	Tomography mode Silhouette mode Minimum mode Inversion mode Sono-AVC
Megacystis	Tomography mode Silhouette mode Minimum mode Inversion mode Surface mode
Multicystic und polycystic renal dysplasia	Tomography mode Silhouette mode Minimum mode Inversion mode Sono-AVC
Horseshoe kidney, pelvic kidney	Tomography mode Omniview mode
Renal agenesis	Tomography mode Glass-body mode
Genital anomalies	Surface mode Tomography mode

18.5 Conclusions

Examination of the intrathoracic and intraabdominal organs, including the gastrointestinal and renal systems, can be performed with both multiplanar and volume rendering modes. From a clinical point of view, the most important tool for documenting abnormalities in these regions is the tomography mode, which can be used to visualize the lesion examined in its extent and with the surrounding anatomy. In addition, volume imaging can provide a more complete spatial representation of the lesion in some specific conditions in fluid-filled organs, such as hydrothorax, ascites, duodenal atresia, hydronephrosis, and cystic kidneys or in anomalies of the body contours, such as omphalocele, gastroschisis, or abnormal genitalia.

19 Fetal Echocardiography in 3D and STIC

19.1 Fetal cardiac scanning in grayscale and color Doppler

According to international guidelines, examination of the fetal heart consists of visualization and documentation of a series of adjacent planes from the upper abdomen to the upper mediastinum. These planes should include the axial section of the upper abdomen, the four-chamber view, the five-chamber view, the pulmonary artery view, and the three-vessel and trachea view. If longitudinal planes are also to be documented, views of the aortic arch, ductal arch, and bicaval veins are visualized. Improved diagnostic accuracy can be achieved by combining grayscale evaluation with color Doppler to visualize diastolic and systolic hemodynamics in the ventricles and great vessels. While atria, ventricles, and atrioventricular valves are visualized simultaneously in the single four-chamber view plane, the great vessels can be assessed only by tilting the transducer to demonstrate their origin and spatial course and relationship. In many places, documentation of a cardiac examination for later evaluation or for a second opinion in a normal or abnormal fetus is still done by storing single images or video clips. This approach has the major limitation that such documentation can only contain what the examiner has seen and recorded. Fetal 3D/4D echocardiography offers important advantages regarding all the above, to be discussed later in this chapter.

19.2 Different acquisitions of cardiac volume data sets

Acquisition of a cardiac volume can be performed using static 3D, STIC, or 4D imaging with a mechanical or electronic transducer (for methodology, see Chapter 1).

19.2.1 Static 3D acquisition

This technique of 3D acquisition is fast and has high resolution. However, wall and valve movements are the major limitation in fetal heart studies because they produce movement artifacts. Despite this limitation, a volume with a good resolution often shows acceptable information about the anatomy of the ventricles and great vessels, provided that the information needed does not depend on wall movements and cardiac cycle depending events. In static 3D, the size of the cardiac structures, their relationships to each other and the fetal situs can be reliably assessed (Fig. 19.1). Static 3D cannot be reliably combined with color Doppler because the direction of blood flow depends on the phase of the cardiac cycle. The authors prefer the use of unidirectional power Doppler in static 3D acquisition because it provides a uniform color display, especially for the demonstration of the course of the vessels. For a combination with color Doppler, acquisition of a STIC volume is preferable.

https://doi.org/10.1515/9783111249513-019

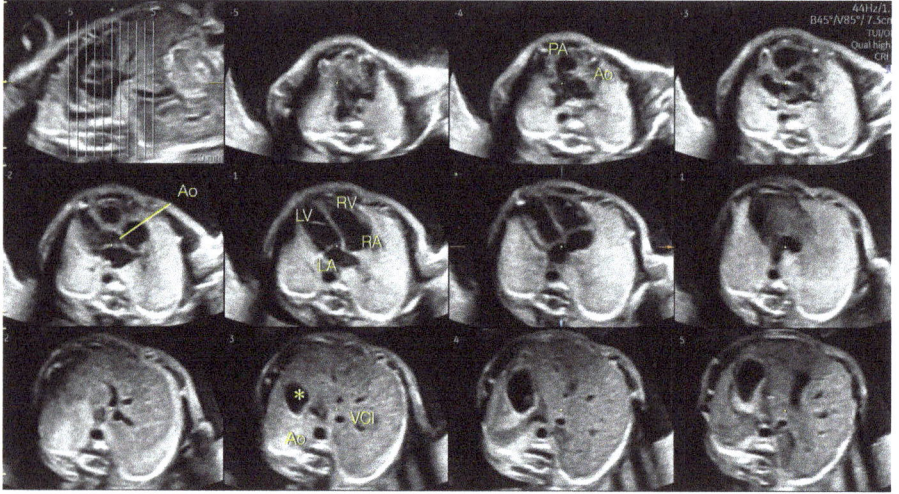

Fig. 19.1: Tomographic mode of a static 3D volume of the heart and upper abdomen. A single image visualizes all the information needed as a normal situs with stomach (*) on the left, heart in four-chamber view and great vessels. Aorta (Ao), left atrium (LA), left ventricle (LV), pulmonary artery (PA), right atrium (RA), right ventricle (RV), vena cava inferior (VCI).

19.2.2 STIC/eSTIC volume acquisition

The best cardiac volumes are acquired using the STIC/eSTIC technique and can be ideally used for offline assessment of fetal cardiac structures and movements (see also Chapter 1). STIC volume acquisition can be performed in combination with grayscale (Fig. 19.2), color (Fig. 19.3), power Doppler, high-resolution bidirectional flow Doppler, and B-flow modes. Prior to volume acquisition, it is recommended that the examiner optimizes the grayscale or color Doppler presets to clearly visualize the flow events in the heart and vessels (see Chapter 1). The starting plane for acquisition depends mainly on the question of interest and the expected image view. Volumes for visualizing cardiac cavities are best acquired from the four- or five-chamber plane, whereas volumes for assessing the position of the great vessels and their course are acquired from an axial plane of the upper mediastinum. For the acquisition of the aortic or ductal arch or abdominal vessels, longitudinal or oblique insonation is recommended. With an electronic matrix transducer, the acquisition of an eSTIC is similar; in this case, the acquisition time is shorter and volume resolution higher.

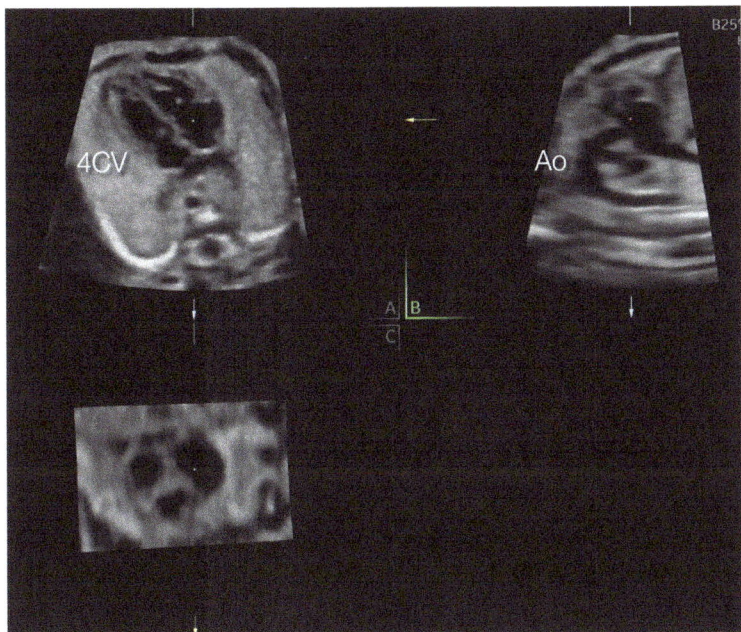

Fig. 19.2: STIC volume of a heart shown in the three orthogonal planes A, B and C. In (A), the four-chamber view (4CV) in diastole with opened atrioventricular valves is clearly visible and in (B) the aortic arch (AO) is reconstructed.

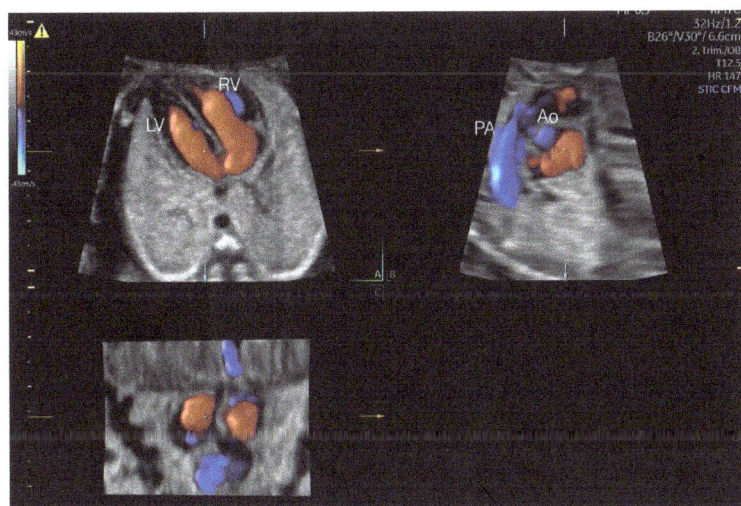

Fig. 19.3: STIC volume in color Doppler shown in the three orthogonal planes A, B, and C. The diastolic phase of the cardiac cycle is shown in the upper left panel with the filling of the right (RV) and left (LV) ventricles. The orthogonal plane in the upper right panel also shows flow in the aorta (Ao) and pulmonary artery (PA).

19.2.3 Real-time 4D acquisition with an electronic matrix transducer

With this transducer, 4D examination can be performed almost in real time with the display of 19–30 volumes per second. The result of such 4D examination can be displayed in orthogonal or tomographic modes, but also in 3D volume rendering. Combination with color Doppler is possible, but the frame rate is often too low. 4D with a matrix probe can be used for examining fetuses with arrhythmias. The combination of 4D with different 3D rendering modes, such as surface, color Doppler, glass-body or inversion mode may make this technique interesting for new applications in the future. The combination with VCI-A (Fig. 19.4) (see Chapter 4 and Chapter 14) is interesting, where – instead of a large 4D volume – a high-contrast image is displayed as the result of a thin-slice acquisition, whose thickness can be adjusted freely.

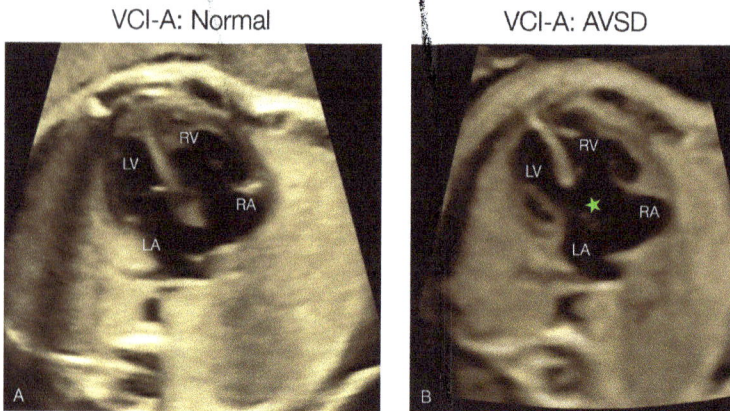

Fig. 19.4: The electronic matrix transducer allows real-time 4D scanning in VCI-A. VCI-A provides increased contrast by using a thin 3D layer of information. In the left image (A), a normal four-chamber view in diastole is shown with both open atrioventricular valves clearly visible. The right image (B) shows a heart with atrioventricular septal defect (AVSD) with the defect (star) well recognized. Left atrium (LA), left ventricle (LV), right atrium (RA), right ventricle (RV).

19.3 Fetal heart in 3D and STIC with multiplanar reconstruction

As stated in the introduction, a comprehensive examination of the fetal heart consists of imaging several adjacent, cross-sectional planes that should contain the typical structures of interest. These planes can also be generated from an acquired 3D volume and visualized either in orthogonal mode (Figs. 19.2, 19.3), tomographic mode (Figs. 19.5, 19.6), or using a few selected Omniview planes (Figs. 19.7, 19.8). In addition, combination with color Doppler allows assessment of systolic and diastolic events in the ventricles and great vessels (Fig. 19.6). Any cross-sectional plane can be reconstructed from a good quality STIC volume.

In a STIC volume, one single hypothetical cardiac cycle is stored as an infinite loop. If required, such a loop can be displayed in slow motion and paused at any time, allowing detailed analysis of the specific phase of the cardiac cycle (Fig. 19.9).

Intracardiac hemodynamic changes can be analyzed particularly well in STIC volumes acquired in combination with color Doppler (Fig. 19.6). Since the entire heart is contained in a digital volume, each sectional plane ("plane of interest") can be reconstructed offline. This way, the typical planes extracted from the volume as well as the desired cardiac examination can be performed virtually. The extracted images can be displayed in one of the multiplanar rendering modes as single (Fig. 19.9), orthogonal (Fig. 19.2), tomographic (Figs. 19.5, 19.6) or Omniview planes (Figs. 19.7, 19.8). The quality

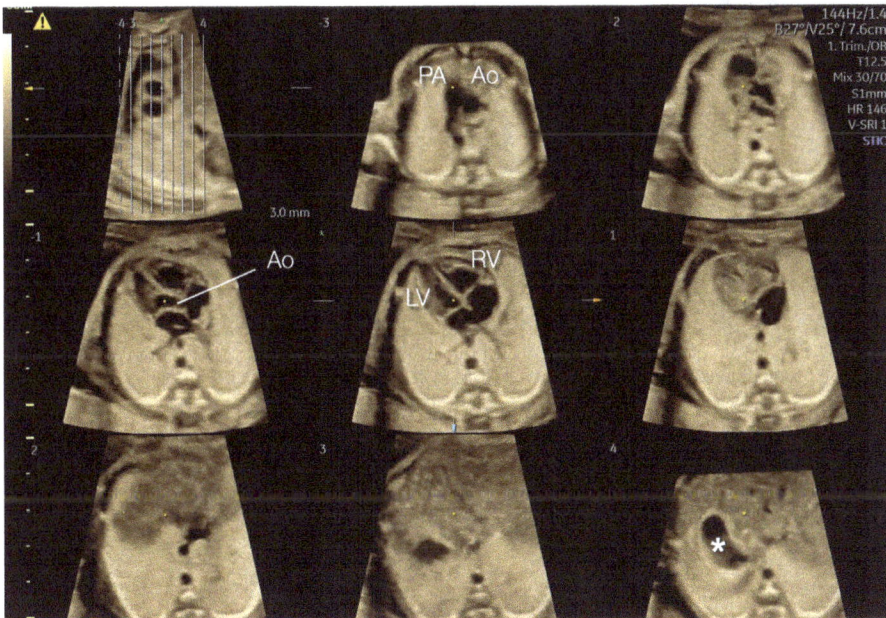

Fig. 19.5: STIC volume in tomographic view with different planes, such as abdomen with stomach (*), heart in four-chamber view and aorta (Ao) with pulmonary artery (PA) in upper mediastinum; left ventricle (LV), right ventricle (RV).

and contrast of the reconstructed images in grayscale can be improved by adding VCI or SRI tools (see Chapter 4). With the latest software version, it is possible to apply VCI also to color Doppler volumes, giving the color a more spatial aspect, as shown in Figure 19.6 (see also Chapter 4). Figures 19.10 to 19.16 show some examples of normal and abnormal hearts in different multiplanar display modes.

STIC volumes can be used to simulate a cardiac examination since the examiner can retrieve the typical sectional planes. This approach enables the examiner to work also off-line on volume samples of fetuses with cardiac abnormalities. Several clinical studies have shown that such volume data sets provide a reliable offline diagnosis of a cardiac abnormality and can therefore be used to reassess the fetal heart or to obtain a remote second opinion from an expert, e. g., by transmitting the volume data set via the Internet. The use of volume data sets in teaching fetal echocardiography has more implications than simply demonstrating images or videos.

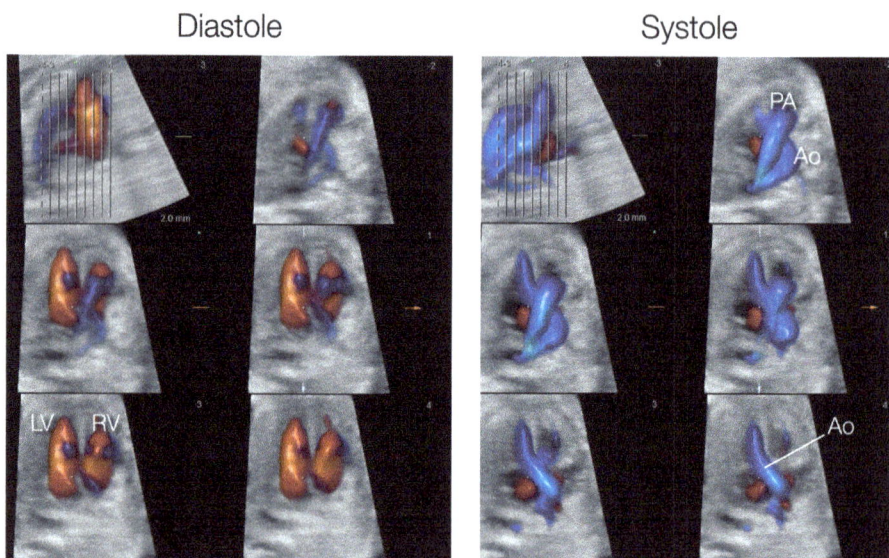

Fig. 19.6: Tomographic mode of a STIC heart volume in color Doppler. Because color Doppler displays systolic and diastolic flow, it is often difficult to reproduce both events within one figure, so we opted to present the same figure during diastole (left) and systole (right) by adding VCI with a slice of 12 mm. VCI in color Doppler enables to provide each plane with a more spatial view of the blood flow than with a glass-body mode. While in diastole, VCI does not add more information (left panel); it shows in systole (right panel) the crossing of both pulmonary artery (PA) and aorta (Ao) over each other.

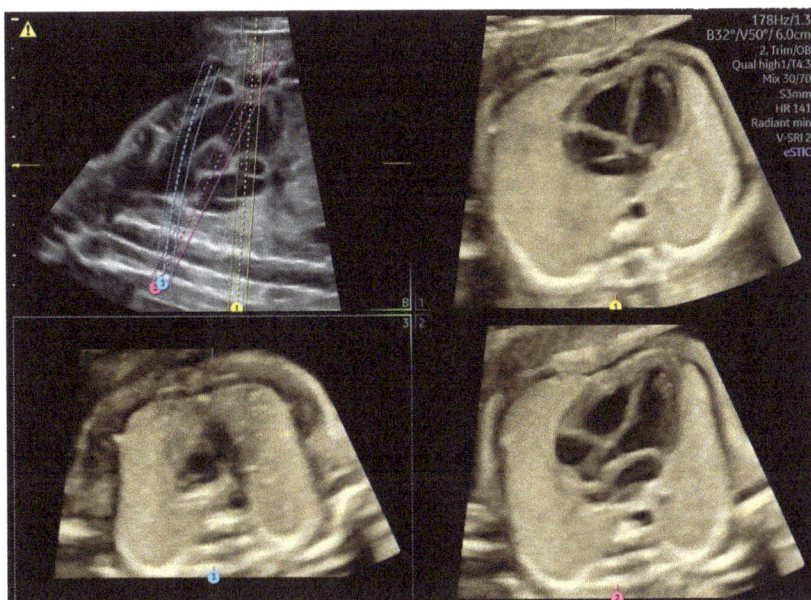

Fig. 19.7: STIC volume in Omniview display. In the reference plane (upper left panel) the heart is seen in a sagittal view and the Omniview lines were placed at typical levels demonstrating the four-chamber-view (plane 1, upper right panel), the five-chamber-view (plane 2, lower right panel) and the three-vessel-view (plane 3, lower left panel).

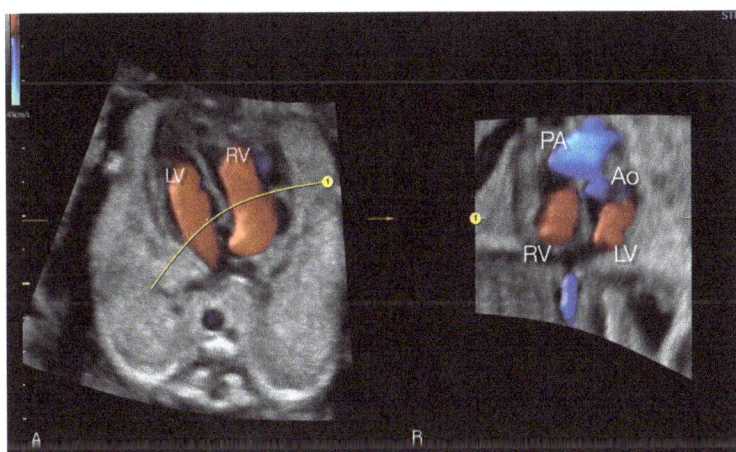

Fig. 19.8: STIC volume in Omniview mode in color Doppler. In (A), a curved line was drawn and placed just in front of the atrioventricular valves (AV) and the great vessels. The effect in (B) shows flow across both AV valves in the right (RV) and left (LV) ventricles. The great vessels are typically located so that the aorta (Ao) is embedded between the two AV valves and the pulmonary artery (PA) anterior to the Ao.

Diastole   Systole

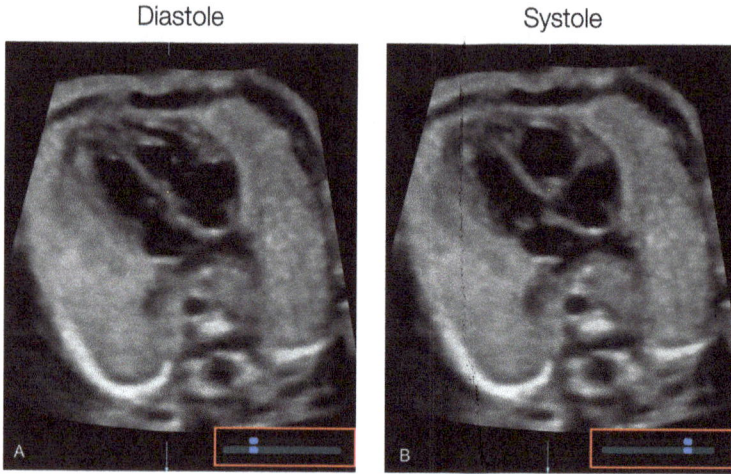

Fig. 19.9: STIC volume showing the four-chamber view. A STIC volume can be used to select any phase of the cardiac cycle and shows here diastole with open valves in (A) and systole in (B).

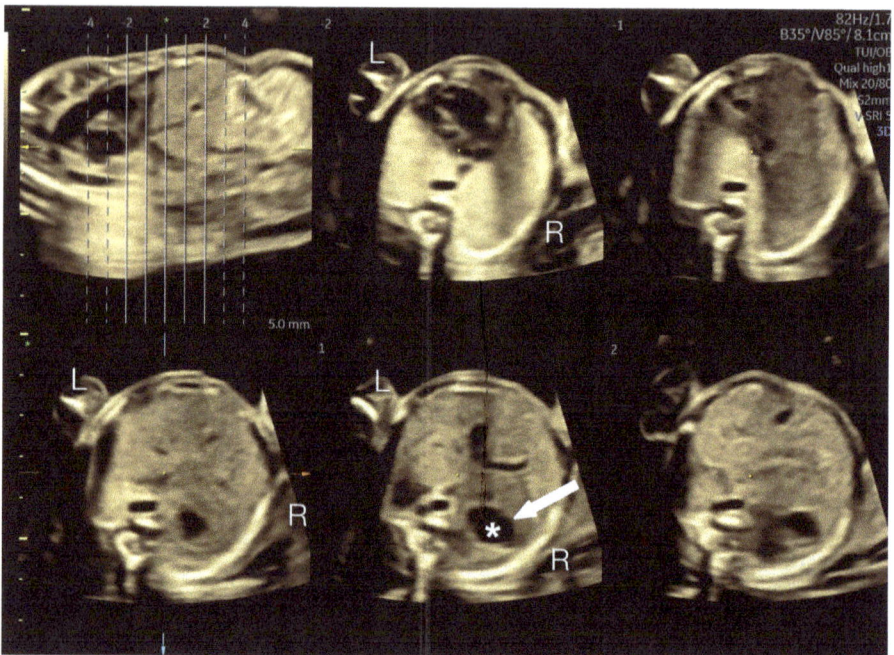

Fig. 19.10: 3D volume in tomographic mode showing a fetus with abdominal situs inversus with stomach (*) on the right side (arrow) and heart on the left side; the cardiac axis is pointing to the left; left (L), right (R).

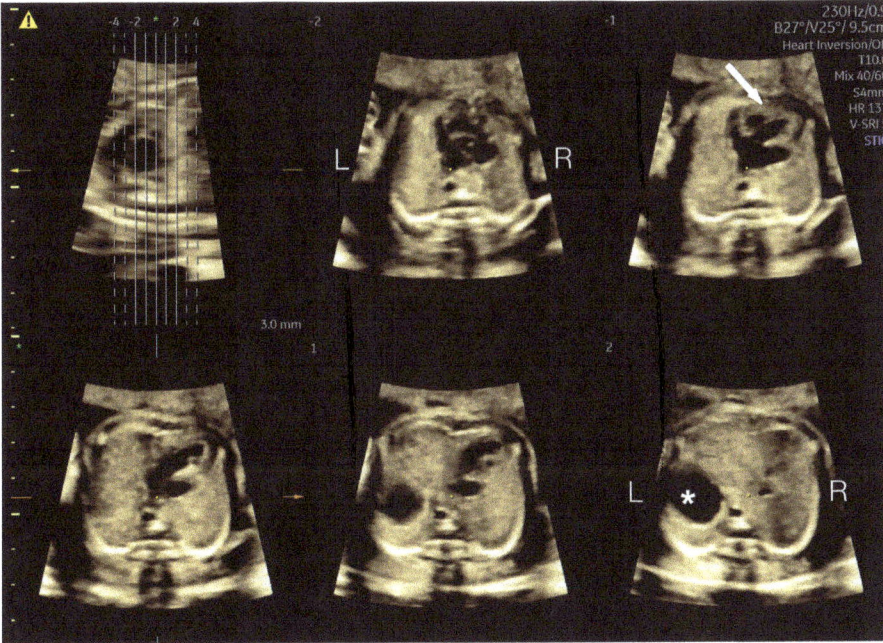

Fig. 19.11: STIC volume in tomographic mode, showing a fetus with dextrocardia with heart on the right (arrow) and stomach (*) on the left, with the heart axis pointing to the right; left (L), right (R).

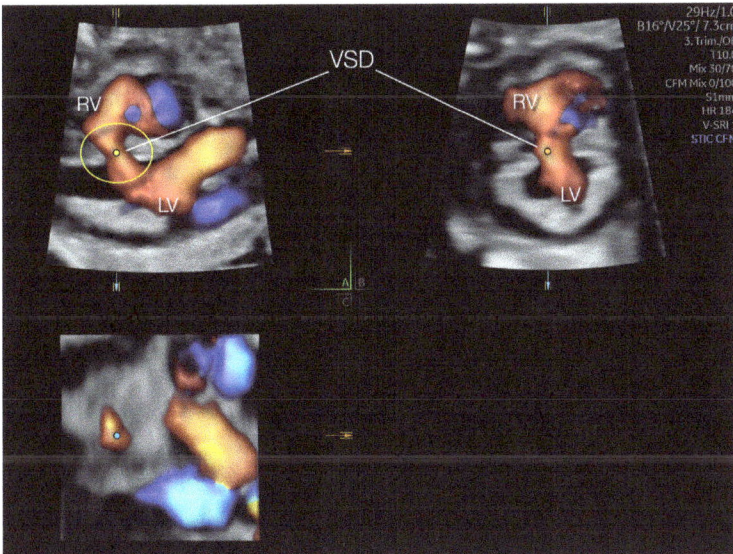

Fig. 19.12: Muscular ventricular septal defect (VSD) shown on 3D ultrasound in orthogonal plane view with VCI in color (slice 1 mm). The dot (shown in the circle) represents the intersection of the three planes. The dot is located on the VSD in (A) (transverse view at the level of the four-chamber view) and can be seen in (B) (short-axis view of the ventricles) and (C) (anterior view of the ventricular septum). Left ventricle (LV), right ventricle (RV).

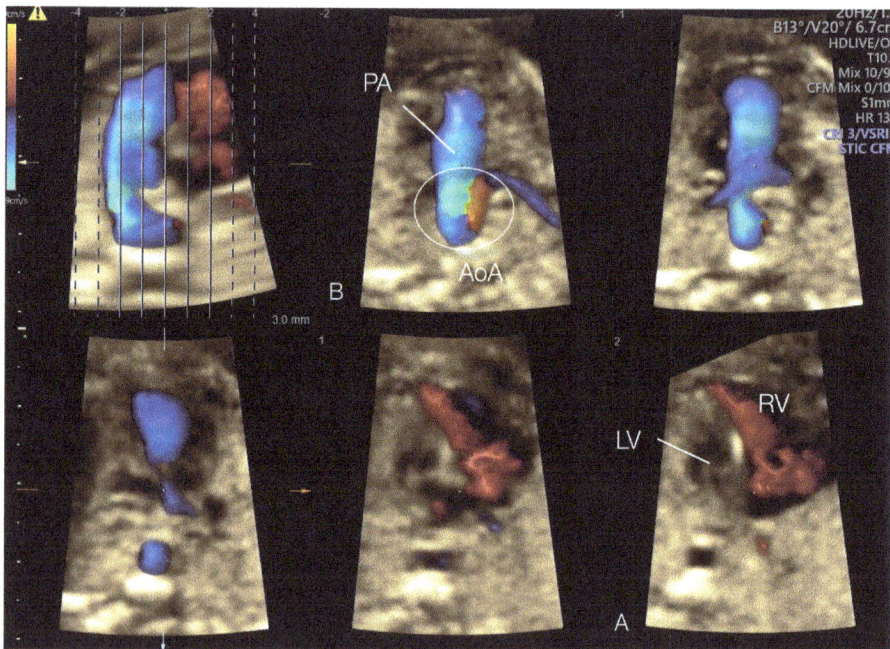

Fig. 19.13: Tomographic mode of a STIC cardiac volume in color Doppler in a fetus with hypoplastic left heart syndrome (HLHS), showing the characteristic features in one image: in the four-chamber view in panel (A), absent flow in the left ventricle (LV) (arrow). In the upper middle panel (B) in the three-vessel trachea view, antegrade flow in the pulmonary artery (PA) (blue) with reverse flow in the aortic arch (AoA) (red).

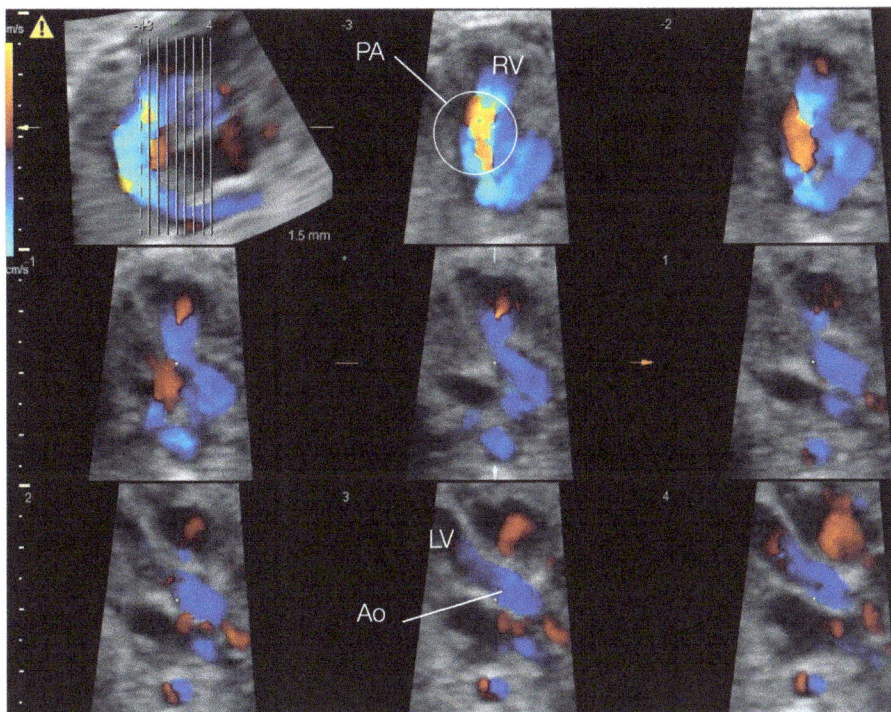

Fig. 19.14: STIC volume in tomographic mode with color Doppler in systole in a fetus with pulmonary stenosis. The aorta (Ao) originating from the left ventricle (LV) shows laminar flow (blue), whereas blood flow in the pulmonary artery (PA) originating from the right ventricle (RV) shows turbulent aliased blood flow (circle) characteristic of pulmonary stenosis.

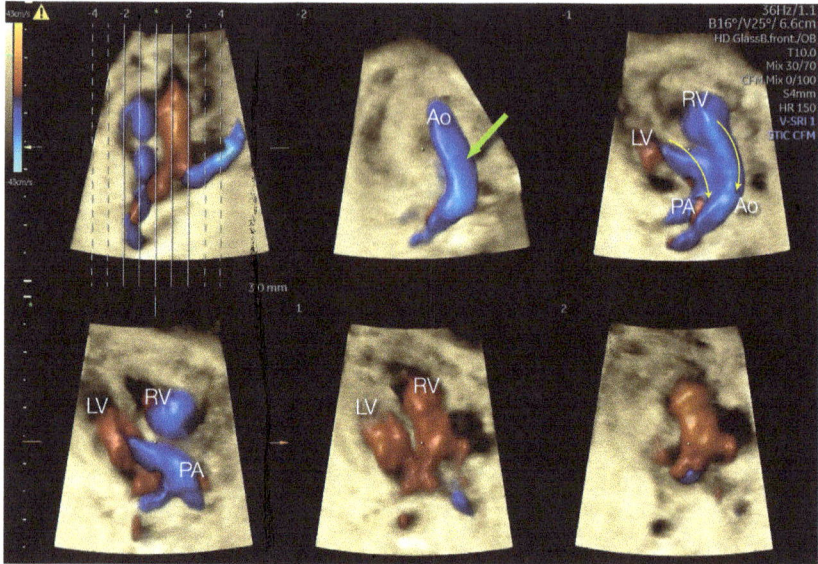

Fig. 19.15: STIC volume in tomographic mode with color Doppler shows transposition of the great arteries in this fetus. This single tomographic plane combines all the necessary information, including the pulmonary artery (PA) arising from the left ventricle (LV), the aorta (Ao) arising from the right ventricle (RV), and the parallel course of the Ao and PA (arrows). Note in the upper mediastinum the aorta as a single vessel (arrow), visible in this plane as a characteristic sign of this anomaly.

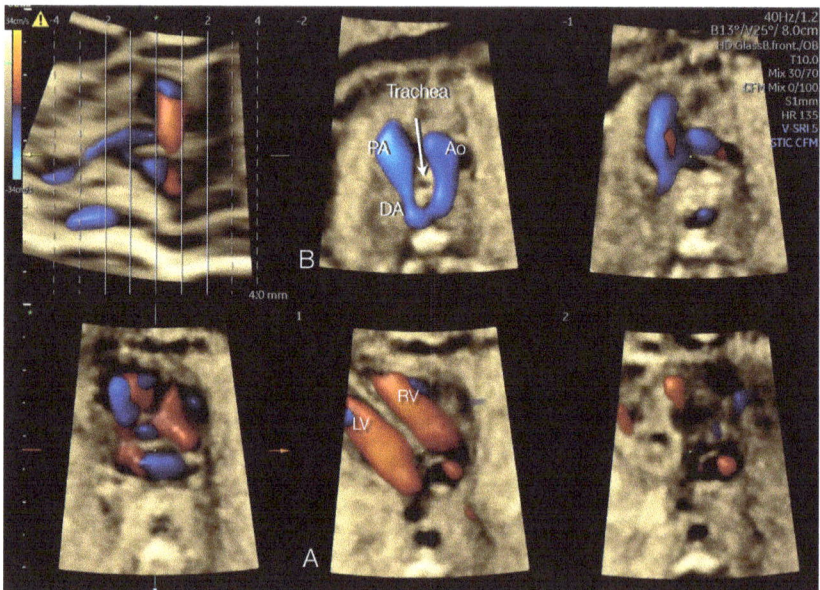

Fig. 19.16: STIC volume in tomographic mode with color Doppler in a fetus with right-sided aortic arch. Whereas the four-chamber view appears normal with filling of both the right (RV) and left (LV) ventricles in diastole (A), the three-vessel trachea view shows a right-sided aortic arch (Ao) and a left-sided pulmonary artery (PA) with ductus arteriosus (DA) and the trachea between both (B).

19.4 Fetal heart in grayscale STIC with rendering

Like the rendering of other fetal structures (see Chapter 7), cardiac volumes can also be displayed in different 3D rendering modes, such as surface, silhouette, minimum, inversion modes and others.

Surface mode: Depending on the question of interest, the rendering may focus on showing the surface of the walls and the lumen in the ventricles and less frequently on the great vessels. Surface rendering can be applied to the fetal heart after STIC volume acquisition by using the interface between the cavities and the heart walls (Fig. 19.17). For ideal visualization of the cardiac cavities, the camera line should be placed within the heart just below the origin of the aortic valve. Figures 19.18 and 19.19 show step by step how to display the four-chamber view with surface mode. A rare approach is to place the rendering line in the atria or in the ventricles facing the valves to visualize the opening and closing movements of the two atrioventricular valves (Fig. 19.20). Another rare application is to focus on the aortic or pulmonary valve to visualize opening movements in normal and dysplastic or stenotic valves. The surface mode of the heart cavities can be enhanced by adding a silhouette tool that highlights the borders of the heart walls and valves (Fig. 19.17D). The surface mode can thus be used ideally to demonstrate typical fetal heart planes providing a 3D view. This 3D view can be used for abnormalities that are present in the four-chamber view. Figure 19.17 shows a normal heart; in comparison, Figures 19.21 to 19.23 show cardiac anomalies with an abnormal four-chamber view in 3D surface mode.

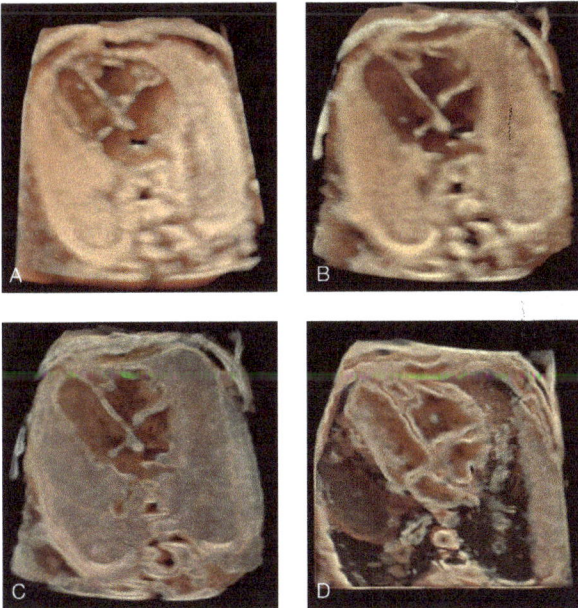

Fig. 19.17: Grayscale surface mode rendering of a STIC volume in the four-chamber view in different display modes: in (A) and (B) in surface mode with different light sources, in (C) and (D) with different levels of silhouette mode.

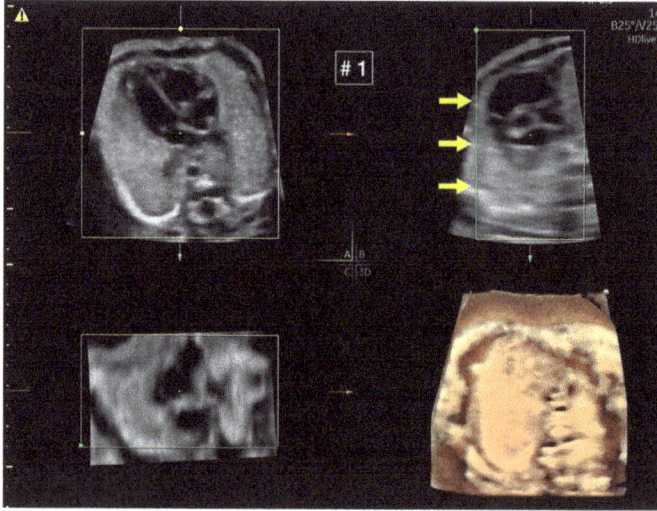

Fig. 19.18: Step by step instructions for rendering a 3D or STIC volume obtained on the plane of the four-chamber view in surface mode. After volume acquisition, the surface volume rendering is activated, and the rendering direction line is selected (front/back) with a view from the upper mediastinum to the heart (short arrows).

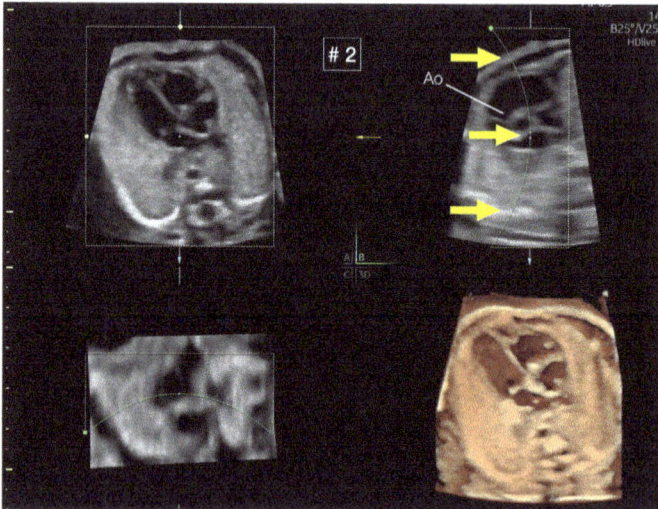

Fig. 19.19: In this second step, reduce the size of the render box by aligning the green line inside the heart, ideally below the aortic root (Ao). Note that a better result can be achieved by selecting a curved line (arrows). See Chapter 3 for more details.

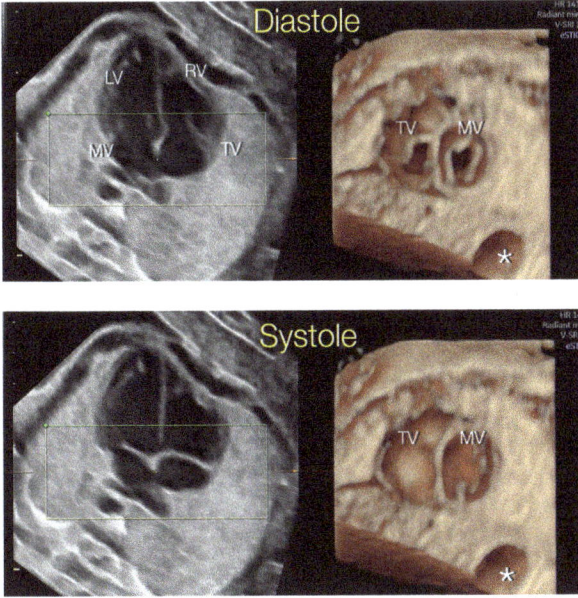

Fig. 19.20: Surface rendering mode of a STIC volume in grayscale obtained at the four-chamber view plane. This is a view of the two atrioventricular valves (AV) as seen from the ventricles. In the upper panel, diastole is shown and the AV valves are seen open in both 2D (left) and 3D (right). In the lower panel, the AV valves are closed in systole and are clearly visible in both 2D (left) and 3D (right). Mitral valve (MV), tricuspid valve (TV).

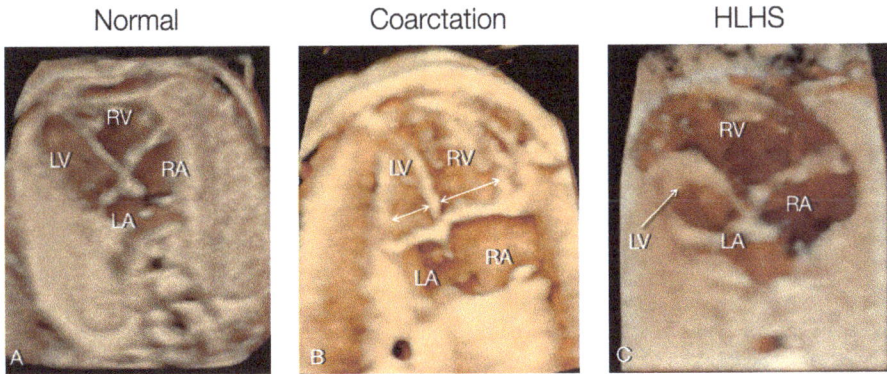

Fig. 19.21: Surface mode of a STIC volume in grayscale in a normal fetus (A) and two fetuses with small left ventricle in aortic coarctation in (B) and in hypoplastic left heart syndrome (HLHS) in (C). Left atrium (LA), left ventricle (LV), right atrium (RA), right ventricle (RV).

Normal

TA - VSD

AVSD

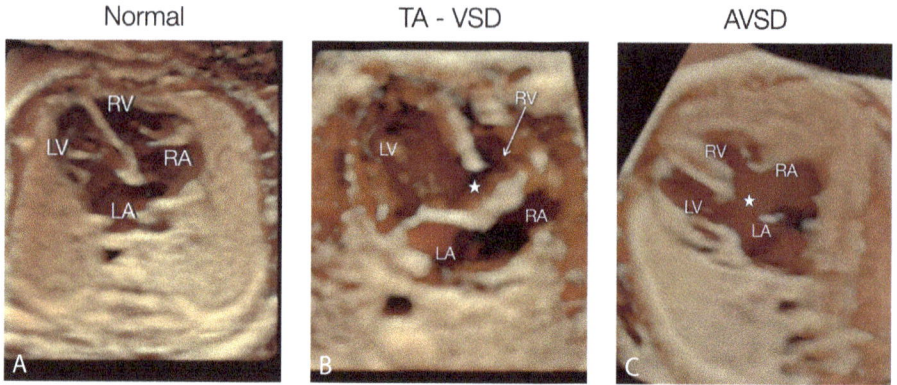

Fig. 19.22: Surface mode of a STIC volume in grayscale in a normal fetus (left) and two fetuses with complex cardiac anomalies: in the middle figure the fetus has tricuspid atresia with ventricular septal defect and in the right figure the fetus has an atrioventricular septal defect. The star in (B) and (C) indicates septal defect. Left atrium (LA), left ventricle (LV), right atrium (RA), right ventricle (RV).

Normal

Rhabdomyoma

Teratoma

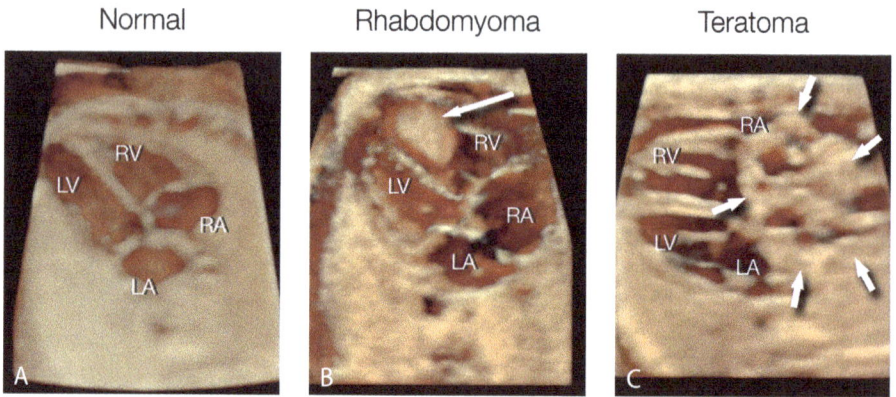

Fig. 19.23: Surface mode of a STIC volume in grayscale in a normal fetus (left) and two fetuses with cardiac tumors: in the middle figure with a rhabdomyoma (long arrow) and in the right figure with a pericardial teratoma (multiple short arrows).

Inversion mode and silhouette mode: A much more spatial image is displayed when inversion mode is used (Fig. 19.24). This mode can be added to a static or STIC acquisition in a rendered display and is explained in detail in Chapter 10. When applied to the fetal heart, fluid-filled spaces, such as the ventricles, appear bright, while heart and vessel walls or lungs disappear. Artifacts that may result from shadowing of the fetal ribs and spine can be removed with the electronic scalpel Magicut (Fig. 10.4). Especially for the spatial course of the vessels, the inversion mode can be beneficial. Figures 10.2 to 10.4 in Chapter 10 show the steps for anatomical display of a rendered volume of the fetal heart in inversion mode. In Figure 19.24, a frontal view of two hearts is shown: on the left, a normal heart with the crossing of the great vessels; on the right, in comparison, a heart with transposition of the great arteries with the parallel course. Other rendering modes include minimum and silhouette modes; while the minimum mode (Chapter 9) is now less used for the heart, the recent introduction of the silhouette mode is promising, as it transparently renders the course and shape of the heart and great vessels (Fig. 19.25).

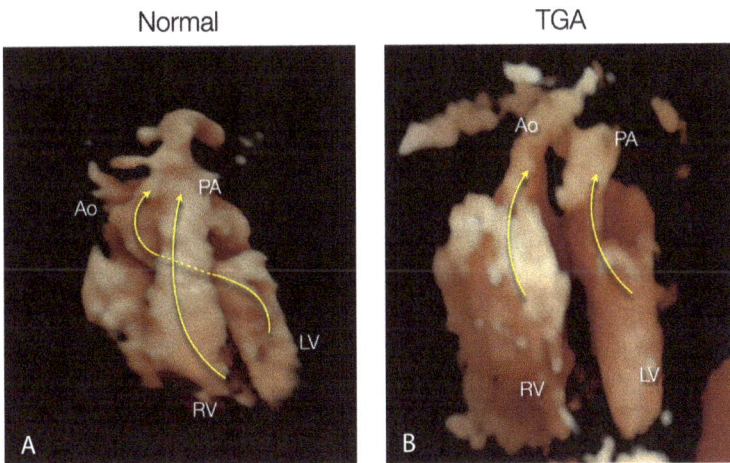

Fig. 19.24: STIC volumes in grayscale in two fetuses with inversion mode showing an anterior view of a normal heart with crossing of the great arteries (left figure) and a heart with transposition of the great arteries (TGA) with parallel course of the great vessels (right figure). Aorta (Ao), left ventricle (LV), pulmonary artery (PA), right ventricle (RV).

Normal

TGA

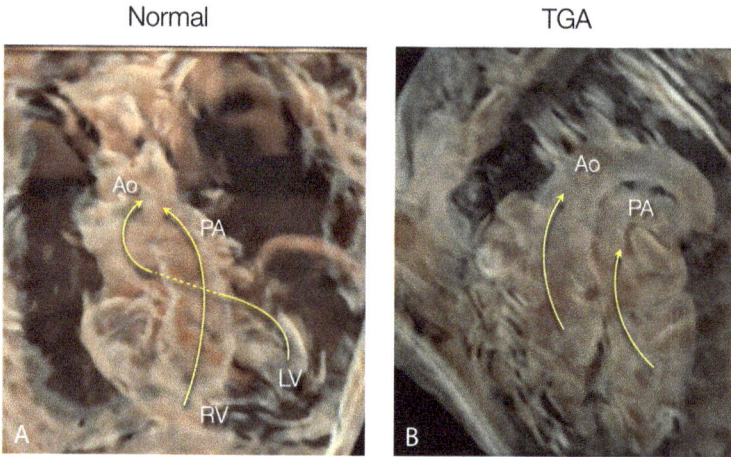

Fig. 19.25: STIC volumes in grayscale in two fetuses with silhouette mode showing an anterior view of a normal heart with crossing of the great arteries in the left figure and a heart with transposition of the great arteries (TGA) in the right figure with parallel course of the great vessels. Aorta (Ao), left ventricle (LV), pulmonary artery (PA), right ventricle (RV).

19.5 Fetal heart in color Doppler STIC with glass-body rendering

The combination of grayscale and color Doppler during a STIC volume acquisition allows the documentation of hemodynamic changes during the cardiac cycle. Cardiac STIC volumes acquired with color Doppler (or power Doppler, HD-Flow, or slow-flow-HD) can be displayed in the glass-body rendering modes, a technique discussed in detail in Chapter 12. Figure 19.26 shows step by step how the four-chamber view and the crossing of the great vessels can be rendered using the glass-body mode.

These display modes make it possible to visualize the blood flow in the heart and in the corresponding vessels particularly clearly. Glass-body mode is helpful in visualizing anomalies at the four-chamber plane (Fig. 19.27), but its main advantage is in showing the spatial course and relationship of the great vessels to each other (Figs. 19.28, 19.29). The best views are obtained either from the upper mediastinum or from a lateral view of the heart (Fig. 19.30).

STIC examination of the fetal heart in early gestation can be used mainly in combination with color or HD-flow Doppler, as shown in Figure 19.31, since 2D resolution is often not reliable enough to provide good STIC images in grayscale.

Step by Step for Color Glass-Body Mode of the Heart

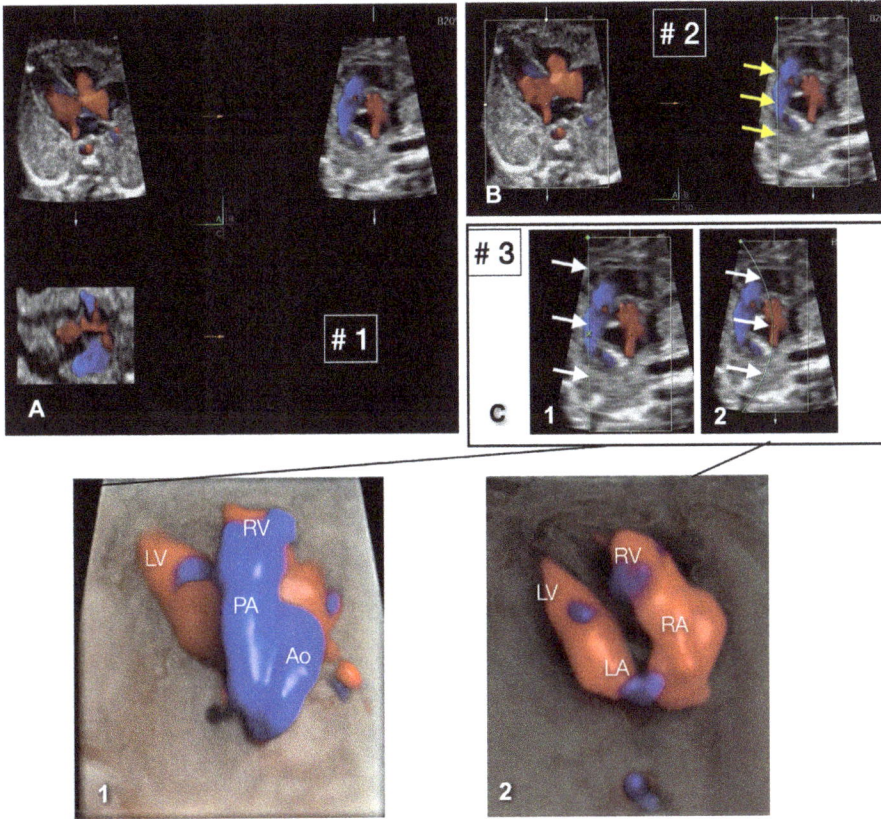

Fig. 19.26: Step by step demonstration of imaging a color Doppler STIC volume with glass-body mode. Step 1 is the acquisition of a volume from the apical four-chamber view (4CV) (A). Step 2 is the activation of render with glass-body mode and selection of HDlive (B). In this step, the rendering direction (yellow arrows) is selected as "front/back" to obtain a view from the upper mediastinum to the heart. In step 3, the user can decide what to include in the final rendered image, either (1) the entire heart with the 4CV and great vessels or (2) only the 4CV by placing the curved render line under the aortic valve. The results are shown in panels 1 and 2 below. Examples of cardiac abnormalities are shown in Figures 19.27 through 19.31. Aorta (Ao), left atrium (LA), left ventricle (LV), pulmonary artery (PA), right atrium (RA), right ventricle (RV).

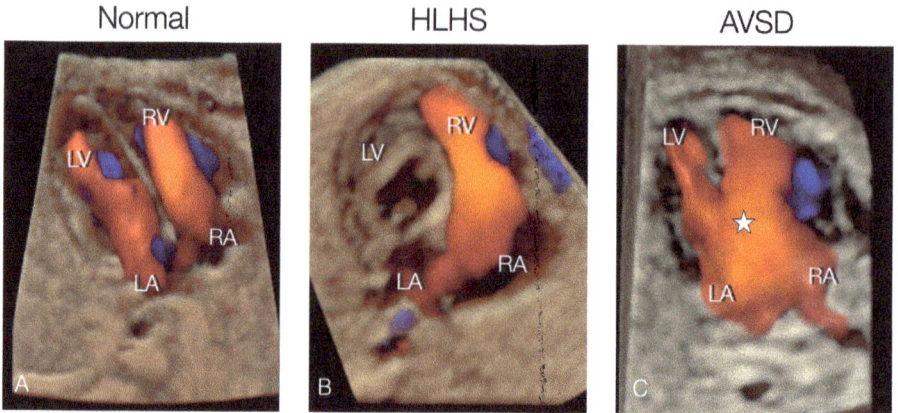

Normal **HLHS** **AVSD**

Fig. 19.27: STIC with color Doppler and glass-body mode rendering of the four-chamber view during dia-stole in a normal fetus (A) and in two fetuses with hypoplastic left heart syndrome (HLHS) and atrioven-tricular septal defect (AVSD), respectively (B) and (C). Note the absence of diastolic flow into the left ventricle (LV) in (B) and the large septal defect (Star) in (C). Left atrium (LA), right atrium (RA), right ventricle (RV).

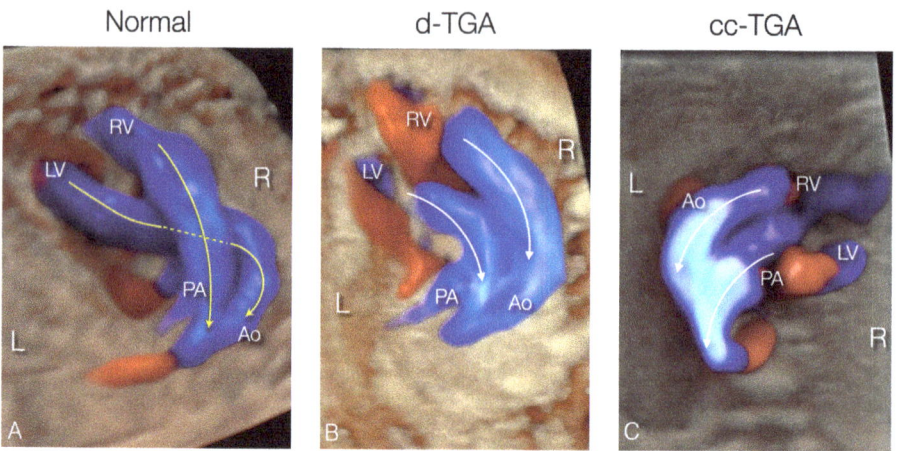

Normal **d-TGA** **cc-TGA**

Fig. 19.28: STIC with color Doppler and glass-body mode of the great vessels during systole in a normal fe-tus (A) and in two fetuses with dextro- (d-TGA) and congenitally corrected transposition of the great arteries (cc-TGA) in (B) and in (C), respectively. Note the crossing of the aorta (Ao) and pulmonary artery (PA) in (A) and the abnormal origin and the parallel course of the Ao and PA in (B) and (C). In d-TGA, the Ao is anterior and to the right of the PA, whereas in cc-TGA it is to the left and anterior. Left (L), left ventricle (LV), right (R), right ventricle (RV).

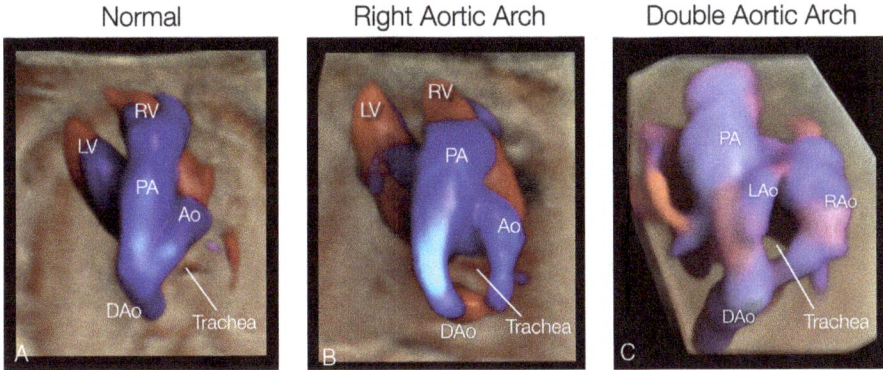

Fig. 19.29: STIC with color Doppler and glass-body mode of the great vessels during systole is shown in a normal fetus (A) and, in comparison, in a fetus with a right (B) and another fetus with a double aortic arch (C), respectively. Note the aorta (Ao) and pulmonary artery (PA) with a course to the left of the trachea in (A), whereas the trachea lies as a vascular ring between the arches in (B) and (C). In general, the trachea is not well seen in this 3D rendering mode. Descending aorta (Dao), left and right aortic arch (LAo, RAo), left ventricle (LV), right ventricle (RV).

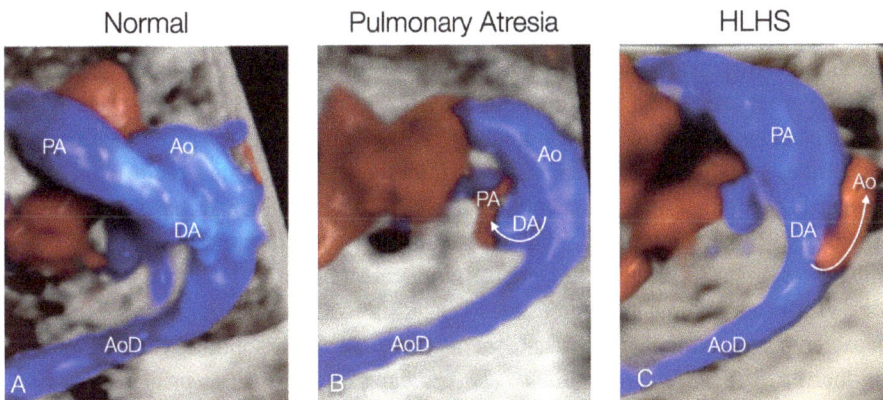

Fig. 19.30: STIC with color Doppler and glass-body mode rendering looking laterally from the left at the great vessels. In (A), a normal heart with the crossing of the aorta (Ao) and pulmonary artery (PA) is clearly visible. In (B), a heart with pulmonary atresia is shown with a reverse flow in the tortuous ductus arteriosus (DA) into the PA. Panel C shows a heart with hypoplastic left heart syndrome (HLHS) with clearly visible reverse flow (curved arrow) in red in the tiny Ao; descending aorta (Dao).

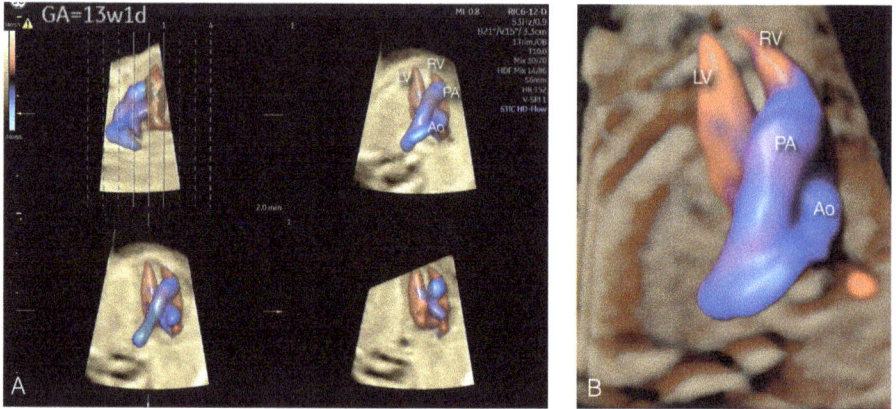

Fig. 19.31: Tomographic mode of a STIC cardiac volume on color Doppler at 13 weeks of gestation. In (A), the VCI thickness of 6 mm allows a view similar to glass-body mode with visualization of the four-chamber view in the background and the crossing of the great vessels in the foreground. In (B), the same STIC volume rendered as glass-body mode. Aorta (Ao), left ventricle (LV), pulmonary artery (PA), right ventricle (RV).

19.6 Automated cardiac volume evaluation and Sono-VCAD

The significant potential of 3D/4D lies not only in the spatial visualization of a heart with the great arteries or the offline manipulation of cardiac volumes. In recent years, efforts have been made to enable automatic recognition of anatomical landmarks within a cardiac volume and to automatically extract the standard planes required in a routine cardiac examination from a volume data set. Alfred Abuhamad (USA) was the first to propose the automation of fetal ultrasound in 3D and to describe this approach, which was initially called *Automated Multiplanar Imaging*. This later evolved into Sono-VCAD for "Volume Computer-aided Diagnosis" with a tomographic display of the extracted planes. A similar approach was later introduced by another group who called the tool *Fetal Intelligent Navigation Echocardiography* (FINE). The principles in both systems are similar. After volume acquisition (3D or STIC), the examiner defines some specific structures on the volume data set (septum, descending aorta and others) to confirm the volume orientation. The automation software then extracts the conventional diagnostic planes from the volume. These techniques have been shown to simplify fetal heart examination and reduce operator dependence. Although many limitations hinder the use of this tool in today's routine examination, we believe this is a step towards automated examination, which may one day be supported by artificial intelligence.

19.7 Other applications of 3D/4D fetal heart examination

It is beyond the scope of this book to discuss the many other applications of 3D to the fetal heart. These include the calculation of volumes using VOCAL or Sono-AVC, which have interesting applications for the calculation of ejection fraction and other volumes. Another application that can be combined with STIC is the calculation of an M-mode tracing, called STIC-M-Mode, which can be applied to both grayscale and color STIC.

19.8 Conclusions

3D/4D examination of the heart has revolutionized fetal echocardiography. The main advantage is both spatial visualization of a heart with the great arteries and offline manipulation of cardiac volumes to reconstruct virtually any desired sectional plane. To expand the use of 3D and STIC on the fetal heart, efforts should be made to facilitate the acquisition and compression of volumes and to improve the automatic detection of landmarks within a cardiac volume.

20 3D in Early Pregnancy

20.1 Introduction

The introduction and widespread acceptance of first trimester screening between 11 and 14 weeks of gestation has led to increased interest in ultrasound screening in early pregnancy. The use of high-resolution transabdominal and transvaginal transducers has opened a new window of opportunity for the diagnosis of fetal malformations before 14 weeks. For the use of 3D, the fetus can be examined transabdominally (Fig. 20.1A), but a much better resolution is achieved with transvaginal ultrasound (Fig. 20.1B).

During the first trimester, 3D imaging of the entire fetus is possible using surface mode and other imaging modes (Figs. 20.2–20.4) which provide additional imaging capabilities, as discussed later in this chapter. From the first sonographic detection of cardiac activity and up to 14 gestational weeks, the entire embryo and fetus can be imaged in vivo, as shown in Figures 20.3 and 20.4. With the high resolution of the transducers, detailed examination of selected organs, such as the brain, heart, face, extremities, and others is possible. The different rendering modes discussed in the previous chapters can all be used in early pregnancy. All cases in this chapter were examined transvaginally, which is a prerequisite for high-resolution 2D and 3D images.

Transabdominal   Transvaginal

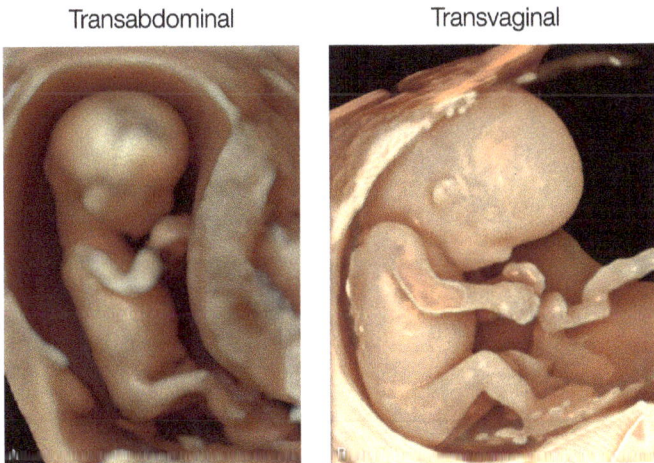

Fig. 20.1: 3D surface mode of two fetuses at 12 weeks of gestation examined with a transabdominal (A) and a transvaginal (B) transducer. The image in (B) has a higher resolution.

https://doi.org/10.1515/9783111249513-020

20.2 3D volume rendering in early gestation

Surface mode is the most commonly used 3D rendering mode in early pregnancy as it allows full visualization of the developing embryo and fetus (Fig. 20.3). Current images of an embryo acquired using the 3D surface mode resemble photographic images and drawings from embryology (Fig. 20.4).

As early as 11 weeks of gestation, the integrity of the fetus and the proportions of the head, trunk, extremities, and other details can be demonstrated reliably. Figures 20.2 and 20.3 show fetuses between 11 and 13 weeks of gestation. Severe anomalies affecting the body surface can be immediately recognized in 3D by both clinicians and patients. However, caution is recommended when relying solely on 3D images before performing a comprehensive assessment in 2D imaging. Figures 20.3 to 20.14 show examples of normal fetuses and fetuses with thickened nuchal translucency (Fig. 20.5), omphalocele (Fig. 20.6), spina bifida (Fig. 20.7), anencephaly (Fig. 20.8), facial anomalies (Figs. 20.9, 20.10, 20.11), as well as arm (Fig. 20.12) and leg (Fig. 20.13) malformations. Figure 20.14 shows that also in fetuses with fluid accumulation in the body, as in the presence of cysts or in megacystis, 3D in combination with silhouette mode can be applied. In other words, 3D ultrasound can play an important role in ruling out major

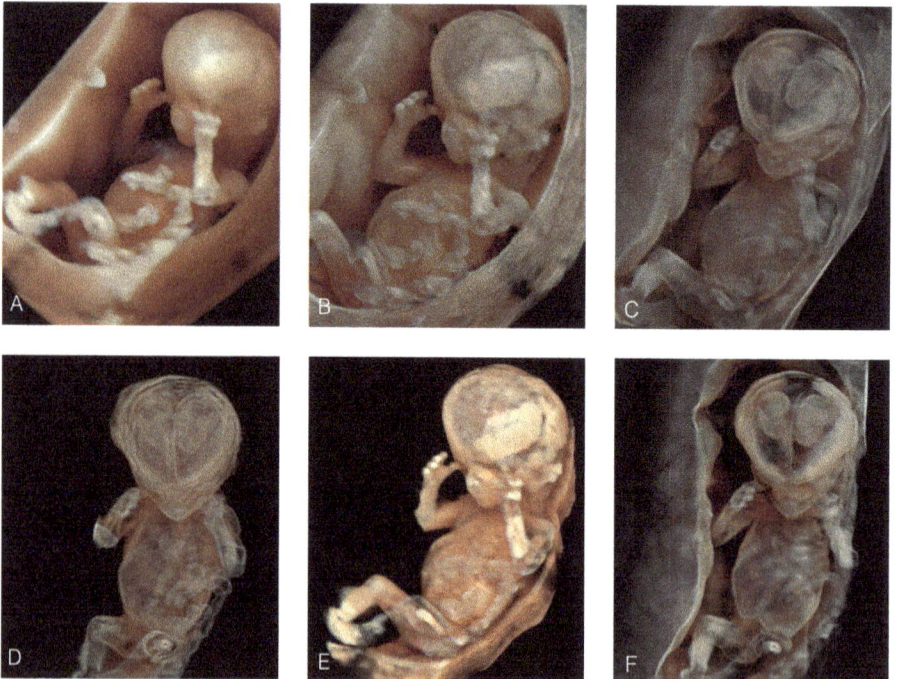

Fig. 20.2: A fetus after transvaginal examination with surface mode (A) and different silhouette rendering tools (B through F) highlighting bones, internal organs, or brain structures depending on the modified presets.

fetal malformations in early pregnancy, especially in pregnant women with a previous history of severe fetal anomalies.

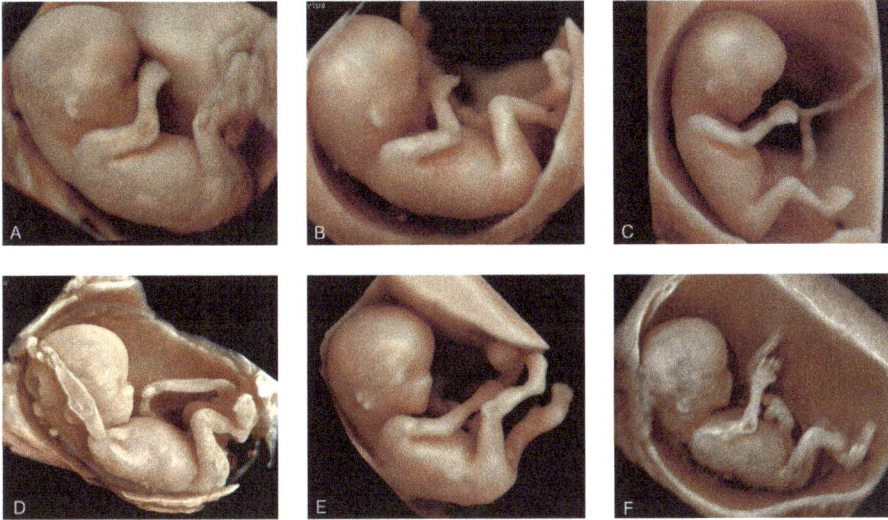

Fig. 20.3: Various fetuses between 11 and 13 weeks of gestation examined transvaginally with the 3D surface mode showing the typical fetal position with the arms often in front of the face in early pregnancy.

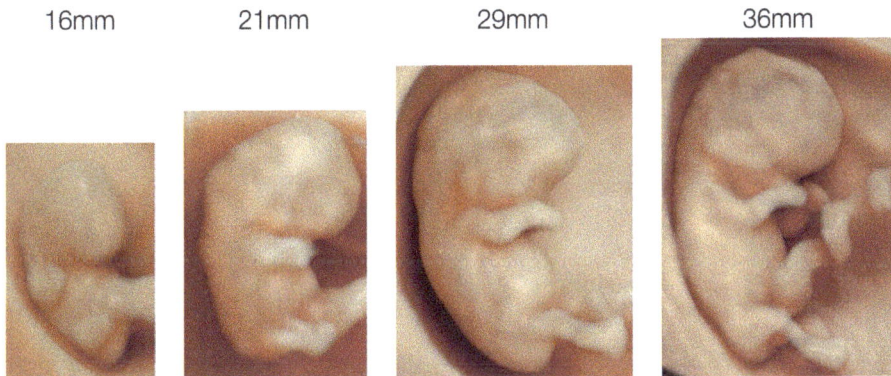

Fig. 20.4: Embryo development between 7 and 10 weeks of gestation with increasing crown-rump length from 16 mm, 20 mm, 29 mm to 36 mm as displayed in 3D surface mode.

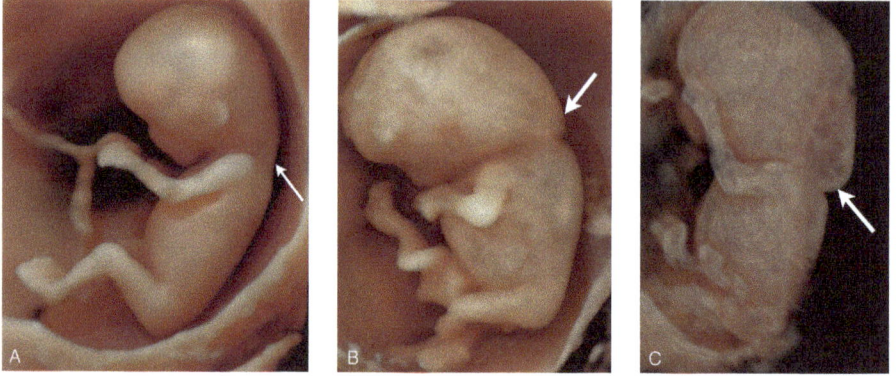

Fig. 20.5: 3D surface mode of a side view of the nuchal region (arrow) showing a normal fetus in (A) and two fetuses with thickened nuchal translucency in (B) and (C).

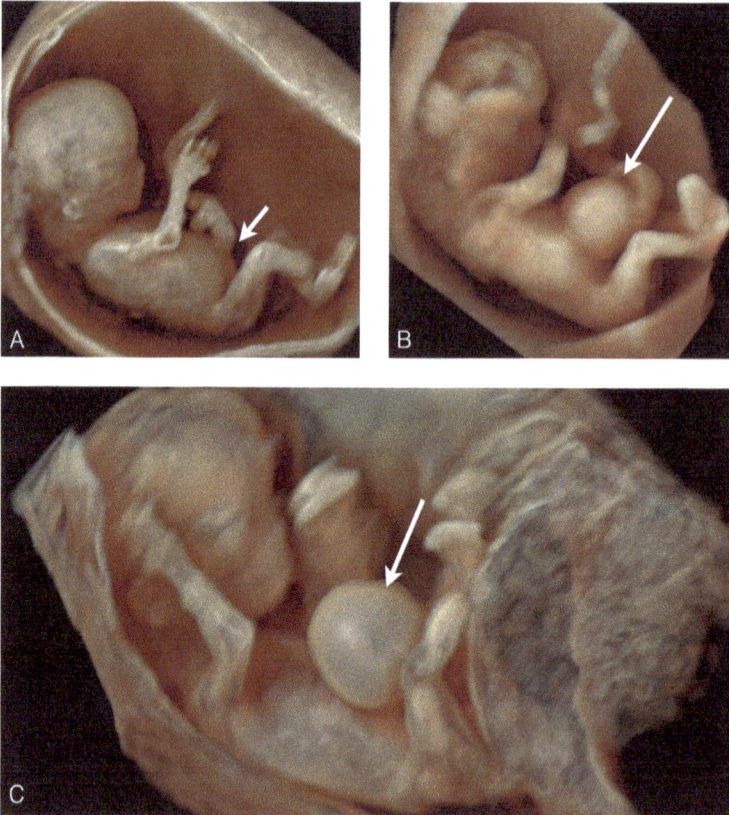

Fig. 20.6: 3D surface mode of a fetus (A) with closed anterior abdominal wall (short arrow) and two other fetuses with an omphalocele in (B) and (C) (long arrows).

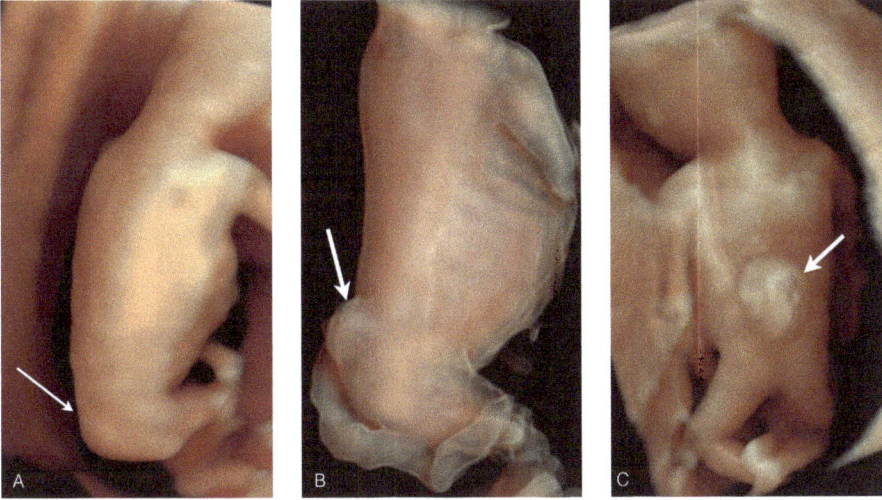

Fig. 20.7: 3D surface mode of the dorsal region of a fetus with closed spine (A) and two fetuses with open spina bifida with a small (B) and a large (C) myelomeningocele.

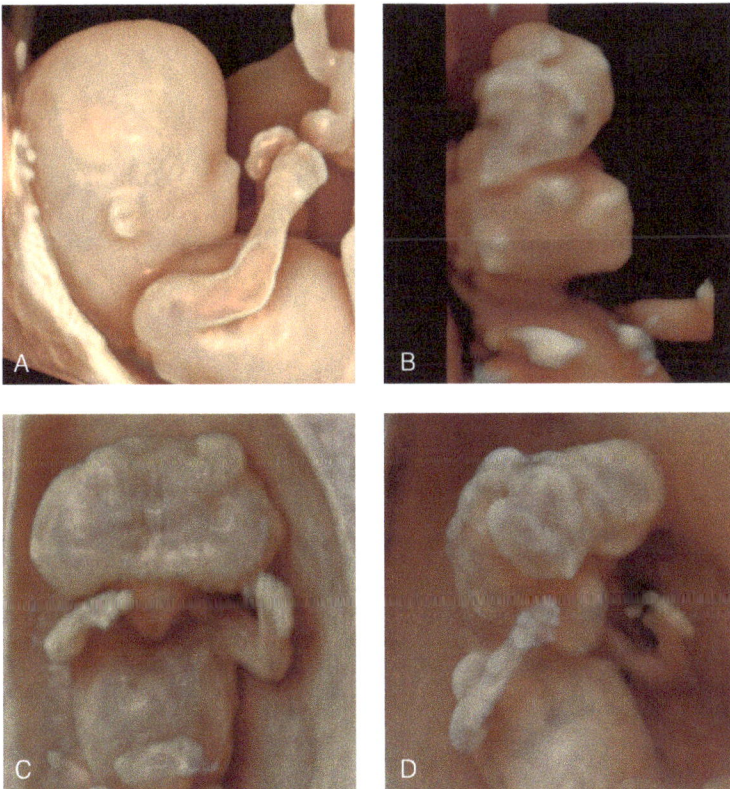

Fig. 20.8: A normal fetal head in (A) and, in comparison, three fetuses (B, C and D) with different types of acrania/exencephaly/anencephaly visualized with a 3D surface mode.

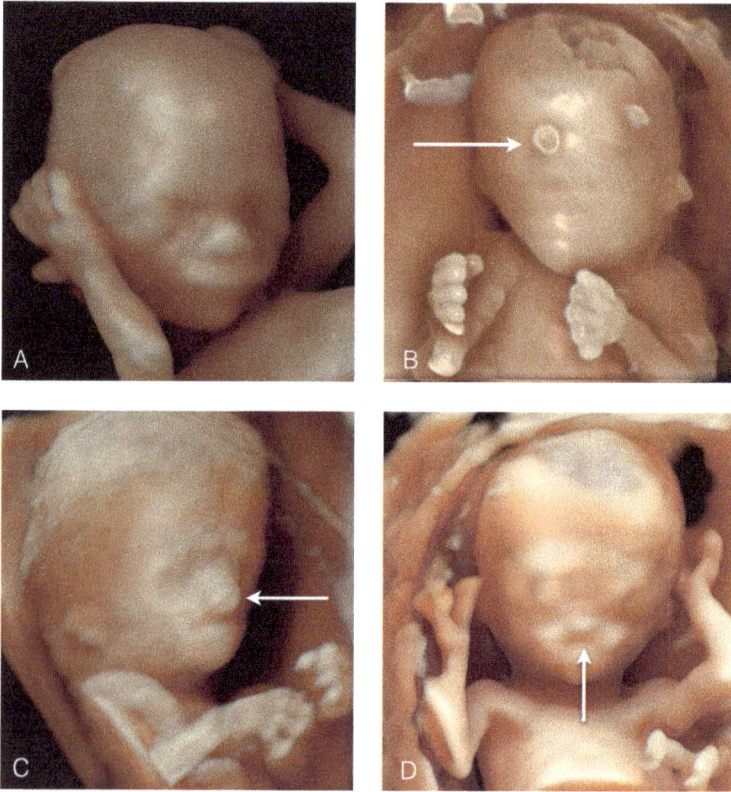

Fig. 20.9: A normal fetal face in (A) and, in comparison, three fetuses (B, C and D) with different types of abnormal faces with holoprosencephaly, visualized with a 3D surface mode. In (B) the fetus shows a proboscis (arrow), in (C) a cebocephaly (arrow), and in (D) a median cleft (arrow) and hypotelorism.

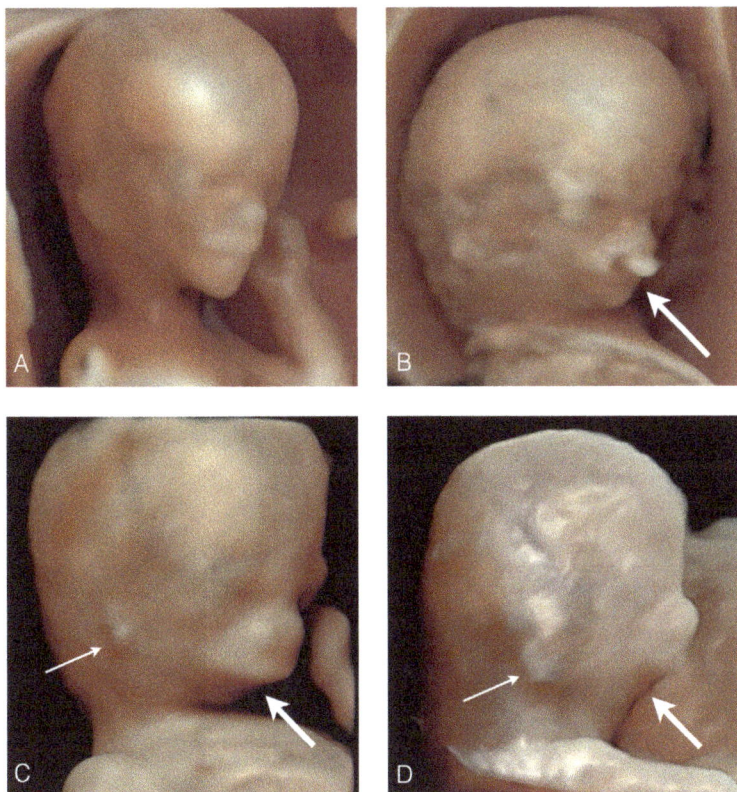

Fig. 20.10: A normal fetal face in (A) and, in comparison, three fetuses with abnormal faces, shown in 3D surface mode. The fetus in (B) has bilateral cleft. The fetus in (C) has Treacher-Collins syndrome with micrognathia and abnormal ears. The fetus in (D) has trisomy 18 with micrognathia and abnormal ears.

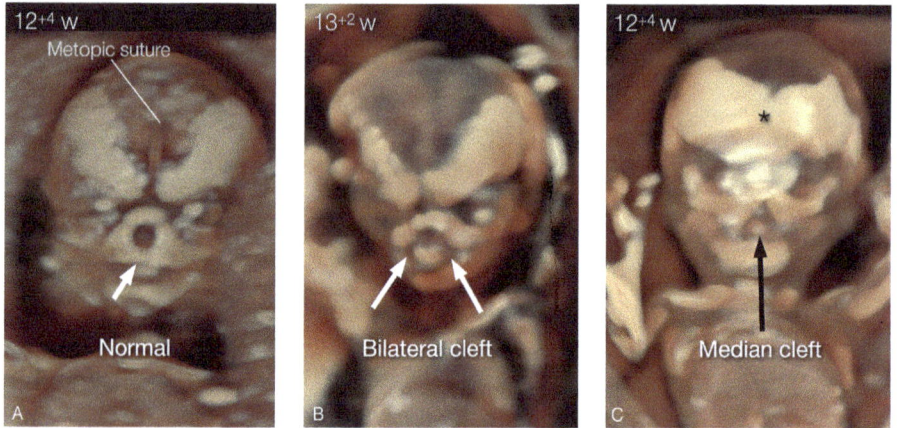

Fig. 20.11: Three fetal faces at 12 and 13 gestational weeks shown in silhouette mode with highlighted facial bones. In (A) a normal fetus with intact maxilla (short arrow), in (B) with bilateral cleft (long arrows), and in (C) with median cleft (black arrow). Note in (A) and (B) the wide-open metopic suture, which is fused in (C) (*), as typically found in fetuses with holoprosencephaly.

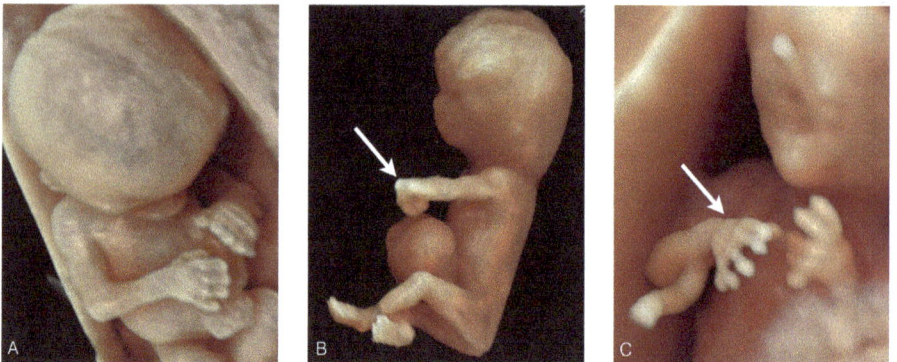

Fig. 20.12: A fetus with a normal hand in (A) and, in comparison, two fetuses with abnormal hands (arrows) (B and C), shown in 3D surface mode. The fetus in (B) has radius aplasia and trisomy 18, while the fetus in (C) has polydactyly and trisomy 13.

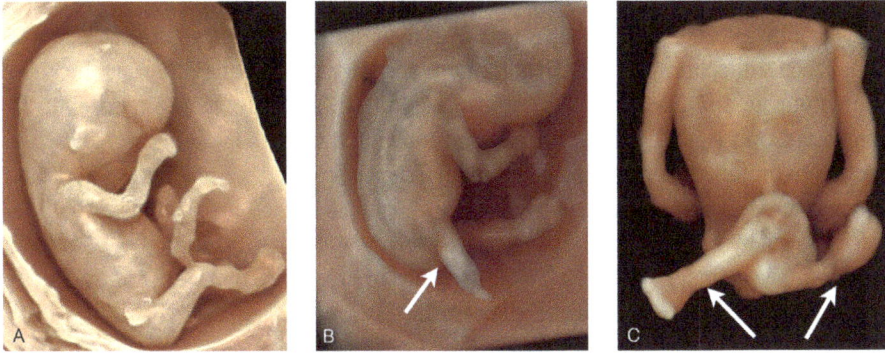

Fig. 20.13: Legs in surface mode; in (A) a fetus with normal legs, in (B) a fetus with a malformed leg (arrow) associated with sacral agenesis (caudal regression), and in (C) abnormal leg position in paralyzed legs in arthrogryposis (arrows).

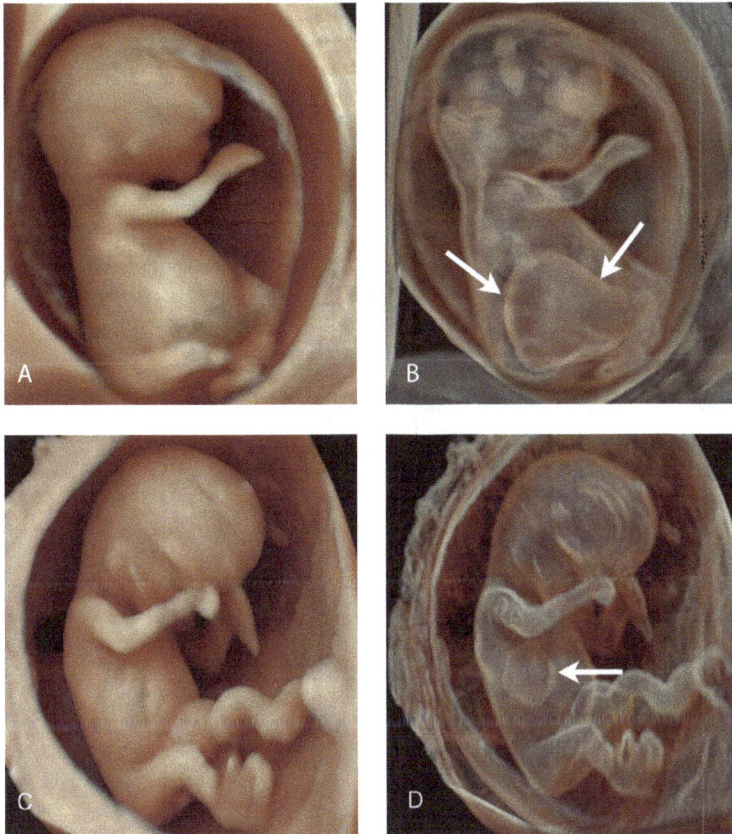

Fig. 20.14: In (A) and (B) a fetus with enlarged abdomen due to megacystis. In (A) the fetus is shown in surface mode and in (B) in silhouette mode. Transparency in (B) allows visualization of the dilated bladder (two arrows). In the lower panel, a normal-appearing fetus is seen in surface mode (C), but an intrahepatic cyst is visible in silhouette mode in (D).

In multiple pregnancies, the fetuses with their surrounding structures can be well visualized. Monochorionic and dichorionic twin pregnancies have different thickness of amniotic membranes (Figs. 20.15 and 20.16) and can be easily distinguished, but the diagnosis is more reliable in 2D ultrasound showing the Lambda- and T-signs. For the parents-to-be, an overview image of both fetuses in 3D is often very important. Furthermore, 3D can be particularly helpful in comparing the proportions of both fetuses, especially in the presence of selective growth restriction. 3D examples of anomalous twin pregnancies, such as a TRAP sequence or conjoined twins are shown in Figure 20.17 and can be diagnosed at a glance using 3D.

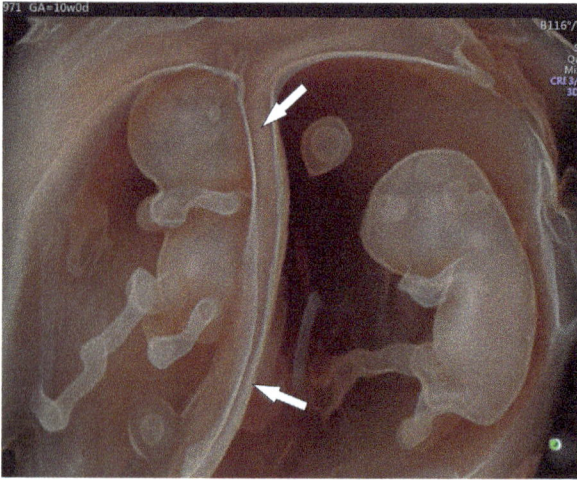

Fig. 20.15: Dichorionic diamniotic twin pregnancy at 10 gestational weeks with a thick separating membrane (arrows) between the two cavities shown in silhouette mode.

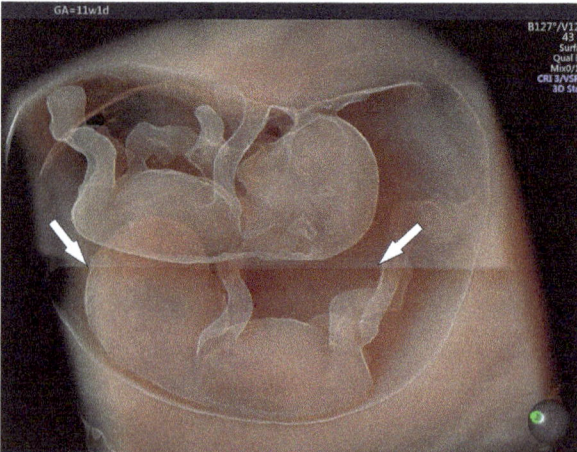

Fig. 20.16: Monochorionic diamniotic twin pregnancy at 11 gestational weeks with a thin separating membrane between the two cavities, shown in silhouette mode.

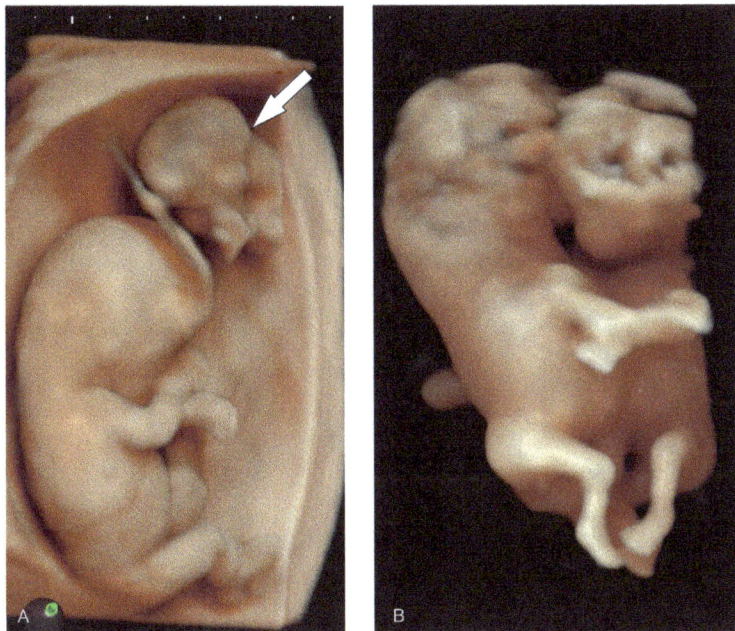

Fig. 20.17: Discordant monochorionic twin pregnancy at 11 gestational weeks, shown in 3D surface mode. In (A): the overview shows a normal twin and an acardiac parasitic twin (arrow) in TRAP sequence, where TRAP is an acronym for Twin-Reverse-Arterial-Perfusion. In (B): typical image of the thoracopagus as a type of conjoined twin.

The maximum mode is rarely used in early gestation because of the lower degree of ossification of the fetal skeleton and the rarity of diagnosis of skeletal disease. Figure 20.18 shows an example of maximum mode with imaging of the spine in a normal and an abnormal fetus. Alternatively, the silhouette mode, which highlights the bones, e. g., the skull, can provide good information about the bones during their ossification as shown in Figure 20.11.

One of the most interesting applications of 3D ultrasonography in the embryonic and early fetal period appears to be the visualization of brain structures under normal and abnormal conditions (Fig. 20.19). While minimum mode is rarely used in these conditions, inversion mode (Fig. 20.20) or the new silhouette mode can be used to visualize the intracerebral ventricular system (Fig. 20.19) (see Chapter 11). We believe that this approach will find more clinical application in the future.

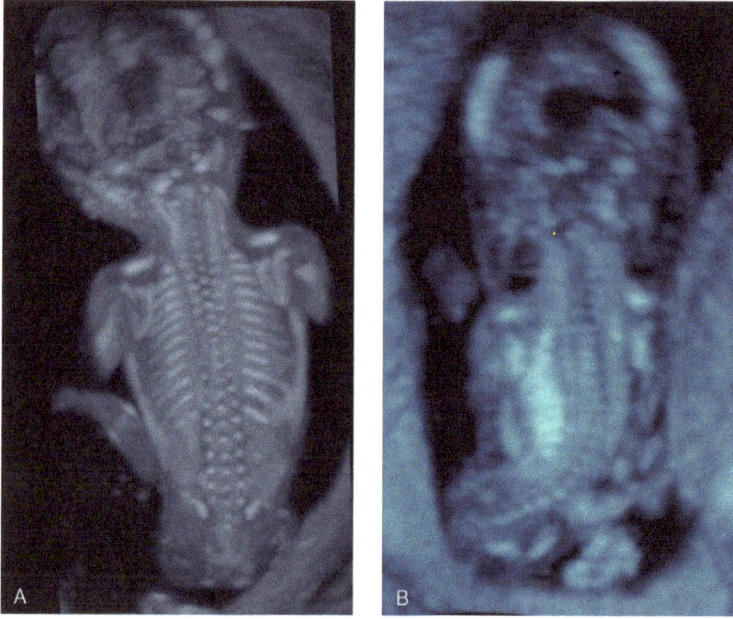

Fig. 20.18: Fetal spine in maximum mode in a normal fetus at 13 weeks (A) and in a fetus at 12 weeks of gestation (B) with deviated spine in a body-stalk anomaly.

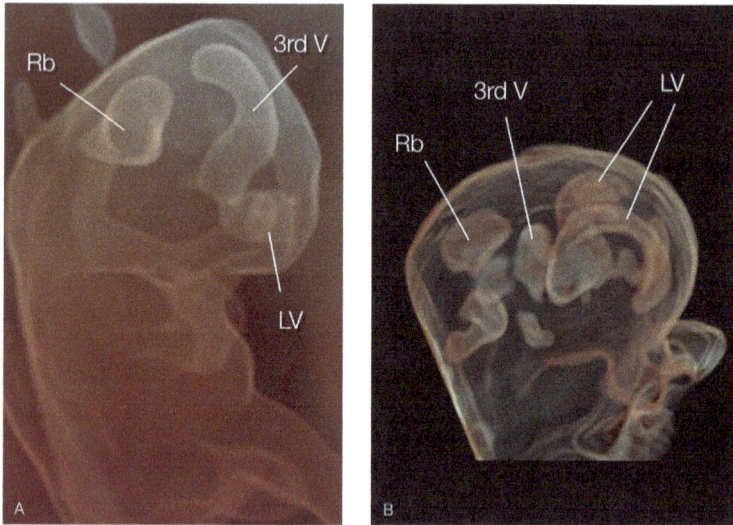

Fig. 20.19: Intracerebral ventricular system of an embryo at 8 weeks (A) and 9 weeks of gestation (B), shown with silhouette mode; lateral ventricle (LV), third ventricle (3rd V.), rhombencephalon (Rb).

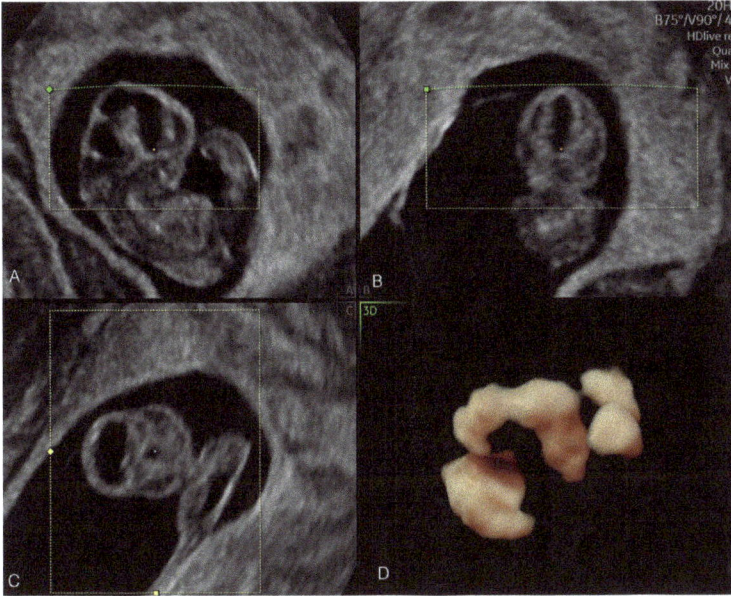

Fig. 20.20: The intracerebral ventricular system of an embryo at 9 gestational weeks shown in orthogonal mode (A, B and C) and in inversion mode (D).

20.3 Multiplanar display in early gestation

If a high-resolution image is needed in early gestation, especially for multiplanar 3D reconstruction, volume acquisition should be performed with a transvaginal approach. Since embryos and fetuses are rarely in an optimal position to visualize all anatomical structures in 2D ultrasound, 3D volume acquisition and plane reconstruction can be of great help. The demonstration of normal anatomy can be then achieved by a static 3D scan with multiplanar, tomographic, or Omniview reconstruction of one or more cross-sectional images. This principle was explained earlier in this book.

For a good overview, the operator can visualize the complete anatomy of the fetus in one image like in the second trimester. Another possibility is to focus on the documentation of selective anatomical regions of the fetus. These can include the intracranial anatomy as shown in Figure 20.21 or the facial region with eyes, nose with maxilla and mandible. Figure 20.22 shows an example of a normal fetus and a fetus with holoprosencephaly as displayed with tomography mode. An important view could be the chest and abdomen with documentation of the heart and abdominal situs with the abdominal organs such as stomach, liver, and kidneys (Fig. 20.23). Figure 20.24 shows an example of a normal fetus and a fetus with a diaphragmatic hernia as displayed with multiplanar mode. The reconstruction of single planes can be also well applied to assess the normal and abnormal posterior fossa (Figs. 20.25–20.27) or to document a normal maxilla or a facial cleft for the fetal facial region (Fig. 20.28). In the presence of thickened nuchal translucency or cystic hygroma, multiplanar reconstruction can provide a reliable image of a midsagittal view to document the severity of the finding.

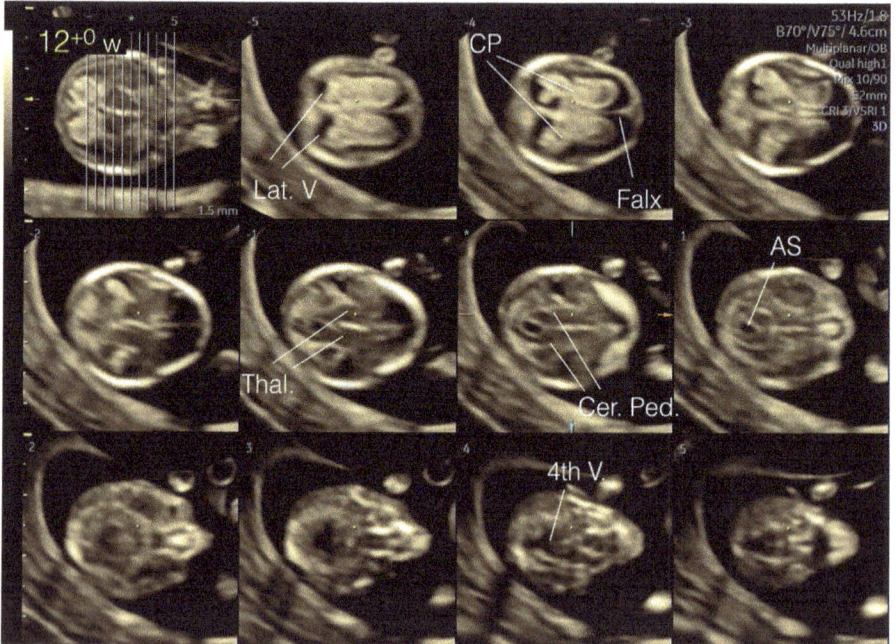

Fig. 20.21: Tomography mode of an axial view of the fetal brain at 12 weeks' gestation, providing an overview of the major landmarks of the brain at this stage of development. These include the large bilateral choroid plexus (CP), the falx cerebri (Falx), the two lateral ventricles (Lat. V), the thalami (Thal.), the cerebral peduncles (Cer. Ped.), the aqueduct of Sylvius (AS), and the fourth ventricle (4th V.).

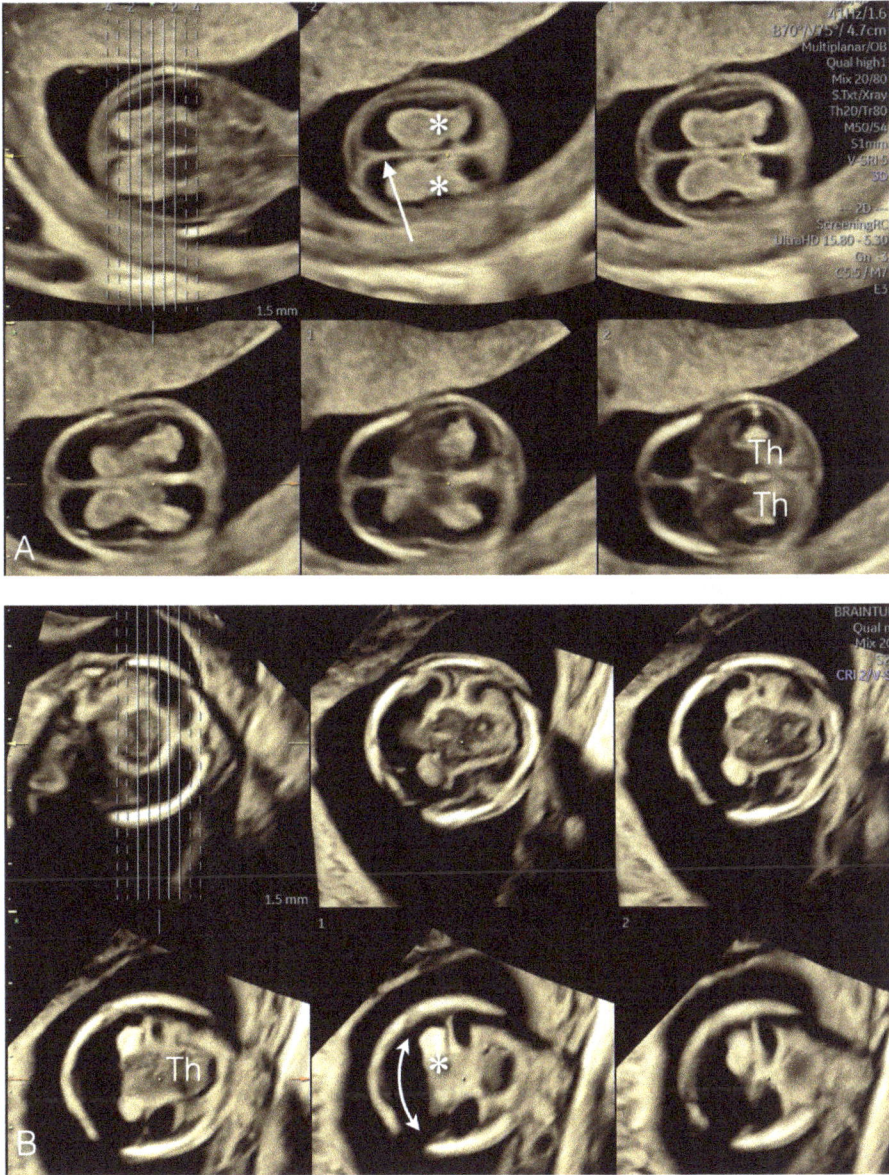

Fig. 20.22: Tomography mode of the brain of a normal fetus (A) showing the clearly visible falx cerebri se-parating the two hemispheres and the bilateral choroid plexuses (*). In comparison, a fetus with holopro-sencephaly (B) showing the absent falx cerebri, fused ventricles (double arrow), fused thalami (Th), and choroid plexus (*).

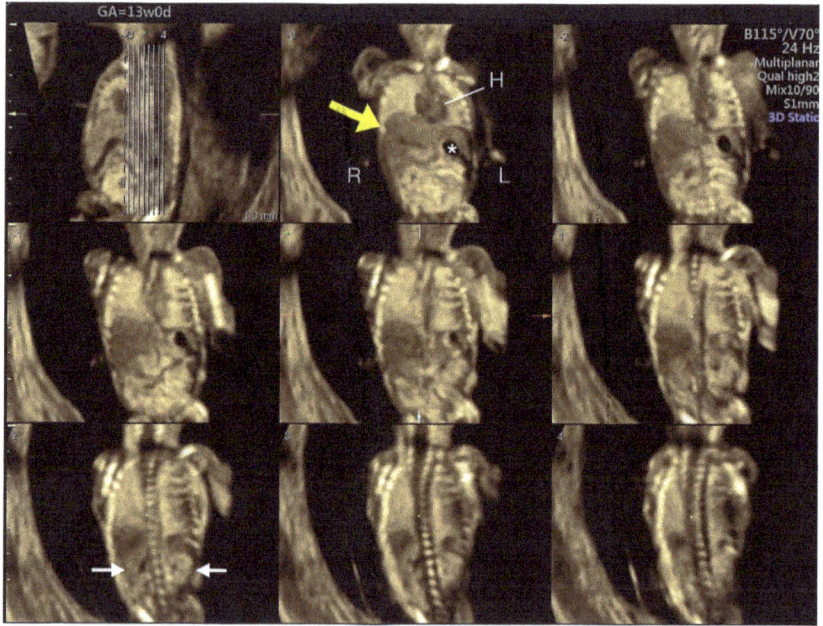

Fig. 20.23: Tomography of the body of a 13-week-old fetus showing the diaphragm (yellow arrow), lungs, liver, stomach (*), kidneys (arrows), and the left-sided heart position; left (L), right (R).

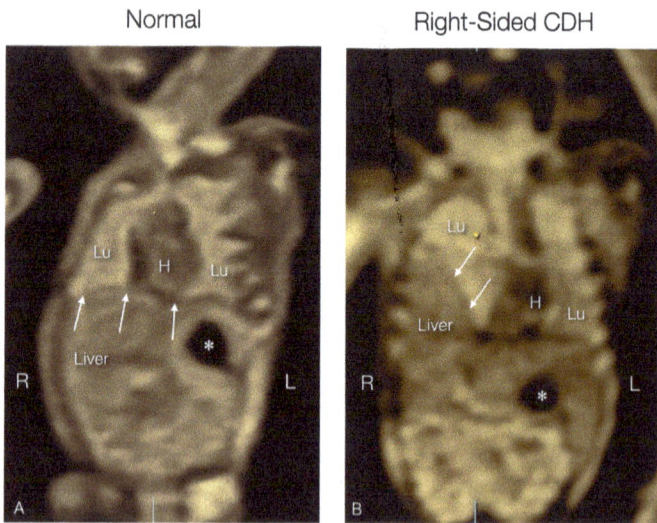

Fig. 20.24: Reconstructed plane in multiplanar mode of thorax and abdomen in a normal fetus (A) and in a fetus with a right-sided congenital diaphragmatic hernia (CDH). In (A) the diaphragm (arrows), separating the liver from the lungs (Lu), is clearly visible and the heart (H) is centrally located. However, in (B) the liver is up on the right side and the heart is slightly shifted to the left. The asterisk indicates the stomach.

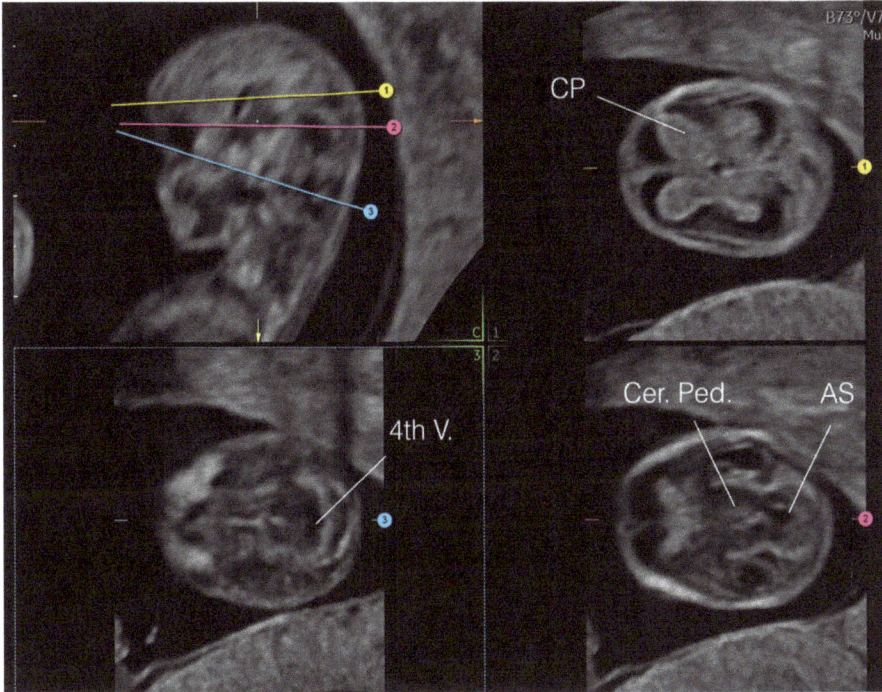

Fig. 20.25: After a lateral static 3D acquisition of a fetal head at 11 weeks of gestation, three Omniview lines were drawn to visualize the three axial planes: line 1 (yellow) the transventricular plane with the two choroid plexuses, line 2 (magenta) the plane at the level of the cerebral peduncles (Cer. Ped) with the Sylvian aqueduct (AS), and line 3 (cyan) at the level of the posterior fossa with the fourth ventricle (4th V.).

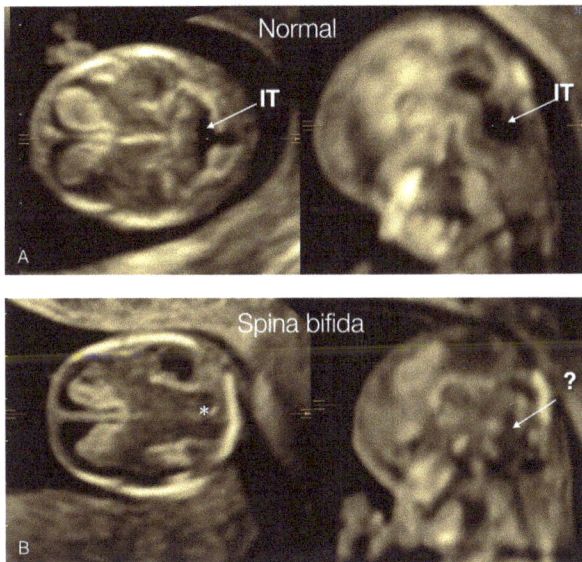

Fig. 20.26: Reconstructed plane in multiplanar mode of a normal fetus (A) showing the posterior fossa with the intracranial translucency (IT), and a fetus in (B) with open spina bifida showing the crash sign (*) and absence of fluid in the IT (?) due to compression of the posterior fossa.

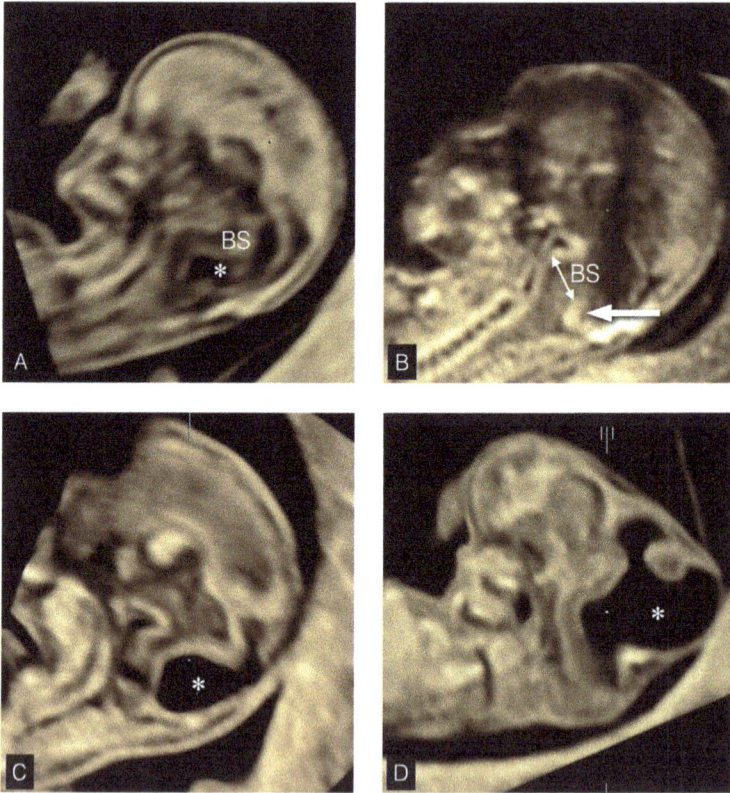

Fig. 20.27: Multiplanar reconstruction of the midline with the posterior fossa in a normal fetus (A) and three fetuses (B, C and D) with abnormal posterior fossa. In (A), the intracranial translucency (*) and thin brainstem (BS) are clearly visible. The fetus in (B) has an open spina bifida with absent fluid in the posterior fossa (arrow) and a thickened BS (double arrow). The fetus in (C) has a chromosomal abnormality and a dilated fourth ventricle (*) resembling a Blake's pouch cyst. The fetus in (D) has a severely dilated fourth ventricle (*) as a developing meningocele in the presence of Meckel-Gruber syndrome.

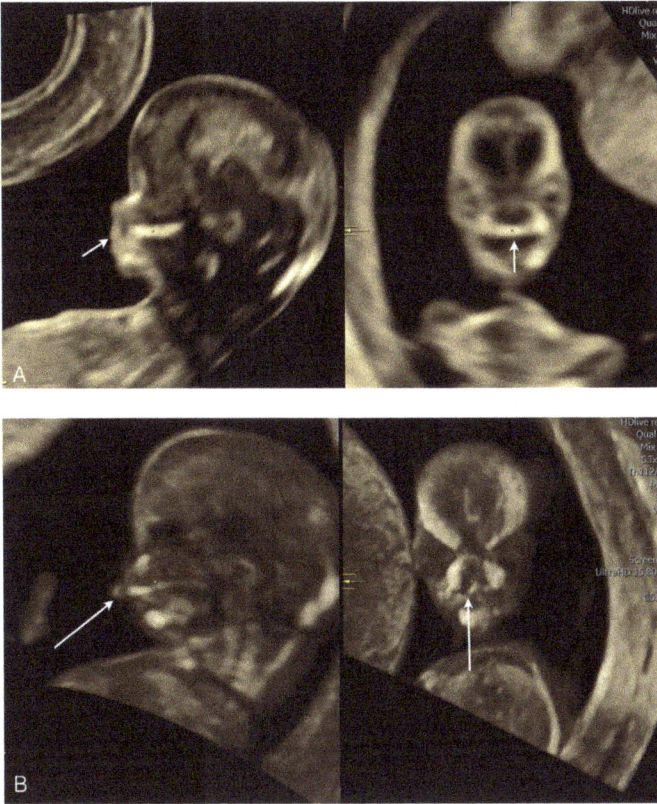

Fig. 20.28: Normal face and maxilla (short arrows) in a fetus at 12 weeks of gestation (A) in orthogonal mode; in (B) a fetus with bilateral cleft (long arrows) with premaxillary protrusion.

20.4 3D Color Doppler in early gestation

In the first trimester, color Doppler can be used to examine the same anatomic regions as in the second trimester. Subsequently, the use of static 3D and STIC can be combined with color Doppler and the volume can be visualized in multiplanar mode or volume rendering mode. The challenge of studying the heart and vasculature in early gestation is the moving fetus during volume acquisition. Acquisition is often slightly longer with color Doppler than without, which is why this method is used less frequently. Typical areas of interest include the heart and the crossing of the great vessels. Figure 20.29 shows a normal heart with the filling of both ventricles in diastole and the crossing of the great vessels in systole. In comparison, Figure 20.30 shows a fetal heart with a single ventricle and the double outlet of the great arteries with a parallel course. Other regions of interest for 3D color Doppler include imaging of the normal and abnormal vessels of the abdomen (Fig. 20.31), particularly the intrahepatic circulation (Fig. 20.32A) or, more recently, the intracerebral circulation (Fig. 20.32B). The potential of using glass-body mode in the first trimester has not yet been fully exploited. Many users are reluctant to use color Doppler in early pregnancy; however, we recommend its use when clearly indicated and in consideration of the ALARA (as low as reasonably achievable) principle.

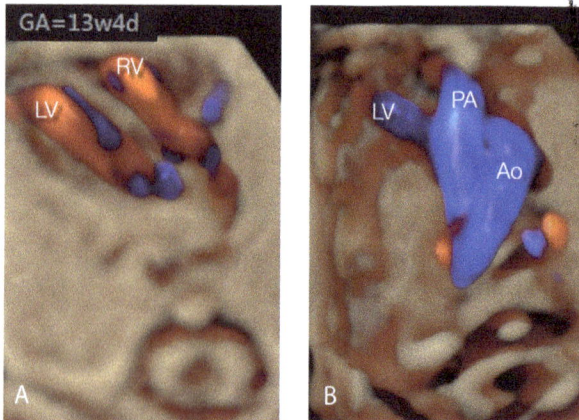

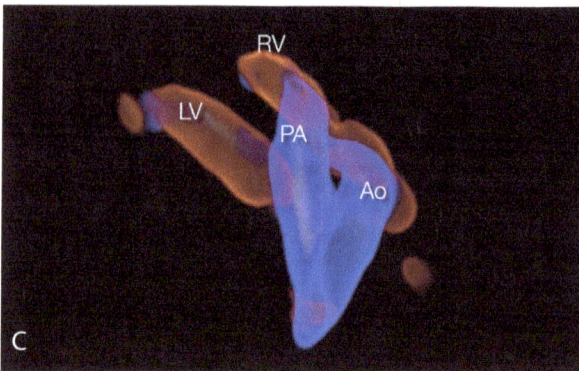

Fig. 20.29: STIC volume of a normal heart at 13 weeks of gestation in glass-body mode showing filling of the right (RV) and left (LV) ventricles in diastole in (A). In (B), a view from the upper mediastinum shows the crossing of the pulmonary artery (PA) and aorta (Ao) in systole. In (C), the grayscale information has been removed and a color silhouette has been activated, showing the filling of the four chambers and the crossing of the great vessels.

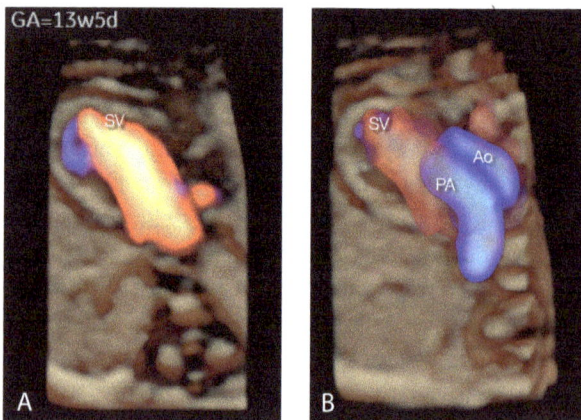

Fig. 20.30: STIC volume of a fetal heart defect in glass-body mode showing in (A) a single ventricle (SV) in diastole and in (B) the abnormal parallel course of the aorta (Ao) and pulmonary artery (PA).

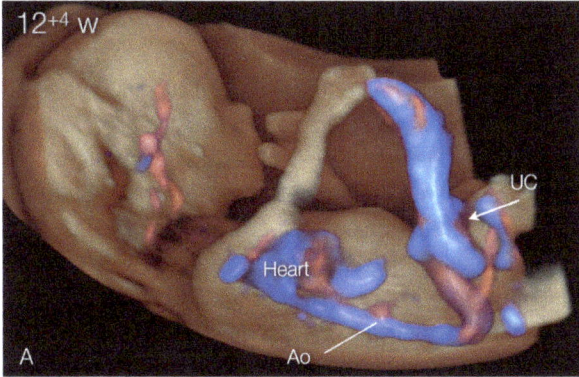

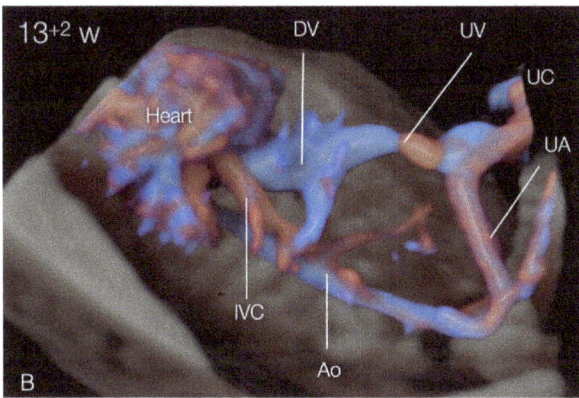

Fig. 20.31: 3D color Doppler glass-body mode of a lateral view of the body. In (A), the complete fetus with the anterior wall and the umbilical cord is clearly visible along with the heart and descending aorta. In (B), another fetus with magnification of the abdominal region showing the umbilical cord (UC), umbilical artery (UA), and umbilical vein (UV). The UV drains to the heart via the ductus venosus (DV) together with the inferior vena cava (IVC).

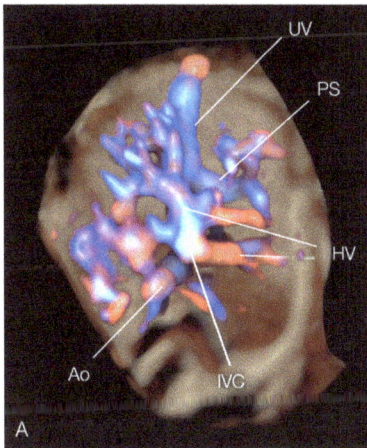

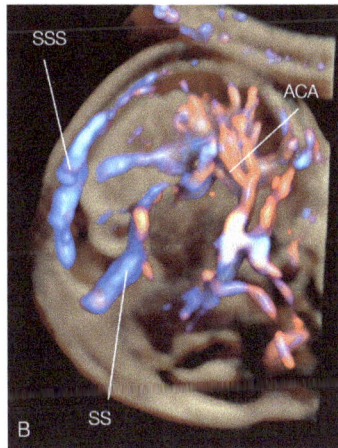

Fig. 20.32: 3D color Doppler glass-body mode of two regions of two fetuses at 12 and 13 weeks of gestation. (A) shows a cranial view of hepatic vascularization with the umbilical vein and portal sinus (PS) in the background and the hepatic veins (HV) in the foreground. (B) shows a midsagittal view of the early cerebral vessels with the anterior cerebral artery (ACA), the great superior sagittal sinus (SSS), and the straight sinus (SS); aorta (Ao).

20.5 Conclusions

3D examination has revolutionized the examination of the early embryo and fetus. The combination of transvaginal ultrasound and 3D has the great advantage of reconstructing any plane and obtaining typical views. The limitations of handling the transvaginal probe can be overcome by combining it with multiplanar 3D reconstruction and different modes of volume rendering. High-resolution images can provide valuable information about the developing embryo and fetus. In particular brain structures can be studied in their embryological development. The external view of the fetus under normal and abnormal conditions can be reliably demonstrated with the surface mode and is ideal for visualizing the external structures, such as the face, limbs, anterior abdominal wall, the back, and others. Accurate examination of the embryo and fetus has improved tremendously since the introduction of 3D ultrasound.

21 Further literature references and sources

Performing a literature search in PubMed end of 2023 with the words "3D, ultrasound, fetal" reveals around 1,800 hits. We found that in such a book, it is impossible to present a comprehensive literature list especially given the fact that this book has been conceived as a practical book. We hereby provide a short list of some literature sources, including some books and journal articles, which partly or completely discuss both technical as well as clinical aspects of 3D ultrasound.

Books
Abu-Rustum RS. A Practical Guide to 3 D Ultrasound. London: CRC Press, Taylor & Francis Group, 2014.
Abuhamad A, Chaoui R. First Trimester Ultrasound Diagnosis of Fetal Abnormalities. Philadelphia, Lippincott Wilkins; 2017.
Abuhamad A, Chaoui R. A Practical Guide to Fetal Echocardiography: Normal and Abnormal Hearts. 4th ed. Philadelphia: Lippincott-Williams Wilkins, 2022.
Gembruch U, Hecher K, Steiner H. Ultraschalldiagnostik in Geburtshilfe und Gynäkologie, 3. Auflage, Heidelberg, Springer-Verlag, 2024.
Khurana A, Dahiya N. 3D and 4D Ultrasound: A text and atlas, Jaypee-JPB Delhi, 2004.
Kurjak A, Azumendi G. The Fetus in Three Dimensions: Imaging, Embryology and Fetoscopy. London: Taylor & Francis, 2007.
Lakshmy RS, Thasleem Z. First and mid trimester ultrasound diagnosis of orofacial clefts. An atlas and guide. Heidelberg, Springer, 2021.
Levaillant JM, Bault J-P, Benoit B. Pratique de l´échographie volumique-Echographie obstetricale. Paris: Sauramps Medical, 2008.
Levaillant JM, Bault J-P, Benoit B, Couly G. Normal and abnormal fetal face atlas. Ultrasonographic features. Heidelberg, Springer, 2017.
Malinger G, Monteagudo A, Pilu G, Paladini D, Timor-Tritsch I: Timor's Ultrasonography of the Prenatal Brain, New York, McGraw-Hill, 2023.
Paladini D, Volpe P. Ultrasound of Congenital Fetal Anomalies: Differential Diagnosis and Prognostic Indicators. London, 2023.
Rama Murthy BS. Imaging of fetal brain and spine. An atlas and guide. Heidelberg, Springer, 2019.
Tonni G, Sepulveda W, Wong A. Prenatal Diagnosis of Orofacial Malformations. Heidelberg, Springer, 2017.
Werner H, Tonni G, Lopes J. 3 D Physical and Virtual Models in Fetal Medicine: Applications and Procedures. Heidelberg, Springer, 2023.

Articles
Abuhamad A, Falkensammer P, Reichartseder F, Zhao Y. Automated retrieval of standard diagnostic fetal cardiac ultrasound planes in the second trimester of pregnancy: a prospective evaluation of software. Ultrasound Obstet Gynecol. 2008;31:30–36,
Abuhamad AZ. Standardization of 3-dimensional volumes in obstetric sonography: a required step for training and automation. J Ultrasound Med. 2005;24:397–401.
Acar P, Dulac Y, Taktak A, Abadir S. Real-time three-dimensional fetal echocardiography using matrix probe. Prenat Diagn. 2005;25:370–375.
Acar P, Hadeed K, Dulac Y. Advances in 3 D echocardiography: from foetus to printing. Arch Cardiovasc Dis. 2016;109:84–86.

https://doi.org/10.1515/9783111249513-021

Achiron R, Gindes L, Zalel Y, Lipitz S, Weisz B. Three- and four-dimensional ultrasound: new methods for evaluating fetal thoracic anomalies. Ultrasound Obstet Gynecol. 2008;32:36–43.

Benacerraf BR, Shipp TD, Bromley B. How sonographic tomography will change the face of obstetric sonography: a pilot study. J Ultrasound Med. 2005;24:371–378.

Benacerraf BR. Inversion mode display of 3 D sonography: applications in obstetric and gynecologic imaging. AJR Am J Roentgenol. 2006;187:965–971.

Benoit B, Chaoui R. Three-dimensional ultrasound with maximal mode rendering : a novel technique for the diagnosis of bilateral or unilateral absence or hypoplasia of nasal bones in second-trimester screening for Down syndrome. Ultrasound Obstet Gynecol. 2005;25:19–24.

Benoit B. The value of three-dimensional ultrasonography in the screening of the fetal skeleton. Childs Nerv Syst. 2003;19:403–409.

Campbell S, Lees C, Moscoso G, Hall P. Ultrasound antenatal diagnosis of cleft palate by a new technique: the 3 D "reverse face" view. Ultrasound Obstet Gynecol. 2005;25:12–18.

Carvalho JS, Axt-Fliedner R, Chaoui R, et al. ISUOG Practice Guidelines (updated): fetal cardiac screening. Ultrasound Obstet Gynecol. 2023;61:788–803.

Caspi Y, de Zwarte SMC, Iemenschot IJ, et al. Automatic measurements of fetal intracranial volume from 3 D ultrasound scans. Front. Neuroimaging. 2022;1:991–998.

Chaoui R, Kalache KD, Hartung J. Application of three-dimensional power Doppler ultrasound in prenatal diagnosis. Ultrasound Obstet Gynecol. 2001;17: 22–29.

Chaoui R, Heling KS, Karl K. Ultrasound of the fetal veins part 2: Veins at the cardiac level. Ultraschall Med. 2014;35:302–18–quiz319–21.

Chaoui R, Levaillant JM, Benoit B, et al. Three-dimensional sonographic description of abnormal metopic suture in second-and third-trimester fetuses. Ultrasound Obstet Gynecol. 2005;26:761–764.

Chaoui R, Heling KS, Kainer F, Karl K. (Fetal Neurosonography using 3-dimensional Multiplanar Sonography) (German). Z Geburtsh Neonatol. 2012;216:54–62.

Chaoui R, Heling K, Karl K. Ultrasound of the Fetal Veins Part 1: The Intrahepatic Venous System. Ultraschall Med. 2014;35:208–228.

Chaoui R, Hoffmann J, Heling KS. Three-dimensional (3 D) and 4 D color Doppler fetal echocardiography using spatio-temporal image correlation (STIC). Ultrasound Obstet Gynecol. 2004;23:535–545.

Chaoui R, Nicolaides KH. From nuchal translucency to intracranial translucency: towards the early detection of spina bifida. Ultrasound Obstet Gynecol. 2010;35:133–138.

Chaoui R, Heling KS. Grundlagen der 3D- und 4D-Echokardiographie beim Fetus unter Nutzung der Spatio-Temporal-Image-Correlation(STIC)-Software. Ultraschall Med. 2006;27:1–7.

Chaoui R, Heling KS. Three-dimensional ultrasound in prenatal diagnosis. Curr Opin Obstet Gynecol. 2006;18:192–202.

Chaoui R, Rake A, Heling KS. Drei- und vierdimensionale fetale Echokardiographie. Gynäkologe. 2006;39:15–24.

Chaoui R, Heling KS. New developments in fetal heart scanning: Three- and four-dimensional fetal echocardiography. Semin Fetal Neonatal Med. 2005;10:567–577.

Chaoui R, Abuhamad A, Martins J, Heling KS. Recent Development in Three and Four Dimension Fetal Echocardiography. Fetal Diagn Ther. 2020;47:345–353.

Chen SA, Ong CS, Hibino N, et al. 3 D printing of fetal heart using 3 D ultrasound imaging data, Ultrasound Obstet Gynecol. 2018;52:808–809.

Chen Z, Ma Y, Wen H, Liao Y, Li S . Sonographic demonstration of sulci and gyri on the convex surface in normal fetus using 3D-ICRV rendering technology Ultraschall Med. 2023;44:123–132.

Conturso R, Contro E, Bellussi F. Demonstration of the pericallosal artery at 11–13 weeks of gestation using 3 D ultrasound. Fetal Diagn Ther. 2015;37:305–309.

Dall'Asta A, Paramasivam G, Basheer SN, et al. How to obtain diagnostic planes of the fetal central nervous system using three-dimensional ultrasound and a context-preserving rendering technology. Am J Obstet Gynecol. 2019;220:215–229.

DeVore GR, Falkensammer P, Sklansky MS, Platt LD. Spatio-temporal image correlation (STIC): new technology for evaluation of the fetal heart. Ultrasound Obstet Gynecol. 2003;22:380–387.

DeVore GR, Polanco B, Sklansky MS, Platt LD. The "spin" technique: a new method for examination of the fetal outflow tracts using three-dimensional ultrasound. Ultrasound Obstet Gynecol. 2004;24:72–82.

Deng J. Terminology of three-dimensional and four-dimensional ultrasound imaging of the fetal heart and other moving body parts. Ultrasound Obstet Gynecol. 2003;22:336–344.

Espinoza J, Kusanovic JP, Goncalves LF, et al. A novel algorithm for comprehensive fetal echocardiography using 4-dimensional ultrasonography and tomographic imaging. J Ultrasound Med. 2006;25:947–956.

Espinoza J, Goncalves LF, Lee W, et al. The use of the minimum projection mode in 4-dimensional examination of the fetal heart with spatiotemporal image correlation. J Ultrasound Med. 2004;23:1337–1348.

Espinoza J, Lee W, Comstock C, et al. Collaborative study on 4-dimensional echocardiography for the diagnosis of fetal heart defects: the COFEHD study. J Ultrasound Med. 2010;29:1573–1580.

Frisova V, Srutova M, Hyett J. 3-D Volume Assessment of the Corpus Callosum and Cerebellar Vermis Using Various Volume Acquisition and Post-Processing Protocols. Fetal Diagn Ther. 2018;43:199–207.

Goncalves LF, Espinoza J, Romero R, et al. Four-dimensional ultrasonography of the fetal heart using a novel Tomographic Ultrasound Imaging display. J PerinatMed. 2006;34:39–55.

Goncalves LF, Romero R, Espinoza J, et al. Four-dimensional ultrasonography of the fetal heart using color Doppler spatiotemporal image correlation. J Ultrasound Med. 2004;23:473–481.

Heling KS, Chaoui R. The Use of the Minimum Mode in Prenatal Ultrasound Diagnostics – Possibilities and Limitations. J Turkish-German Gynecol Assoc. 2008;9:212–216.

Karl K, Heling KS, Chaoui R. Ultrasound of the Fetal Veins Part 3: The Fetal Intracerebral Venous System. Ultraschall Med. 2016;37:6–26.

Kim MS, Jeanty P, Turner C, Benoit B. Three-dimensional sonographic evaluations of embryonic brain development. J Ultrasound Med. 2008;27:119–124.

Kusanovic JP, Nien J, Goncalves, L, et al. The use of inversion mode and 3 D manual segmentation in volume measurement of fetal fluid-filled structures: Comparison with Virtual Organ Computer-aided AnaLysis (VOCAL). Ultrasound Obstet. Gynecol. 2008;31:177–186.

Lee W, Chaiworapongsa T, Romero R, et al. A diagnostic approach for the evaluation of spina bifida by three-dimensional ultrasonography. J Ultrasound Med. 2002;21:619–626.

Lee W, Goncalves LF, Espinoza J, Romero R. Inversion mode: a new volume analysis tool for 3-dimensional ultrasonography. J Ultrasound Med. 2005;24:201–207.

Leibovitz Z, Haratz KK, Malinger G, Shapiro I, Pressman C. Fetal posterior fossa dimensions: normal and anomalous development assessed in mid-sagittal cranial plane by three-dimensional multiplanar sonography. Ultrasound Obstet Gynecol. 2014;43:147–153.

Malho AS, Bravo-Valenzuela NJ, Ximenes R, Peixoto AB, Araujo Júnior E. Antenatal diagnosis of congenital heart disease by 3 D ultrasonography using spatiotemporal image correlation with HDlive Flow and HDlive Flow silhouette rendering modes. Ultrasonography. 2022;41:578–596.

Malinger G, Paladini D, Haratz KK, et al. ISUOG Practice Guidelines (updated): sonographic examination of the fetal central nervous system. Part 1: performance of screening examination and indications for targeted neurosonography. Ultrasound Obstet Gynecol. 2020;56:476–484.

Martinez-Ten P, Perez-Pedregosa J, Santacruz B, et al. Three-dimensional ultrasound diagnosis of cleft palate: "reverse face", "flipped face" or "oblique face" which method is best? Ultrasound Obstet Gynecol. 2009;33:399–406.

Merz E, Abramowicz J, Blaas HG, et al. 3 D imaging of the fetal face – Recommendations from the International 3 D Focus Group. Ultraschall Med. 2012;33:175–182.

Merz E, Pashaj S. Advantages of 3 D ultrasound in the assessment of fetal abnormalities. J Perinat Med. 2017;45:643–650.

Merz E, Welter C. 2 D and 3 D Ultrasound in the evaluation of normal and abnormal fetal anatomy in the second and third trimesters in a level III center. Ultraschall Med. 2005;26:9–16.

Michailidis GD, Papageorgiou P, Economides DL. Assessment of fetal anatomy in the first trimester using two- and three-dimensional ultrasound. The British journal of radiology. 2002;75:215–219.

Moeglin D, Talmant C, Duyme M, Lopez AC. Fetal lung volumetry using two- and three-dimensional ultrasound. Ultrasound Obstet Gynecol. 2005;25:119–127.

Paladini D, Vassallo M, Sglavo G, Lapadula C, Martinelli P. The role of spatio-temporal image correlation (STIC) with tomographic ultrasound imaging (TUI) in the sequential analysis of fetal congenital heart disease. Ultrasound Obstet Gynecol. 2006;27:555–561.

Paladini D, Volpe P, Sglavo G, et al. Transposition of the great arteries in the fetus: assessment of the spatial relationships of the arterial trunks by four-dimensional echocardiography. Ultrasound Obstet Gynecol. 2008;31:271–276.

Paladini D, Giovanna Russo M, Vassallo M, Tartaglione A. The "in-plane" view of the inter-ventricular septum. A new approach to the characterization of ventricular septal defects in the fetus. Prenat Diagn. 2003;23:1052–1055.

Paladini D, Sglavo G, Masucci A, Pastore G, Nappi C. Role of four-dimensional ultrasound (spatio- temporal image correlation and Sonography-based Automated Volume Count) in prenatal assessment of atrial morphology in cardiosplenic syndromes. Ultrasound Obstet Gynecol. 2011;38:337–343.

Paladini D, Malinger G, Birnbaum R, et al. ISUOG Practice Guidelines (updated): sonographic examination of the fetal central nervous system. Part 2: performance of targeted neurosonography. Ultrasound Obstet Gynecol. 2021;57:661–671.

Pashaj S, Merz E. Prenatal Demonstration of Normal Variants of the Pericallosal Artery by 3 D Ultrasound. Ultraschall Med. 2014;35:129–133.

Pilu G, Segata M, Ghi T, et al. Diagnosis of midline anomalies of the fetal brain with the three-dimensional median view. Ultrasound Obstet Gynecol. 2006;27:522–529.

Pilu G, Ghi T, Carletti A, et al. Three-dimensional ultrasound examination of the fetal central nervous system. Ultrasound Obstet Gynecol. 2007;30:233–245.

Platt LD, Devore GR, Pretorius DH. Improving cleft palate/cleft lip antenatal diagnosis by 3-dimensional sonography: the "flipped face" view. Journal of Ultrasound in Medicine. 2006;25:1423–1430.

Pooh RK. Neurosonoembryology by three-dimensional ultrasound. Semin Fetal Neonatal Med. 2012;17: 261–268.

Pooh RK, Kurjak A. Novel application of three-dimensional HDlive imaging in prenatal diagnosis from the first trimester. J Perinat Med. 2015;43:147–58.

Pooh, RK: Sonoembryology by 3 D HDlive silhouette ultrasound – what is added by the "see-through fashion"? J Perinat Med. 2016;44:139–48.

Ruano R, Benachi A, Aubry MC, Dumez Y, Dommergues M. Volume contrast imaging: A new approach to identify fetal thoracic structures. J Ultrasound Med. 2004;23:403–408.

Tonni G, Grisolia G, Sepulveda W. Second trimester fetal neurosonography: reconstructing cerebral midline anatomy and anomalies using a novel three-dimensional ultrasound technique. Prenat Diagn. 2014;34:75–83.

Tonni G, Pinto A, Bianchi A, Pisello M, Grisolia G: 3 D ultrasound angioscan with MV-Flow™: Enhancing fetal brain low-flow microvascular neuroimaging. J Clin Ultrasound. 2023;20:1–5.

Veronese P, Bogana G, Cerutti A, et al. A propective study of the use of fetal intelligent navigation echocardiography (FINE) to obtain standard fetal echocardiography views. Fetal Diagn Ther. 2017;41:89–99.

Vinals F, Munoz M, Naveas R, Giuliano A. Transfrontal three-dimensional visualization of midline cerebral structures. Ultrasound Obstet Gynecol. 2007;30:162–168.

Volpe P, Campobasso G, Stanziano A, et al. Novel application of 4 D sonography with B-flow imaging and spatio-temporal image correlation (STIC) in the assessment of the anatomy of pulmonary arteries in fetuses with pulmonary atresia and ventricular septal defect. Ultrasound Obstet Gynecol. 2006;28:40–46.

Wataganara T, Rekhawasin T , Sompagdee N, et al. A 10-Year Retrospective Review of Prenatal Applications, Current Challenges and Future Prospects of Three-Dimensional Sonoangiography. Diagnostics. 2021;11:1511–1526.

Werner H, Lopes J, Ribeiro G, et al. Three-dimensional virtual traveling navigation and three-dimensional printing models of a normal fetal heart using ultrasonography data. Prenat Diagn. 2019;39:175–177.

Xiong Y, Chen M, Chan LW, et al. Scan the fetal heart by real-time three-dimensional echocardiography with live xPlane imaging. Journal of Maternal-Fetal and Neonatal Medicine. 2012;25:324–328.

Yeo L, Romero R, Jodicke C, et al. Four-chamber view and "swing technique" (FAST) echo: a novel and simple algorithm to visualize standard fetal echocardiographic planes. Ultrasound Obstet Gynecol. 2011;37:423–431.

Yeo L, Romero R. Intelligent navigation to improve obstetrical sonography. Ultrasound Obstet Gynecol. 2015;47:403–409.

Yeo L, Luewan S, Romero R. Fetal intelligent navigation echocardiography (FINE) detects 98 % of congenital heart disease. J Ultrasound Med. 2018;37:2577–2593.

Register

www.ingramcontent.com/pod-product-compliance
Lightning Source LLC
Chambersburg PA
CBHW062012210326
41458CB00075B/5318